Emotion Dysregulation and Outbursts in Children and Adolescents: Part II

Editors

MANPREET K. SINGH
GABRIELLE A. CARLSON

CHILD AND ADOLESCENT PSYCHIATRIC CLINICS OF NORTH AMERICA

www.childpsych.theclinics.com

Consulting Editor
TODD E. PETERS

July 2021 • Volume 30 • Number 3

ELSEVIER

1600 John F. Kennedy Boulevard • Suite 1800 • Philadelphia, Pennsylvania, 19103-2899

http://www.theclinics.com

CHILD AND ADOLESCENT PSYCHIATRIC CLINICS OF NORTH AMERICA Volume 30, Number 3
July 2021 ISSN 1056–4993, ISBN-13: 978-0-323-76256-4

Editor: Lauren Boyle
Developmental Editor: Arlene Campos

Child and Adolescent Psychiatric Clinics of North America (ISSN 1056-4993) is published quarterly by Elsevier Inc., 360 Park Avenue South, New York, NY 10010-1710. Months of issue are January, April, July, and October. Business and Editorial Offices: 1600 John F. Kennedy Boulevard, Suite 1800, Philadelphia, PA 19103-2899. Periodicals postage paid at New York, NY and additional mailing offices. Subscription prices are $348.00 per year (US individuals), $844.00 per year (US institutions), $100.00 per year (US & Canadian students), $388.00 per year (Canadian individuals), $899.00 per year (Canadian institutions), $446.00 per year (international individuals), $899.00 per year (international institutions), and $200.00 per year (international students). International air speed delivery is included in all *Clinics* subscription prices. All prices are subject to change without notice. **POSTMASTER:** Send address changes to *Child and Adolescent Psychiatric Clinics of North America*, Elsevier Health Sciences Division, Subscription Customer Service, 3251 Riverport Lane, Maryland Heights, MO 63043. **Customer Service: 1-800-654-2452 (U.S. and Canada); 314-447-8871 (outside U.S. and Canada). Fax: 314-447-8029. E-mail:** JournalsCustomer Service-usa@elsevier.com **(for print support) or** journalsonlinesupport-usa@elsevier.com **(for online support).**

Reprints. For copies of 100 or more of articles in this publication, please contact the Commercial Reprints Department, Elsevier Inc., 360 Park Avenue South, New York, New York 10010-1710 Tel.: 212-633-3874; Fax: 212-633-3820, E-mail: reprints@elsevier.com.

Child and Adolescent Psychiatric Clinics of North America is covered in *MEDLINE/PubMed (Index Medicus), ISI, SSCI, Research Alert, Social Search, Current Contents,* and *EMBASE/Excerpta Medica.*

Contributors

CONSULTING EDITOR

TODD E. PETERS, MD, FAPA
Vice President/Chief Medical Officer (CMO), Chief Medical Information Officer (CMIO),
Sheppard Pratt Health System, Consulting Editor, *Child and Adolescent Psychiatric
Clinics of North America* Baltimore, Maryland

EDITORS

MANPREET K. SINGH, MD, MS
Associate Professor of Psychiatry and Behavioral Sciences, Director, Pediatric Mood
Disorders Program, Stanford University School of Medicine, Stanford, California

GABRIELLE A. CARLSON, MD
Professor of Psychiatry and Pediatrics, Renaissance School of Medicine, Stony Brook
University, Putnam Hall-South Campus, Stony Brook, New York

AUTHORS

PEVITR S. BANSAL, MS
Department of Psychology, College of Arts and Sciences, University of Kentucky,
Lexington, Kentucky

CHRISTINE M. BARTHELEMY
PediMIND Program, Mclean Hospital, Belmont, Massachusetts; Division of Child
Psychiatry, McLean Hospital, Harvard Medical School, Boston, Massachusetts

RAMAN BAWEJA, MD
Department of Psychiatry, Penn State College of Medicine, Hershey, Pennsylvania

CHRISTOPHER BELLONCI, MD
Chief Medical Officer and Vice President of Policy and Practice, Judge Baker Children's
Center, Assistant Professor, Harvard Medical School, Boston, Massachusetts

JEFF Q. BOSTIC, MD, EdD
Professor, Department of Psychiatry, MedStar Georgetown University Hospital,
Washington, DC

JEFFREY D. BURKE, PhD
Associate Professor, Department of Psychological Sciences, University of Connecticut,
Storrs, Connecticut

EMILIE J. BUTLER, BA
Department of Psychological Sciences, University of Connecticut, Storrs, Connecticut

GABRIELLE A. CARLSON, MD
Department of Psychiatry, Renaissance School of Medicine, Stony Brook University,
Stony Brook, New York

EMMA CHAD-FRIEDMAN, MS
Department of Psychology, University of Maryland, College Park, Maryland

JACLYN DATAR CHUA, DO
Attending Physician, Department of Child and Adolescent Psychiatry and Behavioral
Science, Children's Hospital of Philadelphia, Philadelphia, Pennsylvania

JUDITH A. CROWELL, MD
Division of Child and Adolescent Psychiatry, Department of Psychiatry and Behavioral
Sciences, Stony Brook University, Stony Brook, New York

D. CUNNINGHAM, PhD
Faculty Consultant, Department of Psychiatry, University of Maryland School of Medicine,
Baltimore, Maryland

MELISSA P. DELBELLO, MD, MS
Professor of Psychiatry and Pediatrics, Dr. Stanley and Mickey Kaplan Professor and
Chair Department of Psychiatry and Behavioral Neuroscience, University of Cincinnati
College of Medicine, Cincinnati, Ohio

LENA L.A. DEYOUNG
PediMIND Program, Mclean Hospital, Belmont, Massachusetts; Division of Child
Psychiatry, McLean Hospital, Harvard Medical School, Boston, Massachusetts

DANIEL P. DICKSTEIN, MD
PediMIND Program, Mclean Hospital, Belmont, Massachusetts; Simches Center of
Excellence in Child and Adolescent Psychiatry, McLean Hospital, Harvard Medical
School, Boston, Massachusetts

LEA R. DOUGHERTY, PhD
Department of Psychology, University of Maryland, College Park, Maryland

SPENCER C. EVANS, PhD
Postdoctoral Fellow, Department of Psychology, Harvard University, Cambridge,
Massachusetts; Department of Psychology, University of Miami, Coral Gables,
Florida

ABIGAIL FARRELL, BS
Clinical and Research Program in Pediatric Psychopharmacology and Adult ADHD,
Massachusetts General Hospital, Boston, Massachusetts

MARY A. FRISTAD, PhD
Department of Psychiatry and Behavioral Health, The Ohio State University Wexner
Medical Center, Harding Hospital, Nationwide Children's Hospital Behavioral Health
Pavilion, Columbus, Ohio

ANNA C. GILBERT
Division of Child Psychiatry, Brown University (Prior PediMIND Program Member),
Providence, Rhode Island

REBECCA HU, MD
Resident Physician, Department of Psychiatry and Behavioral Sciences, University of
California, San Francisco School of Medicine, San Francisco, California

SAMANTHA HUBACHECK, MS
Department of Psychology, University of Maryland, College Park, Maryland

JONATHAN C. HUEFNER, PhD
Boys Town Child and Family Translational Research Center, Boys Town, Nebraska

GRACIE A. JENKINS
PediMIND Program, Mclean Hospital, Belmont, Massachusetts; Division of
Child Psychiatry, McLean Hospital, Harvard Medical School, Boston,
Massachusetts

OLIVER G. JOHNSTON, MS
Department of Psychological Sciences, University of Connecticut, Storrs, Connecticut

ELLEN M. KESSEL, PhD
Division of Child and Adolescent Psychiatry, Columbia University, New State Psychiatric
Institute, New York, New York

KERRI L. KIM, PhD
Division of Child Psychiatry, Brown University (Prior PediMIND Program Member),
Providence, Rhode Island

KATHARINA KIRCANSKI, PhD
Staff Scientist, Section on Mood Dysregulation and Neuroscience, Intramural Research
Program, National Institute of Mental Health, Bethesda, Maryland

DANIEL N. KLEIN, PhD
Department of Psychology, Stony Brook University, Stony Brook, New York

ELLEN LEIBENLUFT, MD
Senior Investigator and Chief, Section on Mood Dysregulation and Neuroscience,
Intramural Research Program, National Institute of Mental Health, Bethesda,
Maryland

HEATHER A. MACPHERSON, PhD
Division of Child Psychiatry, Brown University (Prior PediMIND Program Member),
Providence, Rhode Island

RICHARD MATTISON, MD
Professor of Psychiatry, Penn State College of Medicine, Hershey, Pennsylvania

DAVID J. MIKLOWITZ, PhD
Distinguished Professor of Psychiatry, Division of Child and Adolescent Psychiatry at the
UCLA Semel Institute, University of California Los Angeles School of Medicine; Visiting
Professor, Department of Psychiatry at Oxford University, Oxford

CHRISTOPHER O'BRIEN, MA
Prime Home Developmental Disabilities Services, Omaha, Nebraska

TOM OLINO, PhD
Department of Psychology, Temple University, Philadelphia, Pennsylvania

LUIS R. PATINO, MD, MSc
Assistant Professor, Department of Psychiatry and Behavioral Neuroscience, Division of
Bipolar Disorders Research, University of Cincinnati College of Medicine, Cincinnati,
Ohio

PETYA RADOEVA, MD, PhD
Division of Child Psychiatry, Brown University (Prior PediMIND Program Member),
Providence, Rhode Island

TABAN SALEM, PhD
Department of Psychology and Neuroscience, Millsaps College, Jackson, Mississippi

LAUREN SANTUCCI, PhD
Associate, Department of Psychology, Harvard University, Psychologist, McLean Hospital School Consultation Service, Cambridge, Massachusetts

MANPREET K. SINGH, MD, MS
Director, Stanford Pediatric Mood Disorders Program and the Pediatric Emotion and Resilience Lab, Associate Professor, Department of Psychiatry and Behavioral Sciences, Stanford University School of Medicine, Stanford, California

MICHAEL T. SORTER, MD
Director, Division of Psychiatry, Professor of Clinical Psychiatry and Pediatrics, Cincinnati Children's Hospital, University of Cincinnati, Cincinnati, Ohio

CARRIE VAUDREUIL, MD
Clinical and Research Program in Pediatric Psychopharmacology and Adult ADHD, Massachusetts General Hospital, Department of Psychiatry, Harvard Medical School, Boston, Massachusetts

JOSEPH S. VERDUCCI, PhD
Department of Statistics, The Ohio State University, Columbus, Ohio

DENNIS G. VOLLMER, MHD, MBA
Boys Town Residential Treatment Center, Boys Town, Nebraska

KIMBERLY A. WALTERS, PhD
Statistics Collaborative, Inc., Washington, DC

DANIEL A. WASCHBUSCH, PhD
Department of Psychiatry, Penn State College of Medicine, Hershey, Pennsylvania

JAMES G. WAXMONSKY, MD
Department of Psychiatry, Penn State College of Medicine, Hershey, Pennsylvania

JANET WOZNIAK, MD
Clinical and Research Program in Pediatric Psychopharmacology and Adult ADHD, Massachusetts General Hospital, Department of Psychiatry, Harvard Medical School, Boston, Massachusetts

Contents

Development

Emotion regulation (ER) is a complex process that combines inherent as well as environmental and learned components of reactivity and regulation. Elements of ER are present from birth and are elaborated across development. An understanding of emotion dysregulation requires careful examination of all the elements that constitute typical ER so that relevant domains can be therapeutically targeted. This contribution reviews the development of ER in typically developing youth to set the stage for discussion of points of intervention.

Limited research has examined precursors/risk factors for adolescent irritability. In the current study, we examined the continuity of irritability from ages 3 to 15 and identified early childhood antecedents of adolescent irritability. Age 3 irritability predicted self- and mother-reported age 15 irritability. A broad range of age 3 variables, that in many instances differed as a function of either informant or gender, predicted age 15 irritability. Findings point to distinct developmental pathways from early childhood that have the potential to result in irritable phenotype in adolescence and the importance of considering gender and informant in assessments of adolescent irritability.

Interventions

Explosive outbursts (EO) by students are an intensely distressing experience for that student as well as for all school staff and students present during the outburst. These EO are characterized by rapid escalations, usually far out of proportion to precipitating events, may include significant verbal and/or physical aggression, require intensive staff intervention, are often difficult for the student to process, and are typically recurrent. These explosions cross multiple psychiatric and educational diagnostic categories and require diverse interventions to address behavioral, emotional, impulsive, and sensory components. Interventions for each stage of an EO can be used to deescalate these events.

Children hospitalized in inpatient and residential treatment facilities often present with severe emotion dysregulation, which is the result of a wide range of psychiatric diagnoses. Emotion dysregulation is not a diagnosis but is a common but inconsistently described set of symptoms and behaviors. With no agreed upon way of measuring emotion dysregulation, the authors summarize the existing contemporary treatment focusing on proxy measures of emotion dysregulation in inpatient and residential settings. Interventions are summarized and categorized into individual- and systems-level interventions in addressing aggressive behaviors. Going forward, dysregulation will need to be operationalized in a standard way.

Preadolescent children in residential care have treatment needs that are different from adolescents. An intervention was created using developmental theory to inform decisions about the timing, objectives, strategies, and context best suited to preadolescents in an intensive residential treatment center. Aggressive behavior, seclusions, and restraints data for preadolescents during a 32-month period was used in the analysis. There was a significant decrease in aggressive behavior, seclusions, and restraints for preadolescents during the periods when the developmentally appropriate intervention was used versus the times when they received same intervention as the adolescents.

Explosive and aggressive behavior in children can pose safety risks, disturb family functioning, and lead to significant impairments. Pharmacologic management should be based on the first-line treatment of the primary psychiatric diagnoses of the patient and initiated in combination with appropriate psychosocial interventions. Review of the literature suggests that risperidone has the most supporting evidence in the treatment of explosive behavior. Stimulants have been shown to be helpful in the treatment of explosive behavior in attention-deficit/hyperactivity disorder. Medication treatment can be associated with significant side effects and therefore the risks and benefits of medication management must be weighed carefully.

Irritability, anger, and aggression, although not specific for pediatric bipolar disorder (BD), can be a common finding and an important source of distress and impairment in these patients. Over the past 2 decades the diagnostic significance of irritability in pediatric BD has been highly debated. Beyond the debate of its diagnostic significance, the clinical importance of irritability, anger, and aggression in youth with BD has been well established. In this review, the authors discuss evaluation and management strategies of irritability, anger, and aggression in youth with BD.

A Review of the Evidence Base for Psychosocial Interventions for the Treatment of Emotion Dysregulation in Children and Adolescents   573

James G. Waxmonsky, Raman Baweja, Pevitr S. Bansal, and Daniel A. Waschbusch

Many children with a range of psychiatric diagnoses manifest impaired levels of emotion dysregulation (ED). Over the past decade, there has been increasing examination of psychosocial interventions for ED. We found preliminary evidence of positive effects for a wide range of psychosocial treatments that were associated with improvements in emotion recognition, emotional reactivity, and emotion regulation. More studies are needed because results are limited by the small number of controlled trials, heavy reliance on parent ratings, and heterogeneity of the samples.

Preventing Irritability and Temper Outbursts in Youth by Building Resilience   595

Manpreet K. Singh, Rebecca Hu, and David J. Miklowitz

Severe irritability and temper outbursts are risk factors for the onset of serious and lifelong mood disorders. In treating children and adolescents with severe irritability, clinicians should evaluate and address safety issues before acute stabilization of symptoms. Then, clinicians can initiate interventions to prevent the onset or relapses of the undesired behavior and its functional consequences. This review summarizes primary, secondary, and tertiary relapse prevention strategies, with an emphasis on strategies that build resilience in youth that mitigate the onset, recurrence, and progression of emotion dysregulation.

Psychoeducational and Skill-building Interventions for Emotion Dysregulation   611

Taban Salem, Kimberly A. Walters, Joseph S. Verducci, and Mary A. Fristad

Family psychoeducation plus skill building is a class of interventions considered to be well-established for youth with mood disorders or emotion dysregulation. Psychoeducational psychotherapy (PEP) is an example of this class of interventions. PEP provides psychoeducation for parents and children, skill building to help children better regulate emotions and behaviors, and strategies for parents to better facilitate school-based interventions, develop specific symptom management techniques, and generate coping strategies for the entire family. Evidence is summarized supporting the efficacy of PEP for reducing rage, overall mood symptom severity, disruptive behavior, and executive functioning deficits in youth. Long-term benefits of PEP are discussed.

Severe irritability is common in treatment-referred youth, often occurring in externalizing, anxiety, and mood conditions. The best available evidence indicates behavioral parent training and cognitive-behavioral therapy as first-line interventions. Modular approaches (eg, MATCH) can package these strategies in a flexible format, facilitating personalization. Ample evidence supports MATCH's effectiveness generally and initial evidence supports its effectiveness for irritability specifically. We provide an overview of MATCH and its application to severe irritability. Emphasis is placed on behavioral parent training as a likely primary/first-line treatment. Potential benefits and limitations are considered. This approach calls for careful clinical judgment and for further empirical research.

Future

Oppositional defiant disorder (ODD) includes distinct but inseparable dimensions of chronic irritability and oppositional behavior. These dimensions have been identified across age groups and show discriminant associations with internalizing and externalizing psychopathology. The introduction in the DSM-5 of disruptive mood dysregulation disorder and the diagnostic requirement that it take precedence over ODD are not supported by evidence, introduce confusion about the structure and linkages of irritability and oppositional behavior, and obscure the importance of the behavioral dimension in explaining and predicting poor outcomes. A dimensional framework with irritability, oppositionality, callous-unemotional traits, and aggression may more fully describe antisocial outcomes.

Irritability is one of the most common reasons why children and adolescents are brought for psychiatric care. Too often, clinicians feel excluded from research about the brain/behavior mechanisms of irritability due to jargon or other barriers. This article explains some of these research methods, providing brief summaries of what is known about brain/behavior mechanisms in disorders involving irritability, including bipolar disorder, disruptive mood dysregulation disorder, attention-deficit/hyperactivity disorder, and autism. Greater understanding of these methods may help clinicians now and in the future, as such mechanisms translated into improved care, following the example of childhood leukemia.

We focus on irritability, one subtype of emotion dysregulation, place it within the panoply of relevant constructs and present evidence supporting its external validity. Irritability is not a developmental phenotype of bipolar disorder, but is longitudinally and genetically associated with unipolar depression, anxiety, and attention deficit hyperactivity disorder. Tonic and phasic irritability may be dissociable dimensions. It is important to differentiate shared vs. unique pathophysiological mechanisms among irritability, anxiety, and attention deficit hyperactivity disorder. Irritability is amenable to translational research applying frustrative non-reward, a rodent model, to human irritability. Last, we discuss research suggesting a novel exposure-based intervention for irritability.

CHILD AND ADOLESCENT PSYCHIATRIC CLINICS

SERIES OF RELATED INTEREST
Psychiatric Clinics of North America
https://www.psych.theclinics.com/
Pediatric Clinics of North America
https://www.pediatric.theclinics.com/
Neurologic Clinics
https://www.neurologic.theclinics.com/

THE CLINICS ARE AVAILABLE ONLINE!
Access your subscription at:
www.theclinics.com

Preface

Emotion Dysregulation in Children and Adolescents: Part II

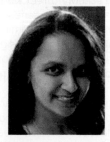 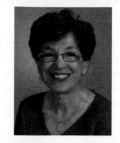

Manpreet K. Singh, MD, MS   Gabrielle A. Carlson, MD
Editors

Part I of this special issue describes the many psychiatric disorders in which explosive outbursts may play an important role. Bipolar disorder, disruptive mood dysregulation disorder, oppositional defiant disorder, posttraumatic stress disorder, or mixtures of diagnoses like co-occurring attention-deficit/hyperactivity disorder (ADHD), oppositional defiant disorder, or autism spectrum disorder are the conditions we describe with case examples. As we noted in Part I, none of these diagnoses are synonymous with or consistently describe the behavior itself. We, in fact, lack a consistent definition of outbursts, and so we lack an outcome measure to identify their severity, duration, and frequency. This complicates our ability to design and conduct clinical trials, which, in the absence of a clinically meaningful outcome measure, may be destined to fail. At this time, youth with outbursts are frequently exposed to multiple psychotropic medications with limited information as to their long-term impact. Nevertheless, medications combined with a collaborative system of care and using a developmental lens can be a blessing if they decrease the risk of escalation and the significant multi-domain impairment that ensues if the problem is untreated. Thoughtful treatment, however, is a challenge especially in globally under-resourced treatment settings.

Whereas Part I focused on psychopathology and treatments of specific conditions, the second part critically evaluates the benefits of existing psychosocial and pharmacologic interventions and makes recommendations for how these interventions can evolve with an improved understanding of behaviors underlying emotion dysregulation, the etiologic factors that contribute to perpetuating the dysregulation, and the various settings in which the dysregulation occurs. We aim to approximate which treatments fit well for which youth, with an exploration of the timing of the interventions along primary, secondary, and tertiary prevention. Thus, a developmentally informed lens focuses on clinically meaningful outcomes and knowing when and in what setting to inform patients and families to seek care.

Child Adolesc Psychiatric Clin N Am 30 (2021) xiii–xiv
https://doi.org/10.1016/j.chc.2021.05.002
1056-4993/21/© 2021 Published by Elsevier Inc.

childpsych.theclinics.com

The first 2 articles introduce the concept that development matters. The first paper by Dr Crowell is a review of normative development of emotion regulation. The second, by Dr Kessel and colleagues, uses multiple methods and informants in a prospective longitudinal design to demonstrate the antecedents and continuity of irritability from early childhood to adolescence. The next series of articles review the extant literature for existing interventions across multiple settings. The first of these articles by Dr Bostic and colleagues characterizes outbursts in a school setting and makes recommendations for interventions that address behavioral, emotional, impulsive, and sensory components across the stages in the evolution of explosive outbursts. The second of the series on interventions across settings is by Dr Chua and colleagues, and reviews the limited extant literature on behaviors that require seclusion or restraint in inpatient settings. The third article by Dr Huefner and colleagues uses data to inform decisions about the timing, objectives, strategies, and contexts best suited to reduce seclusion and restraint in preadolescents in a residential treatment center.

The next two articles review extant pharmacological strategies for explosive and aggressive behavior, first across broad diagnostic groups, by Vaudreuil and colleagues, and second, in bipolar disorders, by Drs Patino and DelBello. We follow these with 4 articles that review psychosocial and preventive interventions for emotion dysregulation, first with a comprehensive review by Dr Waxmonsky and colleagues of a wide range of evidence-supported effective psychosocial interventions, followed by a review by Dr Singh and colleagues of strategies that both prevent onset or progression of emotion dysregulation and build resilience. We have learned that family support is critical to intervening on emotion dysregulation in youth, so additional attention by Dr Salem and colleagues was paid by to the long-term beneficial role of family psychoeducation and skill building in reducing rage, mood symptom severity, disruptive behavior, and associated executive functioning deficits that commonly cooccur. We conclude this series of articles with a modular approach by Drs Evans and Santucci to provide flexible and personalized matches for psychosocial treatment components based on specific clinical presentations.

In the final 2 articles Dr Burke and colleagues first consider the long-term course and outcome of chronic irritability and oppositional behavior, and Dr Dickstein and colleagues review the application of neuroscience tools to evolve mechanistically rooted interventions that target brain-based origins of emotion dysregulation. At the conclusion of this issue, Drs Leibenluft and Kircanski provide a reprise to both parts of this special issue.

Manpreet K. Singh, MD, MS
Department of Psychiatry and
Behavioral Sciences
Stanford University
401 Quarry Road
Stanford, CA, 94305-5719, USA

Gabrielle A. Carlson, MD
Renaissance School of Medicine at
Stony Brook University
Putnam Hall-South Campus
Stony Brook, NY 11794-8790, USA

E-mail addresses:
mksingh@stanford.edu (M.K. Singh)
gabrielle.carlson@stonybrookmedicine.edu (G.A. Carlson)

Development

Development of Emotion Regulation in Typically Developing Children

Judith A. Crowell, MD

KEYWORDS

- Emotion regulation • Development • Typically developing children

KEY POINTS

- Emotion regulation (ER) is complex.
- ER combines intrinsic, environmental, and learned components of reactivity and regulation.
- ER is observable at birth and continues over development.
- Components of ER can be therapeutically targeted.

Emotion regulation (ER) is a complex construct that characterizes "processes that allow an individual to manage emotional arousal."[1] These processes emerge in the neonatal period and are elaborated and expanded across childhood and adolescence. They involve both inherent characteristics of the individual and social and environmental influences. An understanding of normal development of ER is critical to any clinical understanding of interventions for its opposite, the severe emotion dysregulation (ED), which is the focus of this issue. There are 2 key dimensions of ER, and they are both present from birth: a reactive component and a control or regulatory component.[1]

THE REACTIVE COMPONENT

The *reactive component* refers to (1) the threshold at which the individual responds to stimuli (eg, sounds, touch, sights), that is, how "sensitive" they are; and (2) the level or type of stimuli that elicits negative affect. The reactive component has close parallels to the construct of "irritability," which includes being abnormally sensitive to stimuli (eg, Merriam-Webster), and has synonyms such as "touchy" and "hypersensitive" as well as the dimension of negative affect. Often, definitions in the clinical literature focus on persistent negative affect and proneness to anger and tantrums.[2,3] However, given the link between varying sensitivities that are present in

Putnam Hall- South Campus, Stony Brook University, Stony Brook, NY 11794, USA
E-mail address: Judith.crowell@stonybrookmedicine.edu

Child Adolesc Psychiatric Clin N Am 30 (2021) 467–474
https://doi.org/10.1016/j.chc.2021.04.001
1056-4993/21/© 2021 Elsevier Inc. All rights reserved.

childpsych.theclinics.com

some disorders, for example, autism spectrum disorder or anxiety, it is important to keep the full definition of irritability in mind as developmental processes in ER are considered.

Of note, this definition of reactivity is also similar to temperament qualities of high reactivity, withdrawal/fearfulness, and negativity.[4] These characteristics are the most heritable domains of temperament along with activity level, in contrast to soothability or positive affect.[5,6]

THE REGULATORY COMPONENT

With respect to the regulatory component of ER, Kopp[7] was among the first to describe development of ER in infants and young children. Many others have since expanded on how self-regulatory processes develop. Over the course of development, the regulatory or control dimension becomes more complex and elaborate, and the reactive and control dimensions intertwine and become difficult to parse. **Fig. 1** shows the types and timing of various influences on ER across development.

Infancy

Starting from the neonatal period, infants develop a repertoire of behavioral strategies that may reduce, inhibit, amplify, and balance different emotional responses.[8] From birth to 3 months of age, innate physiologic mechanisms are evident, including sucking, turning away (regulation of attention), and crying.

Infants from 3 to 6 months are increasingly predictable in eating, elimination, and sleeping cycles. This regularity is internally organizing and enables caregivers to better predict infant states.[8] Sleep consolidation in the first year of life is associated with subsequent self-regulatory abilities later in childhood.[9,10]

Infants from 3 to 6 months of age increasingly control their own attention and subsequently their own arousal.[11] This voluntary control of arousal occurs through alerting, orienting, social engagement, habituation, and expanding motor abilities.[12] Positive affect increases and distress decreases with expanding periods of focused attention.[13] Attentional disengagement, that is, the ability to flexibly shift attention to social and nonsocial stimuli, emerges at this age. Development of attentional

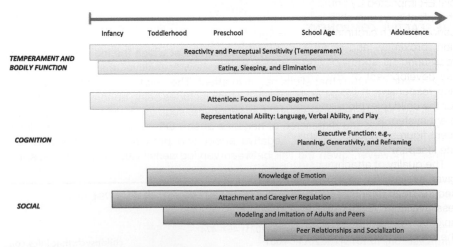

Fig. 1. Influences on the ER across development.

disengagement is typically aided by caregivers and is highly relevant for daily life, adaptation, and learning. It is an aspect of top-down attentional effortful control that improves throughout childhood with brain maturation and increasing functional connectivity across brain regions.[13]

Between 6 and 12 months of age, infants become increasingly active and purposeful, using reaching, retreating, redirecting attention, and self-soothing in a flexible, adaptive manner.[1,14,15] They become adept at social regulation of emotion with preference for, referencing of, and signaling to caregivers. Caregiver-infant interactions help direct the infant's attention away from negative stimuli, thus activating neural connections associated with attention, engagement, and positive mood, rather than negativity or stress, and which has long-term implications for the structure and function of neural systems.[11]

Toddlerhood

Infants are capable of discriminating happy faces from those with other emotions. In toddlerhood, this expands to recognition of anger and sadness.[16] Although toddlers cannot control their emotions independently, they use a variety of strategies to manage affective states.

Aggressive behavior typically peaks at this time, but behavioral control also emerges, and toddlers and young children gain steadily in their ability to comply with parental requests and override their own immediate gratification.[1,7,17] Coinciding with increased control, there is a rapid decline in impulsive anger and aggression over the next 2 years. Greater effortful control (the ability to delay gratification, focus, use a lower voice, and slow motor behavior) begins to emerge at this time. This capacity is associated with the infant's abilities as well as maternal responsiveness to distress and experiences with socialization.[18]

Verbal abilities emerge, and language development is a major step in the development of ER. Parents talk with young children about emotions, and toddlers gain the ability to identify internal states in themselves and others, supporting emotion knowledge and development of theory of mind.[17,19,20] Increased self-awareness allows them to reflect on emotional experience, express needs directly, and understand the feelings and motivations of others.

The attachment system emerges around the first year of life as a key element of social ER impacted by primary caregivers. Attachment behaviors are most evident when the infant or young child is upset, frightened, or uncertain, for example, in a novel situation. In such circumstances, the child orients toward the caregiver, seeking information, proximity, and contact. Contact provides safety, and with respect to ER, is reassuring, is soothing, and restores emotional homeostasis. Caregivers facilitate the development of attachment behavior by being available, sensitive, cooperative, and responsive in times of distress, and supportive and encouraging when it is safe for the child to explore and learn, that is, the secure base phenomenon.[21] The attachment system is continuously operating, and relationship or relationships with attachment figures (typically parents and romantic partners) serve as an ER system across the lifespan.[22]

The quality of attachment in the infant/child varies with respect to the levels of caregiver availability, sensitivity, and responsiveness.[23] The description above is of a secure attachment pattern. Attachment insecurity is linked to a caregiver who is less available, responsive, and sensitive to the child distress and exploration. The anxious-avoidant attachment pattern develops when the caregiver rejects or ignores the infant's distress, discouraging contact, and they may be overly "pushy" in encouraging exploration. The anxious-ambivalent pattern is associated with inconsistent parenting that appears to be driven by parental emotional needs as opposed to those of the infant.

Recent meta-analyses show similar findings of the relation between infant attachment and later ER.[24,25] Children classified as secure in infancy are more positive emotionally, regulate emotions more effectively, and use both cognitive strategies and social supports effectively. Regulatory difficulties were most often seen in children with ambivalent attachment, who show more negative affect in general and in response to stimuli. Children classified as avoidant relied less on social supports for coping and had less positive affect and less effective ER.

The Preschool Period

Preschoolers are keen observers of the behaviors of others, and they model behavioral strategies and planning. The family environment is a major site for ER learning, including parenting behaviors that surround children's emotions as well as the quality of the marital relationship.[26] Sibling relationships are perhaps the most emotionally charged relationships that individuals experience in life, with the frequent expression of pleasure, pride, protectiveness, jealousy, anger, and frustration.[27] Thus, sibling relationships present a unique, critical, and understudied emotional learning environment.

Until the preschool years, the family is the most relevant ER environment. However, at this age, children are increasingly exposed to peers and begin negotiating play, cooperative, and competitive strategies with nonfamily members. Preschoolers show a preference for peers who exhibit high inhibitory control and the capability to regulate negative emotions.[28] They attempt to inhibit negative emotions in social situations, and girls are more effective at this than boys.[29] Whereas automatic ER continues, for example, shifting attention, the ability to willfully control emotions is associated with brain development from 3 to 6 years.[30]

Young children can distinguish between accidental and intentional behaviors and preferentially imitate those that are intended versus those that are not.[31] By preschool, they can understand, discuss, and cope with distressing events that happen "by accident." They respond to adults' interpersonal "scaffolding" (drawing attention to emotions, what they look like, and how they feel) with greater ability to engage in ER.[30] Girls tend to have more advanced understanding of emotions at this age.[32]

The preschool period is the peak period for pretend play, which largely disappears by preadolescence. It is a culturally universal phenomenon, with a set pattern of development, and is observed in many mammalian species, suggesting that it serves an adaptive evolutionary function, quite possibly in the domain of ER.[33] The pretend world has a set of "as-if" rules that are clearly signaled as not being part of the "real" world. Animal models allow for the interruption of the development of play. For example, a rat pup reared with an adult female rather than with its mother and siblings is deprived of the opportunity to play fight. As adults, development of their orbitofrontal and medial prefrontal cortices is impacted, and they are impaired in their ability to read social signals. In human children, play involves complex social understanding, including the symbolism of behaviors and objects, theory of mind, and regulation of emotion.[34]

In support of this hypothesis, a longitudinal investigation of play in 5- to 6-year-old preschoolers indicated that all types led to enhanced social competence.[32] Dramatic play (defined as taking clear social role in play), compared with fantasy play (pretending that objects stand for something else) and rough-and-tumble play or exercise, was most highly associated with mothers' reports of the children's ER, observed positive emotions, and understanding emotions concurrently and over time. Rough-and-tumble play, especially for boys, is associated with positive emotional expression and ER, supporting the idea that this type of play builds the ability to signal emotions clearly as well as modulating them. Fathers often serve as models for managing excitement and more aggressive emotions in the context of play.[35,36]

School Age and Adolescence

School-age children engage in self-distraction and can reevaluate and reframe frustrating/disappointing situations in a positive light. Planning and goal-directed behaviors assist with regulation of arousal. Across the school-age period, ER transitions from that which is more emotionally based, that is, instinctive and intuitive, to that which is more cognitively based and appraising.[37,38]

Although young children learn ER almost entirely through parents' and siblings' responses,[39] peer relationships play an increasingly prominent role in socialization of ER in childhood and adolescence. Children and teens learn that there are social reasons to regulate emotions and behavior in both the short and the long term. That is, negative emotions may have repercussions of damaging relationships and hurting others. Nevertheless, the role of parents remains strong and has enduring implications for the development of ER.[40] For example, mothers' observed negative responses to child negative emotions at age 5 have been linked to parent and teacher ratings of ER in those children at ages 10 and 15 years.

Behavioral inhibition, anger regulation, and goal-setting all improve across adolescence. Although girls start out as more effective in regulating anger and setting goals at age 12, by age 18, there are no gender differences in these abilities.[41]

Adolescence can be a time of some risk because emotional arousal is heightened by hormonal changes and neurodevelopmental progression.[42,43] Teens are not yet as effective in reading emotions as adults.[44] There is an increase in sensation seeking, reckless behaviors, and risk of emotional problems, especially in early adolescence. Nevertheless, well-regulated children tend to be well-regulated adolescents.[45,46] Full biological development of ER does not emerge until the prefrontal cortex is fully developed in the mid-twenties.[37]

Of note, there is emerging literature on gaming and ER abilities in middle childhood and adolescence.[47] There appears to be a curvilinear relationship between gameplaying and ER, with moderate gaming being associated with enhanced ER strategies and emotional intelligence. Identification with a character can also enhance emotional skills. In a study of Norwegian youth, Internet gaming disorder at age 10 was associated with more impaired ER and social skills at age 8, rather than gaming being associated with subsequent reduced ER.[48] In contrast, the evidence of screen time and ER in younger children is limited but suggests that the amount of screen time at age 4 is negatively correlated with both ER and math and literacy scores at ages 6 and 8 years.[49]

SUMMARY

In summary, there are many aspects of ER, with both reactive and regulatory components in evidence from birth. Effective ER develops steadily from infancy to young adulthood, and very likely after that. However, many intentional ER abilities develop in the toddler and preschool years, laying a strong foundation for later success. Inherent abilities are important, such as control of attention, sensitivities to stimuli, and capacity for language and symbolic play. Nevertheless, families, and later, peers, are critical to enhancing those inherent abilities and supplementing them with soothing, teaching, challenging, modeling, and supporting. Historical events and the greater social context, such as pandemics, the Great Depression, the World Wars, and natural disasters, may elicit vulnerabilities in the development of ER. A comprehensive assessment of ED should examine each of the developmental aspects of ER, including the relationships with parents and peers and the broader social context. This careful examination of ER domains can elucidate entry points for effective and tailored interventions, including parent training, attachment-focused therapies, cognitive behavioral and dialectical behavioral strategies, and medication management.

DISCLOSURE

The author has no disclosures or conflicts of interest.

REFERENCES

1. Calkins S, Perry N. The development of emotion regulation: implications for child adjustment. In: Cicchetti D, editor. Developmental psychopathology: maladaptation and psychopathology. Wiley; 2016.
2. Mazefsky C, Day T, Golt J. Autism. In: Roy A, Brotman M, Liebenluft E, editors. Irritability in pediatric psychopathology. 1st edition. Oxford: Oxford University Press; 2019.
3. Mikita N, Hollocks M, Papadopolous A, et al. Irritability in boys with autism spectrum disorder: an investigation of physiological reactivity. J Child Psychol Psychiatry 2015;56:1118–21.
4. Prokasky A, Rudasill K, Molfese V, et al. Identifying child temperament types using cluster analysis in three samples. J Res Personal 2017;67:190–201.
5. Goldsmith H, Lemery K, Biuss K, et al. Genetic analyses of focal aspects of infant temperament. Dev Psychol 1999;35:972–85.
6. Planalp E, Goldsmith H. Observed profiles of infant temperament: stability, heritability, and associations with parenting. Child Dev 2019;91(3):e563–80.
7. Kopp C. Antecedents of self-regulation: a developmental perspective. Dev Psychol 1982;18:199–214.
8. Calkins S. The emergence of self-regulation: biological and behavioral control mechanisms supporting toddler competencies. In: Brownell C, Kopp C, editors. Transitions in early socioemotional development: the toddler years. New York: Guilford; 2010.
9. Bernier A, Beauchamp M, Bouvette-Turcot A, et al. Sleep and cognition in preschool years: specific links to executive functioning. Child Dev 2013;84:1542–53.
10. Williams K, Berthelsen D, Walker S, et al. A developmental cascade model of behavioral sleep problems and emotional and attentional self-regulation across early childhood. Behav Sleep Med 2017;15:1–21.
11. Swingler M, Perry N, Calkins S. Neural plasticity and the development of attention: intrinsic and extrinsic influences. Dev Psychopathol 2015;27:443–57.
12. Posner M, Rothbart M, Rueda R. Developing attention and self-regulation in childhood. In: Nobre A, Kastner S, editors. Oxford library of psychology; Oxford handbook of attention. Oxford Univeristy Press; 2014. p. 541–69.
13. Posner M, Rothbart M, Sheese B, et al. Developing attention: behavioral and brain mechanisms. In: Advances in neuroscience. 2014. p. 9.
14. Haley D, Stansbury K. Infant stress and parent responsiveness: regulation of physiology and behavior during still-face and reunion. Child Dev 2003;74:1534–46.
15. Weinberg M, Tronick E. Infant affective reactions to the resumption of maternal interaction after the still-face. Child Dev 1996;67:905–14.

16. Camacho M, Karim H, Perlman S. Neural architecture supporting active emotion processing in children: a multivariate approach. Neuroimage 2019;188:171–80.
17. Rothbart M, Rueda M. The development of effortful control. In: Mayr U, Awh E, Keele S, editors. Decade of behavior developing individuality in the human brain: a tribute to Michael I Posner. American Psychological Association; 2005. p. 167–88.
18. Kochanska G, Murray K, Harlan E. Effortful control in early childhood: continuity and change, antecedents, and implications for social development. Dev Psychol 2000;36:220–32.
19. Dunn J, Bretherton I, Munn P. Conversations about feeling states between mothers and their young children. Dev Psychol 1987;23.
20. LaBounty J, Wellman H, Olson S, et al. Mothers' and fathers' use of internal state talk with their young children. Soc Dev 2008;17:757–75.
21. Waters E, Kondo-Ikemura K, Posada G, et al. Learning to love: mechanisms and milestones. In: Gunnar M, Sroufe L, Lawrence, editors. The Minnesota Symposia on child psychology: self-processes and development. Erlbaum Associates, Inc; 1991. p. 217–55.
22. Crowell J, Fraley R, Roisman G. Measures of individual differences in adolescent and adult attachment. In: Cassidy J, Shaver P, editors. Handbook of attachment: theory, research, and clinical applications. 3rd edition. New York: Guildford; 2016.
23. Ainsworth MDS, Blehar M, Waters E, et al. Patterns of attachment: a psychological study of the strange situation. Hillsdale, NJ: Lawrence Erlbaum; 1978.
24. Cooke J, Kochendorfer L, Stuart-Parrigon K, et al. Parent-child attachment and children's experience and regulation of emotion: a meta-analytic review. Emotion 2019;19:1103–26.
25. Zimmer-Gembeck M, Webb H, Pepping C, et al. Review: is parent-child attachment a correlate of children's emotion regulation and coping? Int J Behav Dev 2017;41:74–93.
26. Morris A, Silk J, Steinberg L, et al. The role of family context in the development of emotion regulation. Soc Dev 2007;16:361–88.
27. Kramer L. Learning emotional understanding and emotion regulation through sibling interaction. Early Educ Dev 2014;25:160–84.
28. Nakamichi K. Differences in young children's peer preference by inhibitory control and omotion regulation. Psychol Rep 2017;120:805–23.
29. Cole P. Children's spontaneous control of facial expression. Child Dev 1986;57: 1309–21.
30. Grabell A, Huppert T, Fishburn F, et al. Neural correlates of early deliberate emotion regulation: young children's responses to interpersonal scaffolding. Dev Cogn Neurosci 2019;40:100708.
31. Carpenter M, Akhtar N, Tomasello N. Fourteen- through 18-month-old infants differentially imitate intentional and accidental actions. Infant Behav Dev 1998; 21:315–30.
32. Lindsey E, Colwell M. Pretend and physical play: links to preschoolers' affective social competence. Merrill-Palmer Q 2013;59:330–60.
33. Lillard A. Why do the children (pretend) play? Trends Cogn Sci 2017;21:826–34.
34. Lillard A, Kavanaugh R. The contribution of symbolic skills to the development of an explicit theory of mind. Child Dev 2014;85:1535–51.
35. Paquette D. Theorizing the father-child relationship: mechanisms and developmental outcomes. Hum Dev 2004;47:193–219.
36. Cabrera N, Tamis-LeMonda C. The handbook of father involvement: multidisciplinary perspectives. New York: Routledge; 2002.

37. Perlman S, Pelphrey K. Regulatory brain development: balancing emotion and cognition. Soc Neurosci 2010;5:533–42.
38. Stevens F, Hurley R, Hayman A, et al. Anterior cingulate cortex: unique role in cognition and emotion. J Neuropsychiatry 2011;23:121–5.
39. Granic I. Timing is everything: developmental psychopathology from a dynamic systems perspective. Dev Rev 2005;25:386–407.
40. Morris A, Silk J, Morris M, et al. The influence of mother-child emotion regulation strategies on children's expression of anger and sadness. Dev Psychol 2011;47: 213–25.
41. Memmott-Elison M, Mollanen K, Padilla-Walker L. Latent growth in self-regulatory subdimensions in relation to adjustment outcomes in youth aged 12–19. J Res Adolescence 2020.
42. Casey B, Jones R, Hare T. The adolescent brain. Ann N Y Acad Sci 2008;1124: 111–28.
43. Dumonthiel I. Adolescent brain development. Curr Opin Behav Sci 2016;10: 39–44.
44. Thomas L, De Bellis M, Graham R, et al. Development of emotional facial recognition in late childhood and adolescence. Dev Sci 2007;10:547–58.
45. Rafaelli M, Crockett L, Shen Y-L. Developmental stability and change in self-regulation from childhood to adolescence. Lincoln, NE: Faculty Publications, Department of Psychology; 2005. Digital Commons@University of Nebraska-Lincoln.
46. Niv S, Tuvblad C, Raine A, et al. Heritability and longitudinal stability of impulsivity in adolescence. Behav Genet 2012;42:378–92.
47. Villani D, Carissoli C, Triberti S, et al. games for emotion regulation: a systematic review. Games for Health 2018;7:1–15.
48. Wichstrom L, Stenseng F, Belsky J, et al. Symptoms of internet gaming disorder in youth: predictors and comorbidity. J Abnorm Child Psychol 2019;47:71–83.
49. Cerniglia L, Cimino S, Ammaniti M. What are the effects of screen time in emotion regulation and academic achievements? A three-wave longitudinal study on children from 4 to 8 years of age. J Early Child Res 2020.

Early Predictors of Adolescent Irritability

Ellen M. Kessel, PhD[a],*, Lea R. Dougherty, PhD[b], Samantha Hubacheck, MS[b],
Emma Chad-Friedman, MS[b], Tom Olino, PhD[c], Gabrielle A. Carlson, MD[d],
Daniel N. Klein, PhD[e]

KEYWORDS

- Early risk • Development • Irritability • Adolescence

KEY POINTS

- Limited research has examined early precursors/risk factors for adolescent irritability.
- Using multiple methods and informants and a prospective longitudinal design, the authors examined the continuity of irritability from early childhood to adolescence and identified other early predictors of adolescent irritability.
- Across both self-reports and mother-reports, the authors found evidence for continuity of irritability from ages 3 to 15.
- The authors also found that early antecedents of adolescent irritability differ in many instances as a function of either informant or gender.
- The results also suggest that adolescent irritability is characterized by several distinct developmental pathways from age 3 that have the potential to result in an irritable phenotype at age 15.
- They also suggest that self-reported and mother-reported irritability may be capturing distinct underlying constructs, and both should be considered in assessments of adolescent irritability.

In recent years, developmental psychopathology research increasingly has focused on irritability—a transdiagnostic phenotype and frequent clinical concern across development.[1] Unfortunately, tailored treatments are lacking, in part because little still is known about irritability's etiology or how to conceptualize irritability across development. At its root, irritability is characterized by a tendency toward anger and temper outbursts.[2,3] Irritability is a dimensional phenotype spanning the normal-abnormal continuum. It is common, heritable,[4] and relatively stable in community samples of

In Gabrielle A. Carlson & Manpreet K. Singh (Eds.) CAPS Clinics Emotion Dysregulation in Children: Part II.
[a] Division of Child and Adolescent Psychiatry, Columbia University and the New State Psychiatric Institute; [b] Department of Psychology, University of Maryland College Park; [c] Department of Psychology, Temple University; [d] Department of Psychiatry, Stony Brook University School of Medicine; [e] Department of Psychology, Stony Brook University
* Corresponding author.
E-mail address: ellen.kessel@nyspi.columbia.edu

youth. In more severe forms, it is a symptom of at least 10 *Diagnostic and Statistical Manual of Mental Disorders* (*DSM*) psychiatric disorders and is associated with more severe psychopathology and functional impairment, regardless of specific diagnosis.[5]

To better understand the role of irritability in psychopathology, researchers have examined prospective associations between irritability and later psychopathology in clinical and epidemiologic studies, many of which span large age ranges. The leading consensus is that youth irritability specifically predicts internalizing disorders later in life, in particular depression (for a recent meta-analysis, see Vidal-Ribas and colleagues[5]), leading some to speculate that irritability is a mood manifestation that shares common risk factors with depressive and anxiety disorders (eg, see Stringaris and Taylor[1]).

Other studies,[6,7] however, in particular those examining outcomes of very early manifestations of irritability,[8,9] find that irritability predates the emergence of both internalizing and externalizing disorders and their heterotypic comorbidity (ie, the co-occurrence of at least 1 internalizing disorder and at least 1 externalizing disorder).[10] These findings have led other developmental psychopathologists (eg, see Beauchaine and Tackett[11]) to postulate that irritability reflects a nonspecific liability to develop a broad range of psychopathology.

Largely missing from this literature, however, is research examining precursors and risk factors for irritability. Importantly, examining prospective associations between irritability and later psychopathology reduces irritability to a mere risk factor of other conditions rather than a significant clinical concern in and of itself that can require treatment. Expanding irritability research to prospectively examine early risk factors associated with irritability across salient domains of child development at a much younger age not only may deepen understanding of etiology but also create a longer window for prevention/early interventions, and these efforts can begin before the maladaptive processes have crystallized and begun to interfere with normal development.

Additionally, an implicit assumption across studies of youth irritability is that it is a unitary construct across development, which makes reconciling divergent patterns of findings across broad age ranges, as in many of the studies cited previously, challenging. Recent genetic evidence suggests, however, that irritability may be etiologically heterogenous across development. Specifically, earlier and more persistent forms of irritability may be more related genetically to neurodevelopmental conditions, whereas later irritability may be linked more closely to disruptions in mood.[12,13] These findings caution against extrapolating findings in one age group to another and highlight the importance of examining irritability at specific stages of development as opposed to over broad age ranges.

Adolescence is a developmental period when biological, psychological, and social systems undergo rapid changes to meet crucial developmental tasks.[14] Irritability can interfere with core aspects of adaptive functioning during this developmental period, including social affiliation and situationally functional goal-directed behavior, which can have cascading consequences and become more severe in adulthood.[11] Coinciding with these changes is the emergence of many common forms of psychopathology in which irritability is a prominent feature (ie, major depressive disorder, borderline personality features, generalized anxiety disorder, and conduct disorder).[15] Sex differences in the prevalence of internalizing problems also emerge in adolescence, with female adolescents having higher rates of internalizing psychopathology compared with male adolescents.[16] Thus, examining early antecedents of irritability during adolescence may have important clinical implications and help elucidate how sex influences the development of irritability.

The limited research examining prospective associations between prior psychopathology and adolescent irritability suggest that internalizing and externalizing problems can precede adolescent irritability.[17–19] These studies, however, either have lacked baseline measures of irritability or first assessed irritability during late childhood/adolescence, although for many youths, irritability tends to emerge very early in life. Thus, it is unclear whether irritability truly is a consequence of earlier psychopathology or actually a continuation of an earlier problem.

The few other studies that have examined risk factors for irritability have focused mainly on associations between parental psychopathology and very early manifestations of irritability. Across these studies, parental mood disorders consistently emerge as a significant predictor of childhood irritability,[8,20,21] whereas parental anxiety disorders[8] and substance use disorders (SUDs)[21] have emerged as significant predictors in some studies but not others. It is unclear, however, whether the same associations are apparent in adolescence.

No prospective studies have examined psychosocial factors that may be early indicators or contributors to the development of irritability, although cross-sectional studies have identified several factors, such as early adversity and maladaptive parenting practices, that co-occur with irritability.[22–24] Examining the temporal ordering of such factors may help elucidate developmental pathways that may be tractable.

Additionally, research examining irritability in youth has for the most part relied on parent-report measures and, to a lesser extent, self-report measures in older youth. The rates of agreement between parent-reported and child-reported irritability are only moderate ($r = 0.40$)[25]; and studies have shown that self-reported irritability is associated more strongly with other emotional problems, whereas parent-reported irritability is linked more tightly to externalizing problems.[26] Youth may have access to feelings that are not observable to their parents. On the other hand, youth who externalize may be less aware of their mood states. Importantly, recent psychometric research suggests that parent and child measures of irritability may be capturing different underlying constructs.[27] Thus, information from both informants should be considered in studies of youth irritability.

This study examines early antecedents of self-reported and mother-reported adolescent irritability in a community sample of children followed from age 3 to age 15, using a multimethod (interviews, laboratory assessments, and questionnaires) and multi-informant (mother and youth) design. The first aim was to examine the continuity or stability of irritability as reported from age 3 to age 15 and whether it is consistent across self-report and mother-report at age 15. The second aim was to identify other age 3 predictors of age 15 self-reported and mother-reported irritability. The following 5 domains of potential early childhood predictors were assessed: psychopathology, functioning, temperament, parental psychopathology, and the psychosocial environment. In addition to reporting unadjusted analyses, models examining predictors of age 15 mother-reported and self-reported irritability also were adjusted for age 3 irritability to ensure that adolescent irritability was a consequence rather than a continuation of preexisting problems. Whether sex moderated associations between age 3 predictors and adolescent irritability also was examined.

METHOD
Participants

Participants in this study are part of the Stony Brook Temperament Study, a longitudinal study of early childhood temperament and other risk factors in the development of internalizing disorders (N = 559). Since initial recruitment, the families have participated in several waves of assessments involving a range of measures (see Klein and Finsaas[28]). At the age 3 assessment, 541 parents (primarily mothers) completed diagnostic interviews regarding their 3-year-old children (M_{age} = 3.55 years, SD = 0.43). At age 15, of those families, 421 adolescents (M_{age} = 15.24 years, SD = 0.15) and their mothers completed questionnaires assessing the adolescent's irritability. Full information maximum likelihood estimation was used in analyses to account for missing data. Thus, the analytical sample included 541 participants (45.8% female) and with regards to race/ethnicity was 86.6% white/non-Hispanic, 7.8% Hispanic, 2.8% black/African American, 2.0% Asian, 0.2% Native American, and 0.6% other.

Domains of measures

Age 3 Assessment
Psychopathology. Youth psychopathology was assessed at age 3 with the Preschool Age Psychiatric Assessment (PAPA,)[29] a parent-based structured diagnostic interview. Parents were interviewed by phone by advanced graduate students in clinical psychology trained by a member of the group who developed the interview. The PAPA demonstrates good test-retest reliability,[29] and diagnostic interviews with parents regarding their children administered by phone and face-to-face yielded comparable results.[30] Children's symptoms of depression, anxiety, oppositional defiant disorder (ODD), and attention-deficit/hyperactivity disorder (ADHD) occurring in the 3 months prior to the interview were reported by parents and rated by interviewers.

Symptoms of each psychiatric disorder (depressive, anxiety, ODD, and ADHD) were derived by summing the intensity ratings in each diagnostic category, excluding the items included in the irritability scale, to avoid item overlap (for further description, see Dougherty and colleagues[30]). Coefficient α and interrater intraclass correlation coefficients (ICCs) for symptom scales ranged from 0.54 to 0.89 and 0.98 to 1.00, respectively.

Irritability. Six items from the PAPA interview were used to assess irritability at age 3. Items corresponded to items from the Affective Reactivity Index (ARI), a parent-reported (ARI-mother [M]) and child-reported (ARI-self [S]) chronic irritability scale for older youth.[31] In addition, to assess whether the child experienced irritable mood states for a long time, this criterion was coded as present if the child was rated as having at least a 30-minute duration of irritable mood; being prone to frustration, annoyance or anger; or having difficulty recovering from temper tantrums. The total irritability scale (α = .77) consisted of the sum of the 7 symptoms, coded as present, according to the intensity, frequency, and duration criteria described in Dougherty and colleagues.[8]

Functioning. Functional impairment was assessed using the PAPA interview. The PAPA interviewer rated impairment across several domains (parental relationship quality, household and recreational activities, sibling and peer relationships, and school life) on 5-point scales, ranging from 0 (no impairment) to 4 (severe impairment). Ratings were summed across domains for a total impairment score (ICC = 0.91).

Receptive and expressive vocabulary skills were assessed with the Peabody Picture Vocabulary Test[32] and Expressive One-Word Picture Vocabulary Test,[33] respectively. In order to assess social competence, mothers were interviewed when children were aged 3 using the Vineland Adaptive Behavior Screener socialization subscale[34] by a trained research assistant. The Vineland evaluates children's social skills required for everyday life, including interpersonal interactions and sensitivity, manners, and responsibility ($\alpha = 0.51$).

Child temperament. At age 3, each child and a parent visited the laboratory for a 2-hour observational assessment of temperament that included a standardized set of episodes selected to elicit a range of temperament-relevant behaviors. Tasks were selected from the Laboratory Temperament Assessment Battery (Lab-TAB).[35] The episodes were selected to elicit several affective dimensions, including positive emotionality, fear, anger/frustration, and sadness. Coding procedures followed those reported in a previous study.[36] Coefficient α and ICCs for positive emotionality, fear, anger/frustration and sadness scales ranged from 0.63 to 0.89 and 0.64 to 0.92, respectively.

Parental psychiatric history. Biological parents of children participating in the study were interviewed regarding their psychiatric history with the Structured Clinical Interview for *DSM* (Fourth Edition), nonpatient version,[37] upon their child's entry into the study at age 3. Interviews were conducted by phone by an advanced doctoral student in clinical psychology and a master's-level clinician supervised by a licensed clinical psychologist.[38] Parental lifetime history of depressive disorder, anxiety disorder, and SUD were marked as present if one or both parents had the disorder and as absent if neither parent had the disorder (ICCs ranged from 0.91 to 1.00).

Psychosocial environment. At age 3, salient features of the early environment that have been shown to have lasting consequences across development were assessed and included maternal parenting, early childhood stress, marital satisfaction, and parental education as an index of socioeconomic status. Mothers completed the 37-item Parenting Styles and Dimensions Questionnaire[39] to assess authoritative (ie, warmth and involvement, reasoning and induction, democratic participation, and good-naturedness), authoritarian (ie, verbal hostility, corporal punishment, nonreasoning and punitive strategies, and directiveness), and permissive (ie, lack of follow through, ignoring misbehavior, and low self-confidence) parenting styles. The factors' internal consistencies (authoritative: $\alpha = .82$; authoritarian: $\alpha = .75$; and permissive: $\alpha = .74$) were acceptable.

Early childhood stress was assessed using the PAPA interview. The PAPA includes an assessment of 41 stressful and traumatic events involving the child and immediate family members, including illness, injury, loss of a loved one, and extended separations. Events occurring from the time the child was born until the age 3 assessment were summed to create a total stress score.

Marital satisfaction was assessed at 3 using the 7-item abbreviated Dyadic Adjustment Scale[40] ($\alpha = .86$).

Finally, parental education was assessed when children were 3 years old and included as an index of socioeconomic status (in 67.7% of the families at least one parent graduated from college).

Age 15 Assessment
Irritability. Youth irritability was assessed using the ARI 7-item self-report (ARI-S; M = 1.56; SD = 2.00; $\alpha = .85$) and parent-report (ARI-M; M = 1.00; SD = 1.86; $\alpha = .86$) questionnaire that assesses irritability in youth over the past 6 months.[31]

Data analysis

To examine early predictors of adolescent irritability, the authors first conducted zero-order correlations between age 3 predictors and age 15 self-reported and mother-reported irritability. Age 3 predictors included irritability and variables from each of the following 5 domains: child psychopathology, functioning, temperament, parental psychopathology, and the psychosocial environment.[a] Point-biserial correlations were used to assess the associations between dichotomous and continuous variables. To examine whether the magnitude of the association between age 3 and age 15 irritability differed across informant, the authors conducted a z-test on their β coefficients, calculated by regressing self-reported and mother-reported irritability on age 3 irritability in two separate models while imposing an equality constraint on their residual variance. Next, the authors conducted a series of regression analyses in which self-reported and mother-reported irritability were regressed in separate models on age 3 predictors, while controlling for age 3 irritability to ensure that the subsequent development of, rather than the continuation of, preexisting irritability at age 15 was examined. To explore sex-specific effects, the authors reran each model, including interactions between each age 3 predictor and child sex. Regression models examined variables from each domain separately to elucidate domain-specific main and interaction effects with sex. Because these analyses were exploratory, there were no corrections for multiple comparisons. Continuous variables were centered and cross-product terms were created to test interaction effects. Simple slope terms were tested to probe significant interactions.[41]

RESULTS

There was only modest agreement between age 15 ARI-S–reported and ARI-M–reported irritability ($r = 0.23$; $p < .001$). From ages 3 to age 15, irritability showed modest but significant within construct associations, and the association was significantly weaker for self-reported irritability compared with mother-reported irritability ($t = -3.93$; $p < .001$). Other significant bivariate age 3 predictors (**Tables 1–5**) of ARI-S at age 15 include early childhood anxiety and depressive symptoms, functional impairment, social competence, Lab-TAB anger, parental mood disorder, less parental education, lower marital satisfaction, and permissive parenting. Significant bivariate age 3 predictors of ARI-M at age 15 include early childhood irritability, anxiety, depressive, ODD and ADHD symptoms, functional impairment, Lab-TAB anger, parental anxiety and SUD, early stressors, lower marital satisfaction, and authoritarian and permissive parenting.

Early Childhood Psychopathology

When age 3 predictors were entered simultaneously into each domain-specific multivariate regression model controlling for age 3 irritability, there were no main effects of child psychopathology (anxiety, depressive, and ODD and ADHD symptoms) on either age 15 ARI-S or ARI-M and no main effect of age 3 irritability on age 15 ARI-S. The main effect of early childhood ADHD symptoms on age 15 adolescent-reported irritability, however, was qualified by a significant interaction (see **Table 2**). Girls with higher ADHD symptoms at age 3 reported higher levels of irritability at age 15 ($t = 2.00$; $p < .05$). There was no association between age 3 ADHD symptoms and ARI-S in boys ($t = -0.78$; $p = $ not significant [ns]) (see **Table 1**).

---

[a] All variables were screened for univariate normality. Univariate outliers were winsorized to the next highest value on their respective measure. Kurtosis and skew were high for age 3 irritability (skew = 2.10; kurtosis = 3.85), age 3 depressive symptoms (skew = 3.55; kurtosis = 22.58), and age 15 self-reported (skew = 2.12; kurtosis = 6.04) and mother-reported irritability (skew = 2.98; kurtosis = 10.53), so square root transformations were performed, which brought each of these variables within acceptable parameters. All other study variables were relatively normal, with skewness and kurtosis indices less than ±2.5.

Table 1
Multiple regression model with age 3 irritability, age 3 psychopathology, and sex predicting age 15 self-reported and mother-reported irritability

| | | | | | Age 15 Irritability | | |
| | | Self-Report | | | Mother-Report | | |
Predictors	M (SD)	r	β	SE	r	β	SE
Main effects							
Sex (female)		0.08	0.08	0.05	−0.07	−0.01	0.05
Age 3 irritability	**0.70 (1.30)**	0.10[a]	0.06	0.06	0.36[b]	0.29[c]	0.06
Age 3 anxiety symptoms	**7.61 (6.50)**	0.12[a]	0.07	0.06	0.19[c]	0.08	0.06
Age 3 depressive symptoms	**1.36 (1.71)**	0.14[b]	0.09	0.06	0.18[c]	0.05	0.05
Age 3 ODD symptoms	2.00 (2.00)	0.09	0.01	0.07	0.26[c]	0.05	0.07
Age 3 ADHD symptoms	3.88 (6.22)	0.07	0.03	0.06	0.12[b]	−0.01	0.06
Interactive effects							
Age 3 anxiety symptoms × sex			−0.04	0.06		0.07	0.05
Age 3 depressive symptoms × sex			0.04	0.06		−0.04	0.05
Age 3 ODD symptoms × sex			−0.09	0.06		−0.05	0.06
Age 3 ADHD symptoms × sex			0.13[a]	0.06		0.04	0.06

[a] $p < .05$.
[b] $p < .01$.
[c] $p < .001$.

Table 2
Multiple regression model with age 3 irritability, age 3 functioning, and sex predicting age 15 self-reported and mother-reported irritability

| | | | | | Age 15 Irritability | | |
| | | | Self-Report | | Mother-Report | | |
Predictors	M (SD)	R	β	SE	r	β	SE
Main effects							
Sex (female)		.08	0.08	0.05	−0.07	0.01	0.05
Age 3 irritability	**0.70 (1.30)**	0.10[a]	0.04	0.06	0.36[b]	0.24[c]	0.06
Age 3 functional impairment	**0.84 (1.41)**	0.15[b]	0.18[c]	0.06	0.33[c]	0.23[c]	0.06
Age 3 social competence	**18.91 (3.73)**	0.06	0.10[b]	0.05	−0.05	0.05	0.05
Age 3 receptive vocabulary	102.85 (13.88)	0.02	0.01	0.06	0.08	0.09	0.06
Age 3 expressive vocabulary	100.65 (12.96)	0.01	0.01	0.06	0.04	0.04	0.06
Interactive effects							
Age 3 incapacity × sex			0.02	0.05		−0.03	0.05
Age 3 social competence × sex			−0.06	0.05		−0.06	0.05
Age 3 receptive vocabulary × sex			−0.07	0.06		0.00	0.06
Age 3 expressive vocabulary × sex			0.13[a]	0.06		0.00	0.06

[a] $p < .05$.
[b] $p < .01$.
[c] $p < .001$.

Table 3
Multiple regression model with age 3 irritability, age 3 observed temperament, and sex predicting age 15 self-reported and mother-reported irritability

| | | | | | Age 15 Irritability | | |
| | | | Self-report | | Mother-report | | |
Predictors	M (SD)	r	β	SE	r	β	SE
Main effects							
Sex (female)		.08	0.09[a]	0.05	−0.07	−0.01	0.05
Age 3 irritability	0.70 (1.30)	0.10[b]	0.11[b]	0.05	0.36[c]	0.35[d]	0.04
Age 3 Lab-TAB positive emotionality	−0.03 (1.81)	0.03	0.03	0.06	0.07	0.09[b]	0.05
Age 3 Lab-TAB sadness	0.56 (0.31)	0.03	−0.01	0.06	0.08	0.07	0.06
Age 3 Lab-TAB fear	0.66 (0.35)	−0.03	−0.06	0.05	−0.03	−0.07	0.05
Age 3 Lab-TAB anger	0.57 (0.35)	0.10[b]	0.10[a]	0.05	0.10[b]	0.01	0.05
Interactive effects							
Age 3 Lab-TAB positive emotionality × sex			0.05	0.06		0.01	0.05
Age 3 Lab-TAB sadness × sex			0.10[a]	0.06		0.04	0.05
Age 3 Lab-TAB fear × sex			−0.06	0.06		−0.05	0.05
Age 3 LAB-Tab anger × sex			0.02	0.05		−0.07	0.05

[a] $p < .10$.
[b] $p < .05$.
[c] $p < .01$.
[d] $p < .001$.

Table 4
Multiple regression model with age 3 irritability, parental psychopathology, and sex predicting age 15 self-reported and mother-reported irritability

| | | | | | Age 15 Irritability | | |
| | | | Self-Report | | Mother-Report | | |
Predictors	M (SD)	r	β	SE	r	β	SE
Main effects							
Sex (female)		.08	0.07	0.05	−0.07	−0.02	0.07
Age 3 irritability	0.70 (1.30)	0.10[b]	0.09[a]	0.06	0.36[c]	0.34[d]	0.05
Parental mood disorder, n (%)	247 (46%)	0.14[b]	0.07	0.05	0.10[a]	−0.01	0.05
Parental anxiety disorder, n (%)	261 (49%)	0.10[a]	0.05	0.05	0.15[c]	0.09[a]	0.05
Parental SUD, n (%)	283 (53%)	0.09	0.04	0.05	0.12[b]	0.06	0.05
Interactive effects							
Parental mood disorder × sex			0.00	0.05		0.07	0.05
Parental anxiety disorder × sex			−0.08	0.05		−0.02	0.05
Parental SUD × sex			0.05	0.05		0.02	0.05

[a] $p < .10$.
[b] $p < .05$.
[c] $p < .01$.
[d] $p < .001$.

Table 5
Multiple regression model with age 3 irritability, age 3 psychosocial variables, and sex predicting age 15 self-reported and mother-reported irritability

| | | | Age 15 Irritability | | | | |
| | | | Self-Report | | Mother-Report | | |
	M (SD)	r	β	SE	r	β	SE
Main effects							
Sex (female)		.08	0.06	0.06	−0.07	−0.02	0.05
Age 3 irritability	0.70 (1.30)	**0.10[b]**	**0.09[a]**	**0.05**	**0.36[c]**	**0.31[d]**	**0.05**
Parental education, n (%)	361 (71%)	**−0.18[c]**	**−0.11[b]**	**0.06**	0.01	0.09[a]	0.05
Marital satisfaction	15.96 (3.79)	**−0.12[b]**	**−0.12[b]**	**0.06**	**−0.13[b]**	**−0.11[b]**	**0.05**
Age 3 stress	4.05 (2.78)	0.03	0.01	0.05	**0.12[b]**	0.05	0.05
Age 3 maternal authoritative parenting	61.14 (6.62)	0.06	0.08	0.05	−0.04	0.01	0.05
Age 3 maternal authoritarian parenting	19.98 (4.27)	0.00	−0.07	0.06	**0.22[d]**	**0.11[b]**	**0.05**
Age 3 maternal permissive parenting	10.81 (3.22)	**0.12[b]**	0.10[a]	0.06	0.19[d]	0.10[a]	0.06
Interactive effects							
Parental education × sex			−0.02	0.05		−0.06	0.05
Marital satisfaction × sex			**−0.16[c]**	**0.06**		0.01	0.05
Age 3 stress × sex			0.01	0.05		−0.04	0.05
Age 3 maternal authoritative parenting × sex			−0.02	0.05		−0.02	0.05
Age 3 maternal authoritarian parenting × sex			−0.03	0.06		0.03	0.05
Age 3 maternal permissive parenting × sex			−0.06	0.06		**−0.15[c]**	0.05

[a] $p < .10$.
[b] $p < .05$.
[c] $p < .01$.
[d] $p < .001$.

Functioning

In the multivariate regression model controlling for age 3 irritability, both higher levels of age 3 social competence and functional impairment predicted age 15 ARI-S. In this model, age 3 irritability no longer significantly predicted age 15 ARI-S. Additionally, there was a significant interaction between expressive vocabulary and sex in predicting ARI-S. Girls who rated themselves as more irritable at age 15 had greater expressive vocabulary scores at age 3 at a trend level ($t = 1.63$; $p < .10$). Among boys, there was no association between age 3 expressive vocabulary and age 15 ARI-S ($t = −1.21$; $p = $ ns). Greater age 3 functional impairment continued to predict age 15 ARI-M (see **Table 2**).

Temperament

There were no significant main effects of temperament on age 15 ARI-S after adjusting for age 3 irritability, although Lab-TAB anger continued to predict age 15 ARI-S at a trend level. Greater age 3 Lab-TAB positive emotionality predicted age 15 ARI-M (see **Table 3**).

Parental Psychopathology

There were no significant main effects of parental psychopathology on age 15 ARI-S after adjusting for age 3 irritability. Parental anxiety disorder predicted age 15 ARI-M at a trend level (see **Table 4**).

Psychosocial Environment

Lower parental education and marital satisfaction continued to significantly predict age 15 ARI-S after adjusting for age 3 irritability. There also was trend-level association between permissive parenting and age 15 ARI-S. The main effect of martial satisfaction on ARI-S, however, was qualified by a significant interaction. Among girls, lower marital satisfaction predicted higher levels of age 15 ARI-S ($t = -3.96$; $p < .01$), whereas among boys, there was no association ($t = 0.39$; p = ns). Lower martial satisfaction and maternal authoritarian parenting significantly predicted age 15 ARI-M. There also was a trend-level association between age 3 maternal permissive parenting and age 15 ARI-M that was qualified by a significant interaction (see **Table 5**). Among boys, greater permissive parenting predicted higher levels of age 15 ARI-M ($t = 2.62$; $p < .01$), whereas among girls, there was no significant association ($t = -1.13$; p = ns).

DISCUSSION

Using data from a prospective community study of adolescents from ages 3 to 15, the authors examined early antecedents of adolescent irritability using a multimethod, multi-informant observational design. To the authors' knowledge, this is the first study to characterize adolescent irritability in a community sample while also examining a broad set of predictors of adolescent irritability, including early child psychopathology, functioning, temperament, parental history of psychopathology, and some aspects of psychosocial environment.

In this study, agreement between self-reported and mother-reported adolescent irritability was relatively modest. Consistent with well-known informant discrepancies in developmental psychopathology research,[27,42] the authors' data suggest that self-report and mother-report may be capturing partially distinct underlying constructs of irritability. Across both self-reported and mother-report, the authors found evidence for continuity of irritability from ages 3 to 15, although associations were significantly weaker for self-reported adolescent irritability. The authors also found that antecedents of adolescent irritability differ as a function of informant, as discussed later.

Early Psychopathology

In this sample, early childhood irritability and anxiety and depressive symptoms predicted both self-reported and mother-reported irritability. Additionally, early ADHD and ODD symptoms predicted mother-reported adolescent irritability. After the authors controlled for baseline levels of irritability and simultaneously examined interactions with sex, a somewhat different pattern of findings emerged. Age 3 anxiety and depressive symptoms no longer were associated with either self-reported or mother-reported adolescent irritability, and ODD and ADHD symptoms no longer were associated with mother-reported adolescent irritability. There was an interactive effect between sex and ADHD symptoms on adolescent-reported irritability, however, such that only among girls early symptoms of ADHD predicted later irritability.

These findings suggest that prospective associations between early manifestations of internalizing and externalizing disorders, and later irritability may be solely artifacts of their overlap with co-occurring irritability and are not independent predictors in and of themselves. Early manifestations of ADHD in girls, however, appears to the be exception. It is unclear whether this association reflects a causal relationship—for example, ADHD may interfere with goal-directed functioning over the course of development, increasing the likelihood of failures/goal blockage and ultimately resulting in feelings of frustration and anger.[43] Additionally, compared with boys, girls often are underdiagnosed for ADHD and less likely to receive treatment, hence may have greater functional impairment than boys, more of whose ADHD is treated. Alternatively, ADHD and irritability may be influenced by a shared vulnerability, although family and twin studies typically find that genetic effects account for the overlap between irritability and ADHD in boys, whereas as nonshared environmental factors influence their overlap in girls.[13]

Functioning

Age 3 functional impairment predicted both self-reported and mother-reported adolescent irritability, even after controlling age 3 irritability. When examined simultaneously in the multivariate model with social competence, both higher levels of functional impairment and higher levels of social competence emerged as unique predictors of self-reported adolescent irritability. Additionally, there was a significant interaction between expressive language skills and sex predicting self-reported adolescent irritability, such that among girls, more adept expressive language abilities predicted higher levels of irritability at age 15. Although irritable individuals suffer from a great deal of impairment across multiple domains of functioning, this impairment often is conceptualized solely as a consequence of their irritability. The authors' results suggest, however, that impairments in selective areas of functioning also can precede the development of irritability.

The authors' findings suggest that there may be distinct developmental pathways to later irritability depending on specific areas of functioning, some that are adaptive versus impairing early in development. The prospective associations between greater social competence and among girls, more adept expressive language abilities with later irritability, are somewhat surprising. At age 3, however, social competence is characterized by greater social sensitivity and attunement,[44] which, in line with the notion of differential susceptibility,[45] can render children more susceptible to both adaptive and maladaptive aspects of their social environments. Across development, these children may be particularly vulnerable to interpersonal events that either threaten their personal integrity (eg, bullying) or thwart their affiliative needs (eg, peer exclusion/rejection) and, thus, more prone to anger and irritability.[46] Verbally gifted children, on the other hand, have been shown to have more emotional awareness of themselves and others that make them more skillful in their argumentativeness. These abilities also have been shown to support maladaptive self-speech, like rumination, which is more typical among girls.[47] The specificity of this higher functioning pathway to self-reported irritability also raises the possibility that adolescent-reported irritability may be capturing a behaviorally suppressed manifestation of irritability (ie, anger-in[48]) that may not be observable to another informant because it is accompanied by high levels of self-control and either replaced by socially appropriate expressions or directed toward oneself. This possibility, however, has not yet been tested.

Temperament

Laboratory-observed anger at age 3 predicted both self-reported and mother-reported adolescent irritability. When the authors examined domains of temperament simultaneously, however, while also adjusting for age 3 irritability, laboratory-observed age 3 anger only continued to predict self-reported adolescent irritability at a trend level, and higher levels of observed age 3 positive emotionality emerged as a significant independent predictor of mother-reported adolescent irritability. Translational neuroscientific models of irritability suggest that aberrant frustrative-nonreward underlies irritability.[49] The authors' findings lend support to this model, because both anger and positive emotionality have been linked to greater motivational approach system sensitivity across development.[50,51] Individuals who are higher in approach sensitivity are more likely to be goal-directed and seek out rewards yet also are more likely to experience feelings of frustration and anger when circumstances prevent their desired goals from becoming fulfilled and may be disproportionate or even pathologic in certain contexts.[43] Additionally, the authors' findings suggest that measurements of individual differences in more normative expressions of approach system-related temperament traits may offer incremental validity over using clinical measures alone to predict adolescent irritability.

Parental Psychopathology

Consistent with previous studies,[20] the authors found that lifetime history of a parental mood disorder predicted self-reported and mother-reported adolescent irritability, although its association with mother-reported adolescent irritability was only at a trend-level. Additionally, parental lifetime anxiety disorder and SUD were significant predictors of mother-reported adolescent irritability. In the multivariate model, however, adjusting for age 3 irritability, only parental anxiety continued to predict mother-reported irritability at a trend level, suggesting that parental lifetime mood and SUDS may be etiologically relevant only to adolescent irritability characterized by an earlier onset.

Psychosocial Environment

Developmental psychopathology is, in part, founded on the notion that the early psychosocial environment has lasting consequences on an individual's socioemotional development.[52] Consistent with this, in this study, multiple measures of the psychosocial environment in early childhood were associated with adolescent irritability: both higher levels of permissive parenting and lower levels of marital satisfaction at age 3 predicted higher levels of both self-reported and mother-reported irritability 12 years later. Additionally, higher levels of authoritarian parenting predicted mother-reported adolescent irritability. The effect of lower marital satisfaction on self-reported adolescent irritability, however, was specific to girls, whereas the effect of increased permissive parenting on mother-reported adolescent irritability was specific to boys. Distressed couples are more prone to conflict, which, in addition to being a direct stressor, may socialize children to manage their emotions and interpersonal friction in a manner that is maladaptive and potentially more detrimental to girls, who commonly place a high value on interpersonal relationships.[53] Additionally, the effect of permissive parenting on mother-reported adolescent irritability is consistent with prior research, which suggests that boys may be more likely to have difficulty controlling their own feelings and setting reasonable limits for their behavior if their parents tend to be inconsistent in their approaches to discipline.[54] Finally, lower parental education predicted self-reported adolescent irritability, possibly reflecting the impact of early social disadvantage on neural development.[55]

Limitations

This study is not without limitations. First, because there is no validated measure of irritability in preschoolers, the authors derived their own measure using items from a well-validated diagnostic interview[29] and guided by the content of a well-validated scale for irritability in older youth.[31] Although it was derived ad hoc, the measure has demonstrated predictive validity over a 12-year interval in the current report. Second, although a community sample allows for greater generalization, it may not be readily applicable to children with levels of irritability that present in clinical settings. Thus, future work should attempt to replicate these findings in a clinical sample.

SUMMARY

From ages 3 to 15, irritability is modestly stable across self-report and mother-report. Additionally, a range of variables assessed at age 3, that in many instances differed as a function of either informant or gender, predicted irritability at age 15: functional impairment, greater social competence, lower parental education, and among girls ADHD symptoms, more adept expressive language abilities, and lower marital satisfaction predicted self-reported adolescent irritability; and greater functional impairment, temperamental positive emotionality, maternal authoritarian parenting, lower marital satisfaction, and among boys higher levels of maternal permissive parenting predicted mother-reported adolescent irritability. Taken together, these findings suggest that adolescent-reported and mother-reported irritability may be capturing somewhat distinct underlying constructs of irritability, and both should be considered in assessments of adolescent irritability. If replicated, future research should explore using these predictors to target children for prevention programs.

ACKNOWLEDGMENTS

This work was supported by National Institute of Mental Health grant RO1MH069942 (Klein).

REFERENCES

1. Stringaris A, Taylor E. Disruptive mood: Irritability in children and adolescents. Oxford University Press; 2015.
2. Leibenluft E, Stoddard J. The developmental psychopathology of irritability. Dev Psychopathol 2013;25(4 Pt 2):1473–87.
3. Snaith RP, Taylor CM. Irritability: definition, assessment and associated factors. Br J Psychiatry 1985;147:127–36.
4. Roberson-Nay R, Leibenluft E, Brotman MA, et al. Longitudinal stability of genetic and environmental influences on irritability: from childhood to young adulthood. Am J Psychiatry 2015;172(7):657–64.
5. Vidal-Ribas P, Brotman MA, Valdivieso I, et al. The status of irritability in psychiatry: a conceptual and Quantitative review. J Am Acad Child Adolesc Psychiatry 2016;55(7):556–70.
6. Hawes MT, Carlson GA, Finsaas MC, et al. Dimensions of irritability in adolescents: longitudinal associations with psychopathology in adulthood. Psychol Med 2019;50(16):2759–67.

7. Humphreys KL, Schouboe SNF, Kircanski K, et al. Irritability, externalizing, and internalizing psychopathology in adolescence: cross-sectional and longitudinal associations and moderation by sex. J Clin Child Adolesc Psychol 2019;48(5): 781–9.

8. Dougherty LR, Smith VC, Bufferd SJ, et al. Preschool irritability: longitudinal associations with psychiatric disorders at age 6 and parental psychopathology. J Am Acad Child Adolesc Psychiatry 2013;52(12):1304–13.

9. Wakschlag LS, Estabrook R, Petitclerc A, et al. Clinical implications of a dimensional approach: the normal:abnormal spectrum of early irritability. J Am Acad Child Adolesc Psychiatry 2015;54(8):626–34.

10. Eyre O, Langley K, Stringaris A, et al. Irritability in ADHD: associations with depression liability. J Affect Disord 2017;215:281–7.

11. Beauchaine TP, Tackett JL. Irritability as a transdiagnostic vulnerability trait: current issues and future directions. Behav Ther 2020;51(2):350–64.

12. Riglin L, Eyre O, Cooper M, et al. Investigating the genetic underpinnings of early-life irritability. Transl Psychiatry 2017;7(9):e1241.

13. Riglin L, Eyre O, Thapar AK, et al. Identifying Novel types of irritability using a developmental genetic approach. Am J Psychiatry 2019;176(8):635–42.

14. Steinberg L, Morris AS. Adolescent development. Ann Rev Psychol 2001;52(1): 83–110.

15. Costello EJ, Copeland W, Angold A, et al. Trends in psychopathology across the adolescent years: what changes when children become adolescents, and when adolescents become adults? Journal of Child Psychology and Psychiatry 2011; 52(10):1015–25.

16. Hayward C, Sanborn K. Puberty and the emergence of gender differences in psychopathology. Journal of Adolescent Health 2002;30(4):49–58.

17. Leadbeater BJ, Homel J. Irritable and defiant sub-dimensions of ODD: Their stability and prediction of internalizing symptoms and conduct problems from adolescence to young adulthood. Journal of Abnormal Child Psychology 2015; 43(3):407–21.

18. Mulraney M, Zendarski N, Mensah F, Hiscock H, Sciberras E. Do early internalizing and externalizing problems predict later irritability in adolescents with attention-deficit/hyperactivity disorder? Australian & New Zealand Journal of Psychiatry 2017;51(4):393–402.

19. Savage J, Verhulst B, Copeland W, et al. A genetically informed study of the longitudinal relation between irritability and anxious/depressed symptoms. J Am Acad Child Adolesc Psychiatry 2015;54(5):377–84.

20. Krieger FV, Leibenluft E, Stringaris A, et al. Irritability in children and adolescents: past concepts, current debates, and future opportunities. Braz J Psychiatry 2013; 35(Suppl 1):S32–9.

21. Wiggins JL, Mitchell C, Stringaris A, et al. Developmental trajectories of irritability and bidirectional associations with maternal depression. J Am Acad Child Adolesc Psychiatry 2014;53(11):1191–205, 1205.e1191-1194.

22. Dougherty LR, Smith VC, Bufferd SJ, et al. DSM-5 disruptive mood dysregulation disorder: correlates and predictors in young children. Psychol Med 2014;44(11): 2339–50.

23. Pagliaccio D, Pine DS, Barch DM, et al. Irritability trajectories, cortical thickness, and clinical outcomes in a sample enriched for preschool depression. J Am Acad Child Adolesc Psychiatry 2018;57(5):336–42.e336. https://doi.org/10.1016/j.jaac. 2018.02.010.

24. Wiggins JL, Briggs-Gowan MJ, Estabrook R, et al. Identifying clinically significant irritability in early childhood. J Am Acad Child Adolesc Psychiatry 2018;57(3): 191–9.e192.

25. Stringaris A, Vidal-Ribas P, Brotman MA, Leibenluft E. Practitioner review: definition, recognition, and treatment challenges of irritability in young people. Journal of Child Psychology and Psychiatry 2018;59(7):721–39.

26. Stringaris A, Goodman R. Three dimensions of oppositionality in youth. J Child Psychol Psychiatry 2009;50(3):216–23.

27. Dougherty LR, Galano MM, Chad-Friedman E, et al. Using item Response theory to compare irritability measures in early adolescent and childhood samples. Assessment 2020. 1073191120936363.

28. Klein DN, Finsaas MC. The Stony Brook temperament study: early antecedents and pathways to emotional disorders. Child Develop Perspect 2017;11(4): 257–63.

29. Egger HL, Erkanli A, Keeler G, et al. Test-retest reliability of the preschool age psychiatric assessment (PAPA). J Am Acad Child Adolesc Psychiatry 2006; 45(5):538–49.

30. Lyneham HJ, Rapee R M. Agreement between telephone and in-person delivery of a structured interview for anxiety disorders in children. Journal of the American Academy of Child & Adolescent Psychiatry 2005;44(3):274–82.

31. Stringaris A, Goodman R, Ferdinando S, et al. The Affective Reactivity Index: a concise irritability scale for clinical and research settings. J Child Psychol Psychiatry 2012;53(11):1109–17.

32. Dunn LM, Dunn LM, Bulheller S, et al. Peabody picture vocabulary test. MN: American Guidance Service Circle Pines; 1965.

33. Brownell R. Expressive one-word picture vocabulary test: manual. Novato (CA): Academic Therapy Publications; 2000.

34. Sparrow SS, Balla DA, Cicchetti DV, et al. Vineland adaptive behavior scales. Circle Pines (MN): American Guidance Service; 1984.

35. Goldsmith HH, Reilly J, Lemery KS, et al. Preschool laboratory temperament assessment battery. Madison (WI): Unpublished Instrument, University of Wisconsin; 1995.

36. Dyson MW, Olino TM, Durbin CE, et al. The structural and rank-order stability of temperament in young children based on a laboratory-observational measure. Psychol Ass 2015;27(4):1388–401.

37. First MB. SCID-I: clinician version. Washington, DC: American Psychiatric Press; 1997.

38. Olino TM, Klein DN, Dyson MW, et al. Temperamental emotionality in preschool-aged children and depressive disorders in parents: associations in a large community sample. J Abnormal Psychol 2010;119(3):468–78.

39. Robinson C, Mandleco B, Roper S, et al. The parenting Styles and dimensions questionnaire (PSDQ). Handbook Fam Meas Tech 2001;3:319–21.

40. Sabourin S, Valois P, Lussier Y. Development and validation of a brief version of the dyadic adjustment scale with a nonparametric item analysis model. Psychol Ass 2005;17(1):15.

41. Aiken LS, West SG, Reno RR. Multiple regression: Testing and interpreting interactions. Sage; 1991.

42. De Los Reyes A, Kazdin AE. Informant discrepancies in the assessment of childhood psychopathology: a critical review, theoretical framework, and recommendations for further study. Psychol Bull 2005;131(4):483.

43. Carver CS, Harmon-Jones E. Anger is an approach-related affect: evidence and implications. Psychological bulletin 2009;135(2):183.

44. Lionetti F, Aron EN, Aron A, Klein DN, Pluess M. Observer-rated environmental sensitivity moderates children's response to parenting quality in early childhood. Developmental psychology 2019;55(11):2389.

45. Belsky J, Pluess M. Beyond diathesis stress: differential susceptibility to environmental influences. Psychological bulletin 2009;135(6):885.

46. Baumeister RF, Brewer LE, Tice DM, et al. Thwarting the need to belong: understanding the interpersonal and inner effects of social exclusion. Social Personal Psychol Compass 2007;1(1):506–20.

47. Cole PM, Armstrong LM, Pemberton CK. The role of language in the development of emotion regulation. In: Calkins SD, Bell MA, editors. Human Brain Development. Child development at the intersection of emotion and cognition. Washington, DC: American Psychological Association; 2010. p. 59–77.

48. Spielberger CD. The experience and expression of anger: construction and validation of an anger expression scale. Anger hostility Cardiovasc Behav Disord 1985;5–30.

49. Brotman MA, Kircanski K, Stringaris A, et al. Irritability in youths: A translational model. American Journal of Psychiatry 2017;174(6):520–32.

50. Kessel EM, Dougherty LR, Kujawa A, Hajcak G, Carlson GA, Klein DN. Longitudinal associations between preschool disruptive mood dysregulation disorder symptoms and neural reactivity to monetary reward during preadolescence. Journal of child and adolescent psychopharmacology 2016;26(2):131–7.

51. Kujawa A, Proudfit GH, Kessel EM, et al. Neural reactivity to monetary rewards and losses in childhood: longitudinal and concurrent associations with observed and self-reported positive emotionality. Biol Psychol 2015;104:41–7.

52. Sroufe LA, Coffino B, Carlson EA. Conceptualizing the role of early experience: lessons from the Minnesota longitudinal study. Developmental Rev 2010;30(1):36–51.

53. Fincham FD, Grych JH, Osborne LN. Does marital conflict cause child maladjustment? Directions and challenges for longitudinal research. J Fam Psychol 1994; 8(2):128.

54. Miller JM, DiIorio C, Dudley W. Parenting style and adolescent's reaction to conflict: is there a relationship? J Adolesc Health 2002;31(6):463–8.

55. Farah MJ. Socioeconomic status and the brain: prospects for neuroscience-informed policy. Nat Rev Neurosci 2018;19(7):428–38.

Interventions

Explosive Outbursts at School

Jeff Q. Bostic, MD, EdD[a],*, Richard Mattison, MD[b], D. Cunningham, PhD[c]

KEYWORDS

- Explosive outbursts • School mental health • Education

KEY POINTS

- Explosive outbursts by students occur in schools, require intensive intervention, impair student learning and relationships, and exert a heavy burden on school staff.
- Explosive outbursts by students occur across multiple diagnostic categories and often include rapid and dramatic escalations, reactions out of proportion to events, significant difficulty with redirection or deescalation, difficulty recalling and processing these events accurately, and difficulty controlling these events.
- Schools may use interventions to anticipate and respond to behavioral, emotional, impulsive, and sensory components of explosive outbursts.
- Measures such as monitoring frequency, duration, pervasiveness, severity, and the student's response after the explosive outburst as well as office disciplinary referrals and suspensions may help clarify subtypes of explosive outbursts and impacts of interventions for explosive outbursts.
- Amid the cycle of a student explosive outburst, interventions specific to each stage of outburst may diminish the intensity, length, and distress of these events.

SCHOOL INTERVENTIONS FOR EXPLOSIVE OUTBURSTS AT SCHOOL

Students may explode at school, flying into rages far beyond that of a temper tantrum, and escalate to screaming, throwing furniture, verbally assailing others, and even physically assaulting staff and students or destroying property. These events are not uncommon and deplete school resources (instructional time and staff involvement) to respond and address these events. Explosive outbursts (EO) most often manifest as aggressive, defiant events, which account for nearly half of all office disciplinary referrals (ODR). About one-third of students with such behaviors fail to graduate from high school on time and remain at high risk for later life dysfunction.[1]

[a] Department of Psychiatry, MedStar Georgetown University Hospital, 2115 Wisconsin Avenue, Northwest, Suite 200, Washington, DC 20007, USA; [b] Penn State College of Medicine, Hershey, PA, USA; [c] Department of Psychiatry, University of Maryland School of Medicine, Baltimore, MD, USA
* Corresponding author.
E-mail address: jeffrey.q.bostic@gunet.georgetown.edu

Child Adolesc Psychiatric Clin N Am 30 (2021) 491–503
https://doi.org/10.1016/j.chc.2021.04.003
1056-4993/21/© 2021 Elsevier Inc. All rights reserved.

DEFINITION OF EXPLOSIVE OUTBURSTS

EO here refer to student episodes that arise most often when students are frustrated or distressed and resemble the temper tantrums of younger children.[2,3] However, these outbursts escalate very rapidly (seconds to minutes) and appear far out of proportion to the circumstances. The episodes often last 30 to 45 minutes during which the student does not respond to adult requests or redirection and require significant postevent time (often 10–20 minutes or more) before the student can reengage with academic or typical school tasks. The explosive episodes described here are not planned or anticipated maneuvers, so imposing consequences rarely slow the EO, and EO are not brief reactions of student frustration. These events are not unexpected reactions to medications (or substance abuse) or medical conditions (eg, seizure disorders), or intellectual disabilities that yield erratic behaviors unrelated to the school task or interaction with others at school.

No measures to identify students with EO currently exist, and schools have more commonly focused on responding to these events rather than characterizing them.[4] The Child Behavior Checklist *Dysregulation Profile* (CBCL-DP),[5] which integrates the CBCL syndrome scales of Anxious/Depressed, Aggressive Behavior, and Attention Problems, has been used to approximate disruptive mood dysregulation and EO and relies on input from multiple informants (including teachers). The CBCL-DP has shown good model fit for factor structure across parents and teachers,[6] suggesting that teacher observations will have important research and clinical value as investigations into EO progresses.[7] Spring and Carlson[7] devised the Irritability Inventory (IRRI) to better characterize EO, and a follow-up anchored measure (IRRIAM) has now been devised to monitor a student's progress with EO management at school (see Appendix 1).

SCHOOL RESPONSES TO EXPLOSIVE OUTBURSTS
Office Disciplinary Referrals and Suspensions

The current school response to EO often leads to *ODR* and *suspensions*, with higher rates of suspensions for those students receiving special education, especially those classified as emotional or behavioral disordered (EBD). In a study of well-recorded ODR of middle school students,[8] 41% had at least one ODR, mostly for disobedience, conduct interference, disrespect, and fighting, and usually leading to reprimands or suspensions, although rarely expulsion (0.3%). Students who met criteria for an EBD were significantly more likely to have received an ODR and suspension than other regular or special education students. ODR have also been shown to predict later school dysfunction, as sixth graders referred for fighting continued to have more ODR in eighth grade, and sixth grade boys referred *twice* for such behaviors were found at risk for not finishing high school.[9] ODR for fighting and nonviolent behaviors in sixth grade coupled with low GPA predicted enduring ODR into seventh and eighth grades, which were associated with suspensions in ninth grade. Thus, verbal and physical aggressions (cardinal EO features) are among the most common reasons for ODR in elementary and middle school, as well as for subsequent suspensions.

Similarly, although suspensions occur in approximately 5% of students in public elementary and secondary schools,[10] more than 9% of students with disabilities had at least one suspension, and this may reflect more complex symptoms but may also indicate lack of appropriate resources or consistent staff responses. The percentage of students suspended has increased from 7% to 9%, especially among students with the special education classification of EBD.[11,12] The most common behaviors leading to suspension are fighting, disobedience, and conduct interference. Because ODR and suspensions appear to be associated with more school dysfunction, both short term and long term, ODR and suspensions may add a mechanism to follow the course of students and of treatment impacts on students having EO at school.

Special Education Category of Emotional/Behavioral Disorders

EO can often be difficult for schools to deal with in a regular classroom setting because of persistent ODR and/or suspensions, which can lead to the need for more intensive interventions through special education services. Boys 6 to 11 years old in special education classified with EBD have been found to have significantly more impairing symptoms on parent and teacher checklists than comparison groups of inpatients, outpatients, and the general population.[13] The boys with EBD showed clinically significant scores in externalizing and total problems, with aggressive behaviors the highest.[14] In a cohort of middle school special education students classified EBD, 63% received at least one ODR, 37% had at least one suspension, and on average missed 11 days of school. The most common reason for suspension was physical aggression toward peers and/or staff (45%).[15]

Despite the predominance of externalizing psychopathology (especially attention-deficit/hyperactivity disorder [ADHD]) in students classified EBD, depressive disorders also occur in more than a third of these students. In addition, comorbidity was found in approximately one-half, especially ADHD with conduct or depressive disorders.[14] Abuse and learning disorders (LD) also appear commonly in students categorized as EBD. Most EBD students have a history of maltreatment (60%), especially physical abuse (38.7%).[14] LD has also been reported in more than 50%, and LD remain persistent,[16] as well as neuropsychological deficits, especially in attention/executive functions (EF) and language.[17]

When 151 students with EBD were followed more than an average of 8 years, approximately 50% showed overall success in their educational careers. The most significant enrollment predictors for *unsuccessful* educational outcome (73%) were, in descending order, later enrollment age, presence of conduct or oppositional-defiant disorder, verbal IQ significantly lower than performance IQ, and absence of a depressive or anxiety disorder.[18] Students who begin school later, and who show conduct/behavioral symptoms, and who struggle with reading/writing tasks appear at greater risk for poor outcomes.

RESPONDING TO STUDENTS WITH EXPLOSIVE OUTBURSTS FROM A PSYCHIATRIC VIEWPOINT

EO occurs across multiple *Diagnostic and Statistical Manual of Mental Disorders* (Fifth Edition) (*DSM-5*) psychiatric disorders. Of those students diagnosed with a psychiatric disorder, approximately 75% have been diagnosed with ADHD, although they often also have comorbid oppositional defiant disorder; internalizing disorders such as anxiety, depression, or disruptive mood dysregulation; trauma exposure; language or learning disorders.[19] EO is perhaps currently better characterized as a syndrome rather than a specific separate psychiatric disorder. Little is known about students with EO, and schools identify students with EO differently than *DSM* diagnoses, as schools more often use codes for autism or developmental delay, emotional disturbance (ED; sometimes also designated as severe emotional disturbance [SED], emotional behavioral disturbance [EBD], or emotional disturbance/behavioral disturbance [EDBD]), other health impaired (OHI, frequently used for ADHD), or (maladaptive) behavioral disturbance. **Table 1** shows how students with EO may be categorized in the school setting.

For a student to be identified as one in need of special education services, the student must be identified with a disability. Although school psychologists most

Table 1
Diagnostic and Statistical Manual of Mental Disorders (Fifth Edition) criteria associated with explosive outbursts in youth

DSM-V Disorder	*DSM-V* Criteria Associated with Explosive Outbursts	Educational Category	Factors Associated with Explosive Outbursts at School
Anxiety	Excessive worry; excessive fears; avoidance; fight/flight/fear reactions	ED	Inappropriate feelings/behaviors under normal circumstances; tendency to develop physical symptoms or fears associated with personal or school problems
Attention deficit	Reluctant to engage in tasks that require sustained mental effort; runs about/climbs; blurts out, cannot wait, interrupts/intrudes	Other health impaired	Limited strength, vitality, or alertness, including a heightened alertness to environmental stimuli, that results in limited alertness
Autism	Failure to respond to social interactions; inflexible adherence to routines, difficulties with transitions, rigid thinking patterns; highly restricted, fixated interests; hyperreactivity/hyporeactivity or unusual reactions to sensory input/aspects	Developmental delay (ages 3–9 y-old), or autism	Repetitive activities, resistance to environmental changes or in routine; unusual responses to sensory experiences (and not better explained by an ED)
Bipolar disorder	Explosive irritability; grandiosity, pressured speech; increased activity/psychomotor agitation; excessive involvement in activities without regard for painful consequences	ED	Inability to build/maintain satisfactory interpersonal relationships with peers/teachers; inappropriate behavior/feelings under normal circumstances; general pervasive mood of unhappiness or depression
Conduct disorder	Hostile behavior; destruction of property; assaultive behavior/speech	ED	(may be excluded if perceived "socially maladjusted"); inability to build/maintain satisfactory interpersonal relationships with peers/teachers; inappropriate behavior/feelings under normal circumstances
Depressive disorders	Irritable mood; worthlessness; lack of energy to do school tasks; poor concentration	ED	Inability to build/maintain satisfactory interpersonal relationships with peers/teachers; inappropriate behavior/feelings under normal circumstances; general pervasive mood of unhappiness or depression

(continued on next page)

DSM-V Disorder	DSM-V Criteria Associated with Explosive Outbursts	Educational Category	Factors Associated with Explosive Outbursts at School
Disruptive mood dysregulation disorder	Severe temper outbursts out of proportion to events/age; irritable between outbursts	ED	Inability to build/maintain satisfactory interpersonal relationships with peers/teachers; inappropriate behavior/feelings under normal circumstances; general pervasive mood of unhappiness or depression
Intermittent explosive disorder	Nonpremeditated verbal or physical aggression, grossly out of proportion to events (symptoms not better explained by another disorder, such as bipolar, depression, DMDD, substance abuse, head trauma)	ED	(May be excluded if perceived "socially maladjusted"); inability to build/maintain satisfactory interpersonal relationships with peers/teachers; inappropriate behavior/feelings under normal circumstances
Oppositionality	Loss of temper; easily annoyed, angry, resentful, actively defies/refuses rules or requests	ED	(May be excluded if perceived "socially maladjusted"); inability to build/maintain satisfactory interpersonal relationships with peers/teachers; inappropriate behavior/feelings under normal circumstances
Trauma	Distress at reminders of trauma; frightening dreams or flashbacks; dissociation; avoids others or situations that could remind of past traumatic events; irritable, angry; reckless, self-destructive, exaggerated startle response	ED	Inability to build/maintain satisfactory interpersonal relationships with peers/teachers; inappropriate behavior/feelings under normal circumstances; general pervasive mood of unhappiness or depression
Psychosis	Misinterpret stimuli or events; distrust others; seek to escape situations or others perceived dangerous or frightening	ED	Inability to build/maintain satisfactory interpersonal relationships with peers/teachers; inappropriate behavior/feelings under normal circumstances

Table 1
(continued)

commonly identify disabilities, child psychiatrists can also be helpful by providing specific diagnoses in their reports, and by avoiding rule-out diagnoses, even if diagnoses change over time. Child psychiatrists can be helpful by providing in their reports specific diagnoses and indicators of clinical severity/impairment to help school staff plan for a student's intervention needs. Although schools strive to keep students included within the school whenever feasible under the "least restrictive environment" for delivery of needed services, sometimes the student having EO requires greater density of services and access to supports than can occur in the regular classroom. Clinicians are tasked with identifying the interventions to help diminish EO and to contribute to the school team's recognition of where (eg, separate classroom) and how (eg, therapeutic staff are regularly available to intervene) this can occur for students having EO. To receive an individualized educational program (IEP) through the Individual with Disabilities Education Act, the student must also (a) *exhibit a lack of* educational progress (academically or social-emotionally) and (b) require specialized instruction (beyond just counseling at school; so identified school interventions to manage the student are helpful for developing a behavioral plan to respond to EO). Schools in some states make sharp distinctions between *DSM-5* diagnoses and how they are coded for educational services. For example, in some school districts, in the case of EO, diagnoses such as oppositional defiant disorder and conduct disorder may be categorized as "*maladaptive patterns of behavior*" or attributable to "*socially maladjusted*" and then *excluded* from an IEP or a behavioral plan that affords more supports, which are often needed for students with EO. Thus, clinicians must be familiar with how these disorders are coded in their respective states and school districts.

SPECIFIC INTERVENTIONS FOR EXPLOSIVE OUTBURSTS BY SCHOOL STAFF

The criteria in the preceding section show that EO may result from multiple diagnoses. At least 4 types of circumstances appear to trigger or sustain EO that may help staff focus interventions, given that students may have multiple diagnoses:

1. Behavioral: conduct/oppositional conditions that may include more manipulative, consistently hostile student behaviors surrounding the outbursts, but with limited distress or remorse following an EO
2. Emotional: mood (anxiety, bipolar, depression, disruptive mood dysregulation disorder [DMDD], psychosis, posttraumatic stress disorder [PTSD]) disorders that may include more emotional reactivity to events that spur outbursts, sometimes followed after EO by significant remorse
3. Impulsive: impulse-control difficulties (ADHD, intermittent explosive disorder) conditions that may include difficulties navigating changes or transitions, or rigidity that fuels such outbursts, and difficult to recall/describe after the event
4. Sensory: hypersensitivity to stimuli (autism, PTSD) conditions that may include intense reactivity or triggering by events, and avoidance of others or stimuli-rich environments, and followed by distress and avoidance of others/circumstances after an EO

These aspects can help school staff focus on each individual student's circumstances conducive to EO. The foundation for any effective intervention is for staff to establish a positive and supportive relationship with the student.[20] Student perceptions of teacher support and mutual respect are related to positive changes in the students' academic motivation and engagement.[21] Staff can then provide preparatory and response strategies to impede EO, as shown in **Table 2**.

SCHOOL INTERVENTIONS TO MANAGE AN EXPLOSIVE OUTBURST EVENT USING THE ACTING OUT CYCLE

Although multiple "types" of EO occur based on underlying vulnerabilities and sensitivities, most EO follow a similar course. To better respond to the phases of an EO, clinicians may extrapolate the acting out cycle shown in **Fig. 1** to EO events to clarify

Table 2
Preparing for and responding to different aspects of explosive outbursts in the classroom

Explosive Outburst Aspects	Classroom *Preparation* to Decrease Explosions	School Staff *Response* to Outbursts
Behavioral	Provide specific positive behavioral expectations for student, provide rewards/reinforcement for adherence	Identify positive options, alternative behaviors (to cursing, destruction, and so forth), reasonable limit-setting & consequences
Emotional	Address/minimize student triggers (change readings if about sensitive subjects), provide acceptable options for student becoming emotional (different classroom tasks, breaks, therapeutic staff support)	Provide student alternative places to regroup, staff to support calming techniques, alternative distracting activities (spreading fingers or toes, deep breathing)
Impulsive	Provide clear structure for that day/period; preview transitions and tasks; identify appropriate actions to take if become frustrated	Empathize with distress, provide small number of appropriate options and invite student to choose, support student efforts toward better behavior
Sensory	Optimize classroom stimulation for the student; provide alternative sensory experiences or regulating devices (eg, cushions, headphones, quiet corners, things to squeeze)	Reduce/remove sensory stressors; provide options to decrease (eg, headphones, something to put over distressing color; alternative foods); redirect student to other sensory activity (for example, wash hands, walk in hall)

opportunities to both minimize precipitants for EO and to respond at each stage of an escalation. Students with EO all vary, including how this cycle applies to them, so specific interventions are needed at each stage for students with EO. For students with sensory EO (eg, past trauma), managing triggers and recognizing fight/flight/freeze reactions may be more important. Students with impulsive EO may need familiarity and practice with competing activities when distressed. Students with emotional EO may require more staff to engage them, or counseling techniques (eg, mindfulness, strategies such as evaluating the evidence when they feel badly).

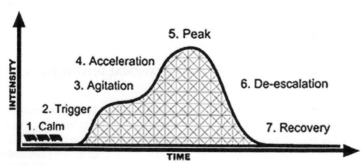

Fig. 1. The acting-out cycle. (Used with permission from Colvin, G., & Scott, T. (2015). Managing the cycle of acting-out behavior in the classroom, Second Edition. Thousand Oaks, CA: Corwin.)

As **Fig. 1** (a roller coaster metaphor) shows, the classroom may initially be in *Calm phase*, although the student may have already arrived at school some days more distressed because of outside school events or circumstances.[22] Amid varying degrees of *calm*, a *Trigger* (eg, comment from a peer, question from a teacher, deviation from the daily schedule, unexpected grade on an assignment, but also nonschool events, such as being hungry/tired, stressful home situation, difficult ride/walk to school) can precipitate ("trigger") an escalation. The *Agitation phase* can percolate as the student disconnects from the classroom interaction, as the student's frustration shifts behavior away from the task, with loss of task focus, often behavioral activation, such as looking around, making sounds or noises, moving in and out of groups, or disengaging from others. Recognition and intervention here by staff are vital to prevent acceleration toward verbal and physical aggression toward others. During the *Acceleration phase*, the student starts gaining momentum down a path toward oppositional, argumentative, resistant, and disengaged disruptive behaviors (and away from adherent, school-task behaviors). School staff may first recognize an explosion building at this point in the cycle, where it may be helpful to redirect the student interaction toward something collaborative, and to reinforce even partial adherence.

At the *Peak phase*, the explosive behaviors have become visibly obvious to everyone and may culminate in physical or verbal assaults, hysterical crying, or property destruction. These peaks can last for varying intervals of time ($\sim$1–20 minutes) and often may seem to slow down but then reignite during this interval, before the student enters the *Deescalation phase* where the student may become less agitated, withdraw, and sometimes feel tired.

This Deescalation phase leads to the *Recovery phase*, where students may avoid discussing what occurred; however, it is important to address the incident rather than reinforce it by leaving the student alone. Unhelpful consequences of not addressing the incident include accrual of secondary gains of teacher or task avoidance from EO. Usually, staff will take steps to get the class back on track and then collaborate with the student in a more "functional behavior assessment" (FBA) approach (described in later discussion) to reduce precipitants, replace dysfunctional behaviors, and remove secondary gains from the EO. The emotional impacts on the class and staff, as well as the student who exploded, may also need to be addressed, with the goal of creating a safer, healthier classroom environment as a result of this EO (ie, "what will we do differently next time to avoid or stop this EO from progressing?"). These stages and student-focused interventions to manage each phase are provided in **Table 3**. In addition, it can be helpful for staff to examine the school/classroom environment, as sometimes changes to the school environment (eg, teacher instruction, positive school climate, arrangement of the classroom environment, teacher skill in responding to student behaviors) can improve student EO.

FUNCTIONAL BEHAVIOR ASSESSMENT AND BEHAVIORAL INTERVENTION PLANNING

Too often, students have repetitive EO, despite the above tactics to impede student escalations to outbursts. If EO are intense and recur at least weekly, the student's school team may complete an FBA, which examines the function of the student's difficult behavior (eg, EO) to then plan more intensive interactions. An FBA explores the precipitants surrounding the target behavior (eg, yelling and throwing items in the classroom) and then the consequences or secondary gain (if any) from such an event. For example, a student may have EO primarily in one class, perhaps because the

Table 3		
Interventions for each phase of the acting out cycle in explosive outbursts		
Phase	**Description**	**Interventions**
1. Calm	Student behavior is goal-directed, calm, adherent, cooperative, responsive to praise	• Teach and reinforce expectations (what will happen if do) • Model desired behaviors (respectful, calm, polite, accepting) • Provide verbal praise • Invite positive communication (seek first to understand) • Provide constructive encouragement (validate effort) • Utilization of routine and consistency in the classroom • Greet students at the door to set a positive tone and assess mood of students
2. Triggering	By: difficult task, transitions, teasing by peers, conflict with teacher; hunger, poor sleep, environmental stressors, traumatic reaction	• Identify what triggers the student and collaboratively make a plan to respond to triggers when student is calm and not in crisis • Discuss triggers and cues of becoming upset • Discuss what he or she can do to deescalate before things get worse • Provide a visual/verbal prompt or reminder • Use problem solving • Use coping/relaxation skills • If possible, remove the trigger from the classroom • Distraction • Use proximity control to help the student control their impulses

3. Agitation	Student is distressed, stopping task, becoming disengaged	• Use coping/relaxation strategies effective for that student
		• Provide the student an opportunity to express what is bothering them and reflect concern
		• Redirect the student or provide options to shift task, such as
		  ○ Work with a partner or the teacher
		  ○ Ask the student if would like assistance (Use "how" or "can" questions, and avoid "yes/no, why, what, didn't, have, are")
		  ○ Change instruction style (staff shifts/stops current interaction)
		  ○ Express interest in something the child likes to shift their attention
		  ○ Suggest use of calming strategies (breathing, preferred positive activities)
		  ○ Provide a precompliance thank you ("Thank you for starting on your assignment.")
		  ○ Offer the student an opportunity to take a break (eg, go get a drink of water; take recycling bin to the office)

(continued on next page)

Table 3 (continued)		
Phase	**Description**	**Interventions**

4. Acceleration	Student shifts away from instructional process and toward arguments and increased disruption	• Acknowledge the student's feelings of frustration, distress
		• Give student time ("several silent seconds") to respond
		• Collaborative problem solving (get student's ideas for how to resolve the issue)
		• Provide 2–3 appropriate options for the student
		  ○ "How about a break in the quiet area or working with someone else?"
		  ○ "Would you like to get a drink or have your snack now?"
		• Provide opportunity to talk with counselor or another trusted adult
		• Provide reinforcement immediately after student begins to respond, even if only reinforcing efforts in the correct or better direction
		  ○ Can be nonverbal (smile or nod) if words are likely to incite conflict
		  ○ Cueing words/phrases, such as "spot," to identify the student should move to a different place in the room
		• Provide flexibility in order to avoid everything becoming a power struggle
		  ○ "Okay, you'd prefer right now to draw...sounds good" (even if not the preferred activity, it's "better than" becoming more disruptive or destructive)

5. Peak	Student out of control, yelling, destructive, unable to calm down	• Decrease stimulation (private conversation instead of comments in front of peers, maintain 3 ft space from student in a nonthreatening stance; avoid touching the student)
		• Maintain safety of all students (by position or moving disruptive student or others)
		• Stay focused on the problem and the student's behavior by valuing the student but not the behavior ("seems you're frustrated about the harder math problems, so you are tearing them up—we can find other solutions")
		• If student is unable to shift, succinctly describe options and consequences available ("if you don't stop throwing books, I will get [another staff person] and contact your caregiver," although these should be framed as helpful options and not threats to the student)
		• Use identified school-specific responses
		  ○ Access administrative or counseling staff
		  ○ Access other teaching staff present to assist
		  ○ Identify acceptable options to reconnect with student (common interests, music, model calmness, quietness to decrease further conflicts)

(continued on next page)

Phase	Description	Interventions
Table 3 (continued)		
		o Move student to identified places for disruptive events o School-specific restraint/seclusion practices • Reinforce even small steps in the correct direction • Reengage student in learning/instruction quickly if possible
6. Deescalation	Student slows down (but could rekindle) and may be tired, worn out; this may take 20+ minutes	• Provide simpler activity immediately to do (read, do mazes, easier math problems) • Classroom resumes instructional activities (calm, productive)
7. Recovery	Student is calm and has regained control and able to have useful conversation	• Debrief briefly about events, clarifying triggers and better options when agitated or accelerating • Debrief with class if necessary (how they can respond and be helpful to each other) • Debrief with teacher and student and a neutral third-party

content is more difficult, or because of teasing from a peer. Also, the EO may lead to avoiding the task, the disliked peers, or instruction/interactions with that teacher, as well as "getting to go home," all of which may sustain or reinforce the EO.

The common steps in an FBA are for the team to (1) identify the target behavior to change; (2) determine how to collect data that will illuminate precipitants and consequences of the behavior, the frequency of the target behavior, what the student is trying to communicate or gain through the target behavior; and (3) develop a hypothesis about the "function" of the behavior and what makes it more or less likely to occur.

The FBA allows for creation of a behavioral intervention plan (BIP) to provide more precision in addressing the targeted behavior.[23] Using the assessment information above, the team typically will plan interventions to alter this cycle (changing precipitants and responses by staff) and evaluate the effectiveness of these interventions.[24] Interventions for a BIP thus address the precipitants, skill difficulties, and consequences through strategies, such as, (1) prevention strategies (eg, classroom adjustment, social stories, video modeling, visual cueing); (2) teaching strategies (skill training, prompting, embedded instruction, functional communication); and (3) response strategies (eg, differential reinforcement, self-management).[25,26] Positive behavioral supports are emphasized to increase expected behaviors, diminish difficult behaviors, improve the quality of life of students with challenging behaviors, while decreasing punitive or punishment-based interventions.[27,28] Commonly, the development of an effective BIP is a process rather than an event, with need for recurrent revision and changes to the interventions as circumstances change for the student (different academic tasks, peers, staff, reactions, and so forth).

SUMMARY

Managing EO occupies substantial time and involvement of school staff. Efforts are underway to better characterize these EO so that more precise interventions can be evaluated, and preferred approaches can be identified when EO occur. Research into understanding the basic characteristics in school of children with EO should improve the understanding of EO in children, and their overall treatment needs and responses. In the context of the above review of EO in schools, several suggestions emerge for child psychiatrists to consider as they assist school staffs in understanding and responding to students with EO:

1. Child psychiatrists can partner with school staff to examine EO from a mental health lens to expand options for children having EO beyond school disciplinary responses.
2. Child psychiatrists can contribute to the mental health assessment of EO by clarifying diagnoses and symptoms contributing to them, including violent or suicidal symptoms, possible substance use, past or current trauma, sensory sensitivity, and impulsivity.
3. Interventions can be devised to both prepare for and respond to circumstances fueling EO.
4. The stages of EO provide intervention points and stage-specific strategies to deescalate EO.
5. Monitoring school interventions for EO by the specific characteristics of EO, as well as frequency and type of ODR, suspensions, and use of FBA or BIP may illuminate effective strategies to reduce EO and their impacts.

DISCLOSURE

J.Q. Bostic: None; R. Mattison: None; D. Cunningham: None.

REFERENCES

1. Waschbusch DA, Breaux RP, Babinski DE. School-based interventions for aggression and defiance in youth: a framework for evidence-based practice. Sch Ment Health 2019;11:92–105.
2. Carlson GA. Presidential address: emotion dysregulation in children and adolescents. J Am Acad Child Adolesc Psychiatry 2020;59:15–9.
3. Colvin G, Scott T. Managing the cycle of acting-out behavior in the classroom. 2nd edition. Thousand Oaks, CA: Corwin; 2015.
4. Stringaris A, Vidal-Ribas P, Brotman MA, et al. Practitioner review: definition, recognition, and treatment challenges of irritability in young people. J Child Psychol Psychiatry 2018;59(7):721–39.
5. Althoff RR, Rettew DR, Ayer LA, et al. Cross-informant agreement of the dysregulation profile of the child behavior checklist. Psychiatr Res 2010;178(3):550–5.
6. Deutz MHF, Geeraerts SB, van Baar AL, et al. The dysregulation profile in middle childhood and adolescence across reports: factor structure, measurement invariance, and links with self-harm and suicidal ideation. Eur Child Adolesc Psychiatry 2016;25:431–42.
7. Spring LM, Carlson GA. The phenomenology of outbursts. Child Adolesc Psychiatr Clin N Am 2021;30(2):307–19.
8. Skiba RJ, Peterson RL, Williams T. Office referrals and suspension: disciplinary intervention in middle schools. Educ Treat Child 1997;20(3):295–315.
9. Tobin TJ, Sugai GM. Using sixth-grade school records to predict school violence, chronic discipline problems, and high school outcomes. J Emotional Behav Disord 1999;7(1):40–53.

10. National Center for Education Statistics. Percentage of students receiving selected disciplinary actions in public elementary and secondary schools, by type of disciplinary action, disability status, sex, and race/ethnicity: 2013-14. Washington, DC: Digest of Education Statistics; 2018. Table 233.28.

11. Krezmien MP, Leone PE, Achilles GM. Suspension, race, and disability: analysis of statewide practices and reporting. J Emotional Behav Disord 2006;14(4): 217–26.

12. Machalicek W, O'Reilly MF, Beretvas N, et al. A review of interventions to reduce challenging behavior in school settings for students with autism spectrum disorders. Res Autism Spectr Disord 2007;1(3):229–46.

13. Mattison RE, Gamble AD. Severity of socially and emotionally disturbed boys' dysfunction at school and home: comparison with psychiatric and general population boys. Behav Disord 1992;17:219–24.

14. Mattison RE. Psychiatric and psychological assessment of emotional and behavioral disorders during school mental health consultation. In: Rutherford RB, Quinn MM, Mathur SR, editors. Handbook of research in emotional and behavioral disorders. New York: Guilford Press; 2004. p. 163–80.

15. Mattison RE. Universal measures of school function in middle school special education students. Behav Disord 2004;29:359–71.

16. Mattison RE, Hooper SR, Glassberg LA. Three-year course of learning disorders in special education students classified as behavioral disorder. J Am Acad Child Adolesc Psychiatry 2002;41:1454–61.

17. Mattison RE, Hooper SH, Carlson GC. Neuropsychological characteristics of special education students with serious emotional/behavioral disorders. Behav Disord 2006;31:176–88.

18. Mattison RE, Spitznagel EL, Felix BC. Enrollment predictors of the special education outcome for SED students. Behav Disord 1998;23:243–56.

19. Baweja R, Mayes SD, Hameed U, et al. Disruptive mood dysregulation disorder: current insights. Neuropsychiatr Dis Treat 2016;12:2115–24.

20. Webster-Stratton C. How to promote children's social and emotional competence. London: Paul Chapman; 1999.

21. Ryan AM, Patrick H. The classroom social environment and changes in adolescents' motivation and engagement during middle school. Am Educ Res J 2001;38:437–60.

22. IRIS Center. Addressing disruptive and noncompliant behaviors (part 1): understanding the acting-out cycle. 2005. Available at: https://iris.peabody.vanderbilt.edu/module/bi1/. Accessed October 14, 2020.

23. Gresham FM. Current status and future directions of school-based behavioral interventions. Sch Psychol Rev 2004;33(3):326.

24. Herzinger CV, Campbell JM. Comparing functional assessment methodologies: a quantitative synthesis. J Autism Dev Disord 2007;37(8):1430–45.

25. Wood BK, Blair KSC, Ferro JB. Young children with challenging behavior function-based assessment and intervention. Top Early Child Spec Educ 2009; 29(2):68–78.

26. Young JF, Mufson L, Gallop R. Preventing depression: a randomized trial of interpersonal psychotherapy-adolescent skills training. Depress Anxiety 2010;27(5): 426–33.

27. Goh AE, Bambara LM. Individualized positive behavior support in school settings: a meta-analysis. Remedial Spec Educ 2012;33(5):271–86.

28. Neitzel J. Positive behavior supports for children and youth with autism spectrum disorders. Preventing Sch Fail Altern Educ Child Youth 2010;54(4):247–55.

Treatment of Childhood Emotion Dysregulation in Inpatient and Residential Settings

Jaclyn Datar Chua, DO[a],*, Christopher Bellonci, MD[b],
Michael T. Sorter, MD[c]

KEYWORDS

- Inpatient • Residential • Aggression • Emotion dysregulation • Restraint • Seclusion
- Outburst

KEY POINTS

- Children hospitalized in inpatient and residential treatment facilities often present with severe emotion dysregulation, which is the result of a wide range of psychiatric diagnoses.
- Both individual-level and systems-level interventions have been effective in addressing emotion dysregulation and aggressive behaviors in inpatient and residential settings.
- Inpatient and residential settings require treatment models that are cost-effective, evidence-based, and generalizable.
- Readily available outcome studies of interventions performed in a variety of settings should outline potential barriers as well as steps required for successful implementation.

INTRODUCTION

Emotion dysregulation, defined as impairment in the psychological processes that maintain a child's emotional and behavioral self-control, may be a result of lagging development skills (ie, trait) or a temporary loss of previously acquired skills (ie, state). During "reactive aggressive" outbursts, behaviors may appear excessive to the triggering event, which is in contrast to "proactive aggression," where aggression is used for specific gain.[1]

Diagnoses, age, and acuity are important to consider in any review of interventions for children with outbursts. For instance, children admitted to a facility for aggressive behavior will have more aggressive behavior in that facility than children admitted for

[a] Department of Child and Adolescent Psychiatry and Behavioral Science, Children's Hospital of Philadelphia, 3440 Market Street, Suite 200, Philadelphia, PA 19104, USA; [b] Judge Baker Children's Center, 53 Parker Hill Avenue, Boston, MA 02120, USA; [c] Cincinnati Children's Hospital and the University of Cincinnati, Cincinnati Children's 3333 Burnet Avenue, Cincinnati, OH 45229, USA
* Corresponding author.
E-mail address: chuaj1@email.chop.edu

Child Adolesc Psychiatric Clin N Am 30 (2021) 505–525
https://doi.org/10.1016/j.chc.2021.04.004
1056-4993/21/© 2021 Elsevier Inc. All rights reserved.

depression or anxiety[2] and are significantly more likely to have externalizing disorder diagnoses. Furthermore, young children have higher rates of aggression than older children and adolescents[2]; hence, age is critical. Finally, the acuity of the setting is important. The goals of an inpatient unit with a length of stay (LOS) of less than a week will not be able to accomplish much in the way of teaching self-regulatory skills. Thus, the goal of an inpatient unit might be to keep the child safe and find a discharge plan that will focus on the triggers and deficits that are complicating the child's life. In reviewing the intervention literature on youth with emotion dysregulation, diagnoses, age, and acuity of treatment setting provide foundational information about the sample in order to adequately assess the appropriateness of a given intervention. In this review, the authors focus on the setting of acuity requiring inpatient hospitalization or residential treatment.

With half of childhood-onset mental illness impacted by trauma, youth with trauma exposure are at a disproportionate risk of hospitalizations.[1,3] Trauma-informed care has been an important focus of treatment. Keeshin and colleagues (Keeshin B, Bryant B, Gargaro E. Aggression and Dysregulation: A Trauma Informed Approach. Child and Adolescent Psychiatric Clinics, 2020, submitted) describe how this meshes with evidence-based treatments for children with externalizing disorders.

Programmatically, the 2 goals in the inpatient management of children with outbursts are to stop or reduce the actual outburst and to treat the underlying condition or deficits that are thought to be instrumental to the problem. Programs aimed to reduce seclusion and restraint (S & R) have addressed the former. Programs focusing on behavior management and/or cognitive behavioral treatment of aggression have tried to address the latter.

The sizable evidence base for treating reactive aggression in outpatients has been summarized by Waxmonsky and colleagues (WAXMONSKY. Child and Adolescent Psychiatric Clinics, submitted) and Evans and colleagues (EVANS. Child and Adolescent Psychiatric Clinics, submitted) in this issue. However, there are no controlled trials for managing the actual outburst. The Agency for Healthcare Research and Quality, in reviewing the data for adults, provided specific recommendations on how to deescalate or prevent outbursts (eg, having a therapeutic milieu where aggression is less likely, using de-escalation techniques, using medication where necessary and seclusion/restraint/holds when those measures fail). Unfortunately, data supporting these guidelines are inadequate to guide policy.[4] There are no data for children other than pointing to situations in which S & R have been reduced but without measuring whether the actual aggression driving these interventions has decreased.

Nevertheless, it is important to review what is known about programs directed at dysregulated children. Thus, the purpose of this review is to (1) summarize existing strategies for the management of emotion dysregulation in inpatient and residential settings, and (2) propose directions for future research and practice.

METHODOLOGY

Because emotion dysregulation is not a diagnosis, the authors used proxy search terms for this review. PubMed and PsycINFO databases were searched with the following MeSH terms: aggress*, inpatient, residential, child, adolescent, management, prevent, externalizing, disruptive, bipolar, attention deficit, and impuls*. The Taylor and Francis publishing database, California Evidence-based Clearinghouse for Child Welfare, and the Center for the Study and Prevention of Violence were also searched to access articles. In addition, citations within the references section of the included papers were reviewed. Exclusion criteria included the following: not specific to children and/or adolescents, lack of specific intervention described to manage dysregulation or aggression, and not occurring in inpatient or residential settings. Studies in international settings were included; however, they must have been in the English language.

INPATIENT AND RESIDENTIAL SETTINGS

Currently, *acute inpatient psychiatric settings* emphasize crisis stabilization and safety while trying to maintain children in the least restrictive environment with recent LOSs decreasing from months to days over the last several decades.[5] There is an emphasis on individualized treatment plans that incorporate strategies to identify triggers, support distress tolerance, teach skills, and manage conflict more effectively.[6,7] The structured environment in *residential facilities* aims to provide an opportunity for the development of life skills necessary to address challenges in children's homes, schools, and/or communities.[8] Treatment can span several service systems, including mental health, child welfare, and juvenile justice.[9]

Outcome literature for inpatient and residential treatments has been hampered by the absence of outcome measures or control or comparison groups, has been limited in the number of studies and small sample sizes, and has given poor attention to sample composition.[5] Often, new models might challenge a longstanding infrastructure and culture with an inability to perform systematic monitoring of results.[10] Other potential challenges include the amount of support from organizational leadership or staff buy-in, financial constraints, staff turnover, or other logistical concerns.[9,11]

REVIEW OF SPECIFIC INTERVENTIONS IN INPATIENT AND RESIDENTIAL SETTINGS

To illustrate the impact that factors such as diagnoses, age, and acuity in terms of LOS have on the intervention, the programs summarized are grouped into the following settings: acute inpatient (LOS <30 days), inpatient in a state hospital, and residential (**Table 1**).

Acute Inpatient Settings

Three acute inpatient programs, with LOSs of 1 to 3 weeks, have used a behavior modification approach to treat children[2] or young adolescents.[6,12] The units with young adolescents[6,12] had fewer aggressive children than the units with children.[2] Although the models differ somewhat (Triple P parenting and Pelham's Summer Treatment Program approach on the child unit; the school-based Positive Behavior Intervention and Supports on the adolescent unit), all have a social-learning theory approach starting with setting clear expectations to the child, using positive reinforcement for desired behaviors with a limit-setting hierarchy, trying to avoid seclusion/restraint but using them in instances requiring safety. Each study uses a historical control to compare measures of interest before and after the intervention. In 2 studies, the intervention was behavior modification.[6,12] In 1 study, it was replacing behavior modification with a verbal deescalation treatment for acute outbursts.[2] Although some measures of success differed, in all 3 studies, children with the behavior modification treatment had fewer seclusions/restraints, and less medication use for agitation. Where it was studied, duration of time in seclusion or restraint was significantly decreased.

The best studied alternative to behavior modification is Collaborative Problem Solving, or "Collaborative Proactive Solutions" (CPS), which is a cognitive-behavioral, trauma-informed approach that reconceptualizes disruptive behaviors by understanding a child's aggression as a result of a lag in their cognitive ability to problem-solve.[13]

Table 1
Review of specific interventions in inpatient and residential settings

Author	Intervention	Demographics	Mean LOS	Sample Size	Treatment Conditions	Measures/Outcome
Acute inpatient						
Dean et al,[6] 2007	Comprehensive Behavioral Management Model based on Triple P	48% child 52% adolescent Mean age = 13.6 y	18 d	151	46% aggression 23% sexual abuse 17% physical abuse	Reduction in S & R, no change in prn use Significant reduction in aggression, injuries, physical restraint, & duration of seclusion
Carlson et al,[2] 2020	BMP modeled after Pelham's Summer Treatment Program	Child only Mean age = 9.6 y	17 d	661	77% with aggression 79.3% DBD 19% trauma	Fewer children had prns when BMP was present (57%) than BMP-absent (74%) Fewer children needed S & R when BMP was present (15%) than BMP-absent (34%) Children when BMP was present needed fewer prns (163 ± 319 per 1000 pd) than BMP absent (483 ± 569 per 1000 pd) BMP present cohorts had fewer S & R (17 ± 58 pd) vs No BMP (65 ± 159 pd)
Reynolds et al,[12] 2016	Modified version of Positive Behavioral Interventions & Supports	Mean age = 13 y 55% female	8 d	1485	39% ADHD, DBD, or PBD 35% depressive	S & R episodes ↓ from 20% to 13% Mean restraint duration ↓ from 20 min to 8 min per episode. prn medication use ↓ from 42% to 30%

Study	Program	Age	Length of stay	N	Diagnoses	Outcomes
Martin et al,[14] 2008	CPS	Mean age = 11 y 64% male	29 d	755	37% PBD 13% hyperactivity 11% MDD	Restraints ↓ (263–7 per year), restraint duration ↓ 41 + 8 min to 18 + 20 min, seclusions ↓ 432–133 per year; episode duration ↓ 27 + 5–21 + 5 min, 92–33 per 1000 pd for seclusion & 40–1 per 1000 pd for restraint. No prn use data or aggression measures
Greene et al,[3] 2006	CPS	Mean age = 9 y (3–14 y) 74% male	14 d	100	95% externalizing 80% trauma	Restraints: 281/9 mo to 1/15 mo. Holds: >100/mo to <10/mo
Tebbet-Mock et al,[15] 2020	DBT	Adolescent (12–17 y) TAU: Mean age = 15 y DBT: Mean age = 15 y	TAU (11 d) DBT (8 d)	TAU (376) DBT (425)	80% affective TAU/DBT: Trauma 2%/5% PBD 36%/33% Externalizing 7%/3%	No significant difference between patients who received DBT vs TAU for patient-to-patient aggression or patient to staff aggression. Restraints per patient lower with DBT (mean = 0.14) vs TAU (mean = 0.16). No significant difference for seclusions
Jonikas et al,[17] 2004	Crisis Prevention Institute	Adolescent	n/r	227	15% conduct disorder 37% depressive	98% decrease in restraints 2 quarters after staff training

(continued on next page)

Table 1
(continued)

Author	Intervention	Demographics	Mean LOS	Sample Size	Treatment Conditions	Measures/Outcome
Inpatient state hospital						
LeBel et al,[20] 2004	6CS	Child & adolescent	n/r	n/r	n/r	S & R episodes: Child 84/1000 pd, teen 74/1000 pd, adult 11/1000 pd. Postintervention ↓ of S & R by 73% on a child inpatient unit and 47% on an adolescent inpatient unit. Hours per episode did not change for children (30 min) but ↓ from 2 to 1 h for teens. Involuntary prns ↓ from ~20/1000 pd to 10/1000 pd in children, 15–10/1000 children, 15–10/1000 pd in teens and 30–10/1000 pd in a mixed unit
Azeem et al,[21] 2011	6CS	Mean age = 14 y	71 d	458	61% DBD 52% mood	79/458 youths needed S & R (17%) and had 276 S & R (3.5 per patient); final 6 mo, 11 children had 31 episodes. Patients involved ≥3 incidents had longer average LOS (85 d) as compared with patients involved in <3 incidents (64 d)

Wisdom et al,[22] 2015	Positive alternatives to restraints & seclusions	Child (0–12 y) & Adolescent (13–17 y) Facility 1 (6 C, 7 A) Facility 2 (2 C, 7 A) Facility 3 (5 C, 5 A)	n/r	Facility 1 (n = 27), facility 2 (n = 17), facility 3 (n = 20)	Total (25 DBD & 39 mood) Facility 1 (41% DBD, 26% mood), facility 2 (12% DBD, 47% mood), facility 3 (60% DBD, 35% mood)	↓ in S & R in 3 facilities by 62%, 86%, & 69%, respectively, after staff training
Donovan et al,[23] 2003	Autonomy, belonging, competence, & doing for others	5–11 y (26%) 12–15 y (37%) 16–18 y (37%) 62% male	~6 mo	Total (442) Child ≤ 12 y (122)	DBD ~30% PBD 4%–14% Mood 24%	Seclusion ↓ ~77–60/1000 pd ($P<.01$) Seclusion duration ↓ 45–40 min Restraints ↓ 54–40/1000 pd ($P<.01$). Restraint duration ↓ ~73–62 min ($P<.01$) Episodes of both per child: 9.2–6.8 ($P<.01$), 100–75/1000 pd; duration ↓ 55–53 min prn use 40% ↑ to 69%, patient injuries from 4% to 8%, and staff injuries 8%–10%

Residential

(continued on next page)

Table 1
(continued)

Author	Intervention	Demographics	Mean LOS	Sample Size	Treatment Conditions	Measures/Outcome
Apsche et al,[1] 2005	MDT	Adolescent CBT (mean age = 15) MDT (mean age = 17 y)	11 mo	40 CBT[16] MDT[18]	CBT (95% externalizing, 37% PTSD) MDT (76% externalizing, 33% PTSD)	Measures: Behavior daily reports, behavior incident reports (serious incidents) of physical or sexual aggression; CBCL and Devereux Rating Scale Reduction of 80.7% (MDT) vs 72.6% (CBT) in physical aggression. 84.5% reduction in sexual aggression vs CBT at 72.0%. CBCL externalizing decreased from T 73.7–65.6 for CBT vs 71.9–50.0 for MDT. Internalizing scores similar
Coleman et al,[30] 1992	Aggression Replacement Training (ART)	Adolescent (12–18 y) Mean age = 15 y	n/r	39 ART[21] Control[12]	64% conduct disorder 10% ODD 3% IQ < 70	Behavior incident report measure did not show change; improvement in social skills knowledge, which included keeping out of fights, dealing with group pressure, and expressing a complaint after 10-wk treatment did not translate into behavioral measures

Fields et al,[25] 2006	Project Re-Education of Children with Emotional Disturbance	Mean age = 10 y 13% female	6 mo	98	92% ADHD 69% conduct or ODD 76% depressive FSIQ Mean = 90	CBCL-externalizing scores: T 69 on admission, T 60 at discharge, T 63 at follow-up 21.4% of youth in the normal range on Behavior Emotional Rating scale
Connor et al,[26] 2002	Principles of the Psychoeducational Model (PEM) of Therapy	82% male Mean age = 13 y	19 mo	87	75% domestic violence exposure 59% sexual/ physical abuse	Teacher-completed Devereux Scales of Mental Disorder showed 68% in deterioration group vs 32% in the no-deterioration/ improvement group at discharge. Conversely, staff-completed Clinical Global Impressions Scale showed 83% of children improved

(continued on next page)

Table 1
(continued)

Author	Intervention	Demographics	Mean LOS	Sample Size	Treatment Conditions	Measures/Outcome
Huefner JC, O'Brien C, Vollmer D. Designing and testing a developmentally appropriate intervention for children in a psychiatric residential treatment facility. Child and Adolescent Psychiatric Clinics, 2020, submitted	Developmentally informed modification of PEM, Jr PEM	Mean age = 10 y	4 mo	76	Behavioral disorder (69%) Mood disorder (29%)	Assaults ↓ 434 per 1000 pd to 210 per 1000 pd; Cohen (d = 1.83), seclusions ↓ 148 per 1000 pd to 53 per 1000 pd; (d = 1.80), and restraints ↓ 138 per 1000 pd to 62 per 1000 pd; (d = 1.72). During Jr PEM months, children had 96.4% fewer restraints and 95.7% fewer seclusions than children during the PEM condition
Miller et al,[27] 2006 Private	Resource Team by an RRC	Child & adolescent (7–19 y) 67% male Mean age = 14 y	11 mo	409 children (276 male; 133 female)	4% developmental disability. All clients were diagnosed with at least 1 *DSM-IV* emotional or behavioral disorder	Measures: Physical restraint defined as any staff person touching a child who is behaving badly; also GAF. North site: 119/1000 pd to 80/1000 pd; south site 142/1000 pd to 60/1000 pd; combined reduction of 59%; GAF from admit to discharge was 41–54

Holstead et al,[28] 2010 Private, nonprofit	Resource Team by an RRC	4 units: Young boys (6–13 y), adolescent boys (13–22 y), girls (6–22 y), & autism (6–22 y)	16 mo	88 (2004) to 125 (2008)	50% abuse/neglect	5000 restraints in 2004 ↓ 786 restraints in 2008. Patient staff injury ↓ 0.199–0.159 injuries per person per year. Patient injury ↓ 307 in 2004 to 145 in 2008
Izzo et al,[31] 2016 State	Children & Residential Experiences Model: creating conditions for change	Male & female (7–18 y)	n/r	n/r	n/r	Compared 12 mo before implementation to 36 mo after. Decreased incident rate ratios (IRR) of aggression toward peers (IRR = 0.91, 95% CI [0.84, 0.99]), property destruction (IRR = 0.88, 95% CI [0.79, 0.99]), and self-harm (IRR = 0.93, 95% CI [0.86, 1.00])
Rivard et al,[32] 2005 State	Sanctuary model	Adolescent (12–20 y) Mean age = 15 y 67% male	n/r	158	33% physical abuse 14% sexual abuse 48% neglect	Aggression was not measured Improved Community Oriented Programs Environment Scale total scale and on the subscales of support, spontaneity, autonomy, problem orientation, and safety No changes in anger

(continued on next page)

Table 1
(continued)

Author	Intervention	Demographics	Mean LOS	Sample Size	Treatment Conditions	Measures/Outcome
Nunno et al,[33] 2003	Therapeutic crisis intervention	90% male unit A (age 6–12 y) Unit B (age 5–18 y) Unit C (age 14–18 y) Unit D (14–18 y)	n/r	350 (11 unit A) (295 unit B) (46 units C + D)	n/r	3 of 4 units took part in the program No change in 2 of them. One unit saw a significant ↓ in aggressive incidents from 101 to 64 and restraints ↓ from 36 to 12 Not clear how units were distinguished
Pollastri et al,[13] 2016	CPS[10]	n/r	n/r	n/r	n/r	Seclusions ↓ 610–29. No data on sample
Jones & Timbers,[34] 2003	Teaching family model	All female (12–18 y)	n/r	9	50% defiance & aggression	Physical restraints ↓ 0.4 per client per month to just >0.1 per client per month (about a 75% reduction)

Hodgdon et al,[35] 2013	Attachment, Self-Regulation & Competency framework	All female (12–22 y) Mean age = 16 y	9-6 mo	126	100% complex childhood trauma	Measures included CBCL, UCLA-PTSD Reaction Index, number of physical restraints. Follow-up every 3 mo. Significant ↓ in overall level of PTSD symptoms, driven by ↓ reexperiencing and hyperarousal symptoms. CBCL T scores: externalizing T 65.4–61.5; internalizing T 66.9–63.6; restraints ↓ ~30–40/mo to 5–15/mo
McCurdy & McIntyre,[36] 2004	Stop-Gap Model	All female (13–18 y)	n/r	25	100% externalizing (conduct and/or ODD often comorbid ADHD)	Reduction from ~2.0–0.5 mean therapeutic holds per resident
van Gink et al,[10] 2019	Nonviolent resistance	Child & adolescent, 8 in each unit (4–18 y)	n/r	n/r	n/r	No information on the sample and the intervention was vague. Over a year, S & R ↓ 215 incidents to 114 incidents in 1 institution for children and ↓ 84–64 in one for adolescents

(continued on next page)

Table 1
(continued)

Author	Intervention	Demographics	Mean LOS	Sample Size	Treatment Conditions	Measures/Outcome
Hambrick et al,[37] 2018	Neurosequential Model of Therapeutics	30% female (5–13 y)	14 mo	62	Majority with developmental trauma with no other diagnostic description provided	Data were not given in a way that allows determination of the amount of aggression or what changed over time Authors state there were significant reductions in reported critical events, such as restraints
Juvenile justice						
Goldstein et al,[29] 2018	Juvenile Justice Anger Management vs TAU	All female Adolescent (14–20 y) Mean age = 17 y	n/r	57	100% externalizing	↓ self-reported feelings of anger measured by Total Anger Scores on the Novaco Anger Scale & Provocation Inventory ($P<.01$) ↓ in reactive aggression measured by the Aggression Questionnaire ($P = .02$)
Gaines & Barry,[38] 2008	Relaxation Breathing Exercise	All male Adolescent Mean age = 14 y	n/r	6	100% externalizing	↓ frequency of curse words & inappropriate behaviors recorded by daily staff checks in 2 children. No data on S & R

Study	Intervention	Population	N	Duration	Diagnoses	Outcomes
Fowler,[39] 2006	Aromatherapy crisis management tool with or without prn medications	Adolescent Primarily male (12–19 y)	45	9–14 mo	n/r; included sex offenders	No effect on use of oral or intramuscular prn or S & R
Atwood and Osgood,[40] 1987	Positive peer culture	All male (13–18 y)	434	12 mo	100% externalizing	Coercive control decreases cooperation. Cooperation leads to attraction to the group & prevents delinquent norms
Van Loan et al,[41] 2015 Wilderness Program	Shifting gears: conflict avoidance through working partnerships	All male Adolescent (12–17 y) Houses ~ 45–55 boys	n/r	6-9 mo	Admitted due to "emotional or behavioral difficulties, substance abuse problems, & sexual offenses"	↓ monthly S & R frequency from 17 to ~6 in 8 mo

Abbreviations: ↓, decrease; ↑, increase; BMP, behavior modification program; CI, confidence interval; DBD, disruptive behavior disorder (ADHD; *DSM-IV*, Diagnostic and Statistical Manual of Mental Disorders (Fourth Edition); ODD, conduct disorder); GAF, global assessment of functioning; MDD, major depressive disorder; n/r, not reported; PBD, pediatric bipolar disorder; pd, patient days; R, restraint; S, seclusion; TAU, treatment as usual; UCLA PTSD, University of California–Los Angeles posttraumatic stress disorder; FSIQ, full scale intelligence quotient.

A meaningful reduction of S & R on a child unit (n = 100, LOS = 14 days), where 95% were admitted for "out-of-control behavior" and 80% had a trauma history,[3] provided a proof of concept. In a better studied sample of 755 children over the age of 4 years,[14] number and duration of S & Rs significantly decreased. It was not clear how many children were admitted with aggression, however, and there were no measurements of as needed (prn) use or rates of aggression reported.

Another conceptual model for inpatient care is dialectical behavioral therapy (DBT), which was used on an adolescent unit with a short LOS for primarily mood-disordered teens to treat mainly self-injurious and suicidal behaviors.[15,16] Compared with a historical control where treatment was mainly CBT or a reward system, DBT did not have a significant impact on rates of aggression.[15,16]

The Crisis Prevention Institute model, where staff identify crisis triggers and teach coping skills, is specifically aimed at preventing or aborting severe outbursts. If outbursts occur, staff are taught restraint techniques that promote safety. Although this approach is widespread, the authors found only 1 paper providing data, and this was for an adolescent unit where 15% of youths had conduct disorder and 37% had depressive disorders. Few data were reported, but restraints significantly decreased.[17,18]

Inpatient Settings in a State Hospital

Reported by the *Hartford Courant's* 1998 series, deaths associated with restraint served as an impetus for agencies to regulate S & R use within psychiatric treatment settings.[19] With S & R rates about 6 times higher in child and adolescent facilities with a greater death rate in comparison to adult patients, initiatives prioritized the reduction and/or elimination of S & R use.[20] One such initiative to reduce S & R includes the six core strategies (6CS) initiative. These strategies are leadership toward organizational change, use of data to inform practice, workforce development, use of S & R reduction tools, improving consumer's role in the inpatient setting, and vigorous debriefing techniques.[20] Applied to 1 child and adolescent inpatient unit (mean age = 14, n = 458) with 61% of the youth presenting with externalizing disorders, 6CS resulted in a significant decrease from the baseline S & R.[21] The use of the 6CS during a positive alternatives to restraints and seclusions project decreased from baseline S & R in 3 state inpatient facilities, although few of those were children with behavior disorders.[22] There is no mention of prn use, except in 1 facility, where prn use increased as S & R decreased.[22] Similarly, the ABCD, or autonomy, belonging, competence, and doing for others, program is a relationship-based intervention that led to a decrease in S & R rates and duration but an increase in prn use when examined on 442 youth, 26% of them in the child unit, with approximately 30% diagnosed with an externalizing disorder.[18,23]

Residential Settings

Mode deactivation therapy (MDT) combines cognitive and DBT techniques as well as focuses on social skills training to decrease aggression in youth who struggle with externalizing behaviors.[1,24] Studied in male adolescents, primarily diagnosed with conduct disorder, cognitive behavioral therapy (CBT) served as a control intervention to examine the use of MDT, which showed a significant decrease of 81% versus 73% in physical aggression and 85% versus 72% in sexual aggression for MDT as compared with CBT groups, respectively.[1]

Three interventions use a psychoeducational treatment model with teacher- or staff-completed measures postintervention. The Project Re-Education of Children with Emotional Disturbance is a 4- to 6-month, strengths-based ecological intervention with a 2-teacher/counselor team that encourages family involvement to ease home transition.[25] Examined with 98 mostly male youth (mean age = 10), diagnosed with attention-deficit/hyperactivity disorder (ADHD; 92%), conduct disorder/oppositional defiant disorder (ODD; 69%), and/or depressive disorders; (76%), half of the youth at borderline or clinical range at baseline were within normal range by discharge, as measured by the Behavioral and Emotional Rating Scale and Child Behavior Checklist (CBCL).[25]

The Psychoeducational Model of Therapy (PEM) uses the following: structured milieu, highly trained staff, group therapy, safety skills, assertiveness and communication training, social problem-solving, academic remediation, and community and family involvement.[26] Examined in youth (LOS = 579 days, mean age = 13) with 59% having a history of sexual and/or physical abuse, the teacher-completed Devereux Scales of Mental Disorder rated 68% in the deterioration group, whereas the staff-completed Clinical Global Impressions Scale reported 83% as improved, which indicates a low level of agreement on youth outcomes at discharge.[26]

Discussed by Huefner and colleagues (Huefner JC, O'Brien C, Vollmer D. Designing and testing a developmentally appropriate intervention for children in a psychiatric residential treatment facility. Child and Adolescent Psychiatric Clinics, 2020, submitted) in this issue, the Junior Psychoeducational Model (Jr PEM) is an adaptation of the above psychoeducational model (PEM) in a residential program serving boys and girls ages 5 to 12. Jr PEM is a developmentally informed program that teaches preadolescents self-control to manage anger and aggression and uses a token economy to promote prosocial life skills (Huefner, 2021). When comparing the use of PEM and Jr PEM for a preadolescent population, the youth were reported to have 97%, 94%, and 96% fewer assaults, restraints, and seclusions, respectively, during the Jr PEM condition, indicating the developmental adaptation of PEM was needed to address the needs of this age group (Huefner, 2021).

In addition, use of a resource team by a restraint reduction committee (RRC) in 1 facility with 3 sites led to a combined reduction of S & R by 59%, whereas 2 other facilities reported decreases in S & R, staff injury, and patient injury by emphasizing leadership, training, staff supervision, data analysis, and clinical case reviews.[27,28]

Admitted for externalizing behaviors, such as impulse control issues, some programs were used in residential juvenile justice facilities in adolescent populations with successful decreases in delinquent behaviors. One program in particular addressed cognitive distortions associated with aggression. Juvenile Justice Anger Management is a cognitive-behavioral approach that lessened self-reported feelings of anger and reactive aggression in 57 female adolescents.[29]

Several studies had 10 or fewer participants or had no clearly reported outcomes, or the interventions themselves were poorly described. Additional programs, including trauma-centered principles, parent management, staff burnout, mindfulness, and use of aromatherapy, are included in the table for completeness, as they were included in the search.

SUMMARY

Managing the risks presented by emotion dysregulation and violent outbursts is seen as a core competency of inpatient and residential programs. Our task was to summarize the literature on the treatment of dysregulated youth in inpatient and residential settings. Despite the prevalence and challenges presented by emotion dysregulation, there is a lack of clarity around standardized approaches to identify, assess, and manage these clinical problems. In addition, the quality and detail of some of the studies were poor, making it difficult to draw clear conclusions from the reported findings. Future research is needed for reliable instruments and techniques to assist clinicians in the early identification, characterization, and severity assessment of emotion dysregulation. Behavioral outbursts and potential violence are frequent with these patients with little understanding of the pathways leading to these episodes. Research of risk identification and effective mitigation strategies for prevention of aggression is required. Appropriate outcome measures are few, are not standardized, and require future study for development and adaptation into clinical practice.

There is an array of specific interventions that have shown some improvements in reducing violence and S & R, but with limited study and replication, there is an inability of the current research to indicate whether behavioral or cognitive-behavioral approaches to aggression are superior.[2] Given sample size differences, the interventions must be developmentally and diagnostically sensitive.[2] There is a need for improved understanding of the dynamics of staff interaction with patients and the elements that promote healing or those that cause conflict and aggression. This requires better understanding of the effects of the care models and the system factors that assist providers with maintaining fidelity to the care program. Expanding the understanding of the core therapeutic factors of these programs is needed. Future study that measures the effectiveness of interventions in inpatient and residential settings, providing both qualitative and quantitative metrics, would enable learning to improve standards of care.

ACKNOWLEDGMENTS

This work was inspired and supported by Dr. Gabrielle Carlson, MD.

DISCLOSURE

J.D. Chua has nothing to disclose. C. Bellonci is a Board Member and past president of the Association of Children's Residential Centers. M.T. Sorter has nothing to disclose.

REFERENCES

1. Apsche JA, Bass CK, Jennings JL, et al. A review and empirical comparison of two treatments for adolescent males with conduct and personality disorder: mode deactivation therapy and cognitive behavior therapy. Int J Behav Consultation Ther 2005;1(1):27.

2. Carlson GA, Chua J, Pan K, et al. Behavior modification is associated with reduced psychotropic medication use in children with aggression in inpatient treatment: a retrospective cohort study. J Am Acad Child Adolesc Psychiatry 2020;59(5):632–41.

3. Greene RW, Ablon JS, Martin A. Use of collaborative problem solving to reduce seclusion and restraint in child and adolescent inpatient units. Psychiatr Serv 2006;57(5):610–2.

4. Gaynes BN, Brown C, Lux LJ, et al. Strategies to de-escalate aggressive behavior in psychiatric patients. Agency for Healthcare Research and Quality: Comparative Effectiveness Reviews; 2016. p. 180.

5. Gathright MM, Holmes KJ, Morris EM, et al. An innovative, interdisciplinary model of care for inpatient child psychiatry: an overview. J Behav Health Serv Res 2016; 43(4):648–60.

6. Dean AJ, Duke SG, George M, et al. Behavioral management leads to reduction in aggression in a child and adolescent psychiatric inpatient unit. J Am Acad Child Adolesc Psychiatry 2007;46(6):711–20.

7. Masters KJ, Bellonci C, Bernet W, et al. Practice parameter for the prevention and management of aggressive behavior in child and adolescent psychiatric institutions, with special reference to seclusion and restraint. J Am Acad Child Adolesc Psychiatry 2002;41(2 Suppl):4S–25S.

8. Holden MJ, Sellers D. An evidence-based program model for facilitating therapeutic responses to pain-based behavior in residential care. Int J Child Youth Fam Stud 2019;10(2–3):63–80.

9. James S, Alemi Q, Zepeda V. Effectiveness and implementation of evidence-based practices in residential care settings. Child Youth Serv Rev 2013;35(4): 642–56.

10. van Gink K, van Domburgh L, Jansen L, et al. The development and implementation of non-violent resistance in child and adolescent residential settings. Residential treatment for Children & Youth 2019;37(3):176-98.

11. Delaney KR. Top 10 milieu interventions for inpatient child/adolescent treatment. J Child Adolesc Psychiatr Nurs 2006;19(4):203–14.

12. Reynolds EK, Grados MA, Praglowski N, et al. Use of modified positive behavioral interventions and supports in a psychiatric inpatient unit for high-risk youths. Psychiatr Serv 2016;67(5):570–3.

13. Pollastri AR, Lieberman RE, Boldt SL, et al. Minimizing seclusion and restraint in youth residential and day treatment through site-wide implementation of collaborative problem solving. Residential Treat Child Youth 2016;33(3–4): 186–205.

14. Martin A, Krieg H, Esposito F, et al. Reduction of restraint and seclusion through collaborative problem solving: a five-year prospective inpatient study. Psychiatr Serv 2008;59(12):1406–12.

15. Tebbett-Mock AA, Saito E, McGee M, et al. Efficacy of dialectical behavior therapy versus treatment as usual for acute-care inpatient adolescents. J Am Acad Child Adolesc Psychiatry 2020;59(1):149–56.

16. Leffler JM. Evaluating the clinical and financial outcomes of implementing dialectical behavior therapy on a psychiatric inpatient unit: a change in practice and culture. J Am Acad Child Adolesc Psychiatry 2020;59(1):40.

17. Jonikas JA, Cook JA, Rosen C, et al. A program to reduce use of physical restraint in psychiatric hospitals. Psychiatr Serv 2004;55:818–20.

18. Delaney KR. Evidence base for practice: reduction of restraint and seclusion use during child and adolescent psychiatric inpatient treatment. Worldviews Evid Based Nurs 2006;3(1):19–30.

19. LeBel J, Goldstein R. Special section on seclusion and restraint: the economic cost of using restraint and the value added by restraint reduction or elimination. Psychiatr Serv 2005;56(9):1109–14.

20. LeBel J, Stromberg N, Duckworth K, et al. Child and adolescent inpatient restraint reduction: a state initiative to promote strength-based care. J Am Acad Child Adolesc Psychiatry 2004;43(1):37–45.

21. Azeem MW, Aujla A, Rammerth M, et al. Effectiveness of six core strategies based on trauma informed care in reducing seclusions and restraints at a child

and adolescent psychiatric hospital. J Child Adolesc Psychiatr Nurs 2011; 24(1):11–5.

22. Wisdom JP, Wenger D, Robertson D, et al. The New York State office of mental health positive alternatives to restraint and seclusion (PARS) project. Psychiatr Serv 2015;66(8):851–6.

23. Donovan A, Plant R, Peller A, et al. Two-year trends in the use of seclusion and restraint among psychiatrically hospitalized youths. Psychiatr Serv 2003;54(7): 987–93.

24. Blake CS, Hamrin V. Current approaches to the assessment and management of anger and aggression in youth: a review. J Child Adolesc Psychiatr Nurs 2007; 20(4):209–21.

25. Fields E, Farmer EMZ, Apperson J, et al. Treatment and posttreatment effects of a residential treatment using a re-education model. Behav Disord 2006;31(3): 312–22.

26. Connor DF, Miller KP, Cunningham JA, et al. What does getting better mean? Child improvement and measure of outcome in residential treatment. Am J Orthop 2002;72(1):110–7.

27. Miller JA, Hunt DP, Georges MA. Reduction of physical restraints in residential treatment facilities. J Disabil Policy Stud 2006;16(4):202–8.

28. Holstead J, Lamond D, Dalton J, et al. Restraint reduction in children's residential facilities: implementation at Damar Services. Residential Treat Child Youth 2010; 27(1):1–13.

29. Goldstein NE, Giallella CL, Haney-Caron E, et al. Juvenile justice anger management (JJAM) treatment for girls: results of a randomized controlled trial. Psychol Serv 2018;15(4):386.

30. Coleman M, Pfeiffer S, Oakland T. Aggression replacement training with behaviorally disordered adolescents. Behav Disord 1992;18(1):54–66.

31. Izzo CV, Smith EG, Holden MJ, et al. Intervening at the setting level to prevent behavioral incidents in residential child care: efficacy of the CARE program model. Prev Sci 2016;17(5):554–64.

32. Rivard JC, Bloom SL, McCorkle D, et al. Preliminary results of a study examining the implementation and effects of a trauma recovery framework for youths in residential treatment. Ther Comm 2005;26(1):83–96.

33. Nunno MA, Holden MJ, Leidy B. Evaluating and monitoring the impact of a crisis intervention system on a residential child care facility. Child Youth Serv Rev 2003; 25(4):295–315.

34. Jones RJ, Timbers GD. Minimizing the need for physical restraint and seclusion in residential youth care through skill-based treatment programming. Families Soc 2003;84(1):21–9.

35. Hodgdon HB, Kinniburgh K, Gabowitz D, et al. Development and implementation of trauma-informed programming in youth residential treatment centers using the ARC framework. J Fam Violence 2013;28(7):679–92.

36. McCurdy BL, McIntyre EK. 'And what about residential…? Re-conceptualizing residential treatment as a stop-gap service for youth with emotional and behavioral disorders. Behav Interv 2004;19(3):137–58.

37. Hambrick EP, Brawner TW, Perry BD, et al. Restraint and critical incident reduction following introduction of the Neurosequential Model of Therapeutics (NMT). Residential Treat Child Youth 2018;35(1):2–23.

38. Gaines T, Barry LM. The effect of a self-monitored relaxation breathing exercise on male adolescent aggressive behavior. Adolescence 2008;43(170):291–303.

39. Fowler NA. Aromatherapy, used as an integrative tool for crisis management by adolescents in a residential treatment center. J Child Adolesc Psychiatr Nurs 2006;19(2):69.
40. Atwood RO, Osgood DW. Cooperation in group treatment programs for Incarcerated adolescents 1. J Appl Soc Psychol 1987;17(11):969–89.
41. Van Loan CL, Gage NA, Cullen JP. Reducing use of physical restraint: a pilot study investigating a relationship-based crisis prevention curriculum. Residential Treat Child Youth 2015;32(2):113–33.

Designing and Testing a Developmentally Appropriate Intervention for Children in a Psychiatric Residential Treatment Facility

Jonathan C. Huefner, PhD[a],*, Christopher O'Brien, BA[b],
Dennis G. Vollmer, MHD, MBA[c]

KEYWORDS

- Residential treatment • Preadolescent • Developmentally informed • Aggression
- Psychoeducational • Seclusions • Restraints

KEY POINTS

- The Junior Psychoeducational Model (Jr PEM) was developed to address the emotional regulatory needs of preadolescents in residential treatment.
- Jr PEM was effective in helping preadolescents decrease their aggressive behaviors.
- Full implementation and fidelity were necessary for the success of the program.
- Very strong treatment effect sizes support the potential use of the program in other clinical settings.

INTRODUCTION

Preadolescent children in residential care have treatment needs that are different from adolescents (ie, 12 and younger vs 13 and older).[1,2] For instance, although preadolescents have a level of verbal ability and independence that allows them to participate in treatment, their relative developmental immaturity may prevent them from fully benefiting from the care they receive.[3] Awareness of these differences has resulted in the call for providing effective treatment for preadolescent children in residential care that accounts for their developmental limitations.[4] Meta-analysis has found strong support for modest effectiveness for cognitive-behavioral therapy

[a] Boys Town Child and Family Translational Research Center, 14015 Flanagan Boulevard Ste 202, Boys Town, NE 68010, USA; [b] Opportunities Inc, 12012 Roberts Road Ste C, La Vista, NE 68128, USA; [c] Boys Town Residential Treatment Center, 14092 Boys Town Hospital Road, Boys Town, NE 68010, USA
* Corresponding author.
E-mail address: Jonathan.Huefner@boystown.org

Child Adolesc Psychiatric Clin N Am 30 (2021) 527–536
https://doi.org/10.1016/j.chc.2021.04.005
1056-4993/21/© 2021 Elsevier Inc. All rights reserved.

(CBT) with youth in residential care settings.[5] Other meta-analyses with juvenile justice populations have similarly found moderate effect sizes for cognitive-behavioral and skill-building programs in reducing recidivism.[6–8] The challenge comes with applying CBT interventions with preadolescents that were designed for and tested in adolescents. Preadolescents in residential care consistently have higher aggression rates than adolescents in those same programs,[1,2,9] and higher use of restraint.[10]

In order to make treatment maximally effective, developmental theory needs to inform decisions about the timing, objectives, strategies, and context best suited to young children.[11,12] Several investigators have summarized the challenges posed by the integration of developmental and cognitive behavioral approaches.[12–14] For instance, preadolescents may respond poorly to traditional forms of CBT because they do not yet have the cognitive, social, or emotional maturity needed to understand and apply the skills being taught in therapy.[3,15] In addition, by focusing on the child, CBT may not give sufficient attention to family and social contexts that can play a key role in the development of externalizing behavior in preadolescents.[13]

Specific suggestions for making CBT developmentally appropriate for preadolescents include proactively teaching social and behavioral skills, making the content child-focused, and making the process experiential.[11,16,17] Tasks and teaching should be brief, active, and fun.[13,18,19] In addition, it is important that some allowance is made for normal, nondisruptive misbehavior as not requiring intervention.[17] Specifically, there is a need to distinguish between normative problem behavior (eg, not doing what they are asked to do, resisting bedtime, low-level defiance) and clinically problematic behavior.[20–22] Although most children occasionally display aggressive behaviors, aggression may indicate psychopathology and be clinically problematic when it is severe, is frequent, or occurs across multiple settings.[13]

The Psychoeducational Model

The Psychoeducational Model (PEM) is an adaptation of the Boys Town Family Teaching Model (itself a CBT model). Boys Town created the PEM to be effective with youth with a variety of severe behavioral and emotional disorders. PEM emphasizes teaching self-control and helps patients learn and use concrete strategies for controlling anger and aggression. It also provides staff with a positive, systematic approach to address these situations effectively.[23]

PEM is a multifaceted combination of treatment strategies for children and adolescents that supplements and supports the more traditional psychiatric and clinical treatment modalities with a consistent behavioral model that is adapted from the Boys Town Teaching Model.[24] The model uses a token economy to reinforce prosocial behaviors and address problem behaviors. Structure, consistency, and a focus on building relationships with the youth during all aspects of the therapeutic day are essential in teaching social, academic, and independent living skills. The Boys Town Teaching Model has proven effective in a variety of child-care settings, including residential treatment centers (RTCs) and psychiatric hospitals.[25]

The PEM program emphasizes comprehensive training and improvement of treatment skills for direct-care staff and the use of behavioral treatment strategies with high positive feedback ratios. In addition, the program provides consistent supervision to ensure model fidelity and maintain high-quality care.

In 2015, the program directors noted that the aggression rate for preadolescents was significantly higher than the aggression rate for adolescents and thought that preadolescents might benefit from a more developmentally appropriate adaptation.

Junior Psychoeducational Model

The Junior Psychoeducational Model (Jr PEM) program is an adaptation of the PEM designed to provide preadolescents with more immediate feedback of positive behaviors. The program is designed to shape behaviors to ensure successful functioning in a normal home or school environment. Children in the program are taught core self-control strategies and prosocial life skills.

An important part of Jr PEM is understanding that a degree of problem behavior is normative for children. Children can be in perpetual motion, have trouble playing nicely with peers, and may have little concept of good table manners. Preadolescents commonly break the rules and test the limits. That is how they learn about which behaviors are acceptable and which behaviors are inappropriate. Identifying normal misbehavior requires knowledge about child development and understanding what is normal for a preadolescents.

Jr PEM has 7 basic components: effective praise, positive teaching, corrective teaching, redirection, setting limits, calm-down time, and follow-up teaching. These components are the means used to support preadolescents in developing emotional regulation and acquiring prosocial skills. A brief description of each of these components follows.

Effective praise

Praise is effective for preadolescents when it occurs at a high and spontaneous rate (4–5 times per hour). Effective praise has 5 steps: provide general praise, label skill, describe specific behavior, provide a rationale/acknowledgment, and give a positive reinforcement. Reinforcement should include a verbal/nonverbal exchange from staff to demonstrate enthusiasm (ie, smiling, high fives, pats on the back, clapping).

Positive teaching

Children at this age require clear and consistent expectations. Engaging children in proactive teaching is an effective and useful tool to communicate staff's expectations and set children up for success. Staff are challenged to use proactive teaching often each day. Positive teaching has 5 steps: introduce skill and provide example of use, review skill steps, provide a rationale/acknowledgment, practice skill, and give a positive consequence.

Corrective teaching

The corrective teaching process consists of 4 basic steps and is designed to decrease the verbal exchange among staff and increase tolerance for "normal" age-appropriate behavior. The steps are redirection, setting limits, calm-down time, and follow-up teaching.

Redirection

The corrective teaching process has a built in "prompt" to redirect normal childhood behavior or initial maladaptive behaviors and provides youth an opportunity to correct the behavior without a response cost or negative consequence. It is important for staff to label a skill and be behaviorally specific when describing what the child is doing incorrectly and describe what the child should do correctly. If the child complies, staff should reinforce the desired behavior with an effective praise (praise with specific detail). If the child continues the undesired behavior, staff will immediately provide the child with a 3-second countdown to engage in the desired behavior.

Setting limits

If the child does not redirect after the 3-second prompt and engage in the desired behavior, staff will set limits by issuing a corrective teaching. Corrective teaching is praising, labeling skill and negative behavior, and delivering a negative consequence (receiving frown faces). If the child accepts and records the frown faces, staff will finish the corrective teaching. If the child continues the undesired behavior and refuses to complete the corrective teaching or accept consequences, staff will immediately move to the third step in the corrective teaching process.

Calm-down time

If the child does not redirect after a 3-second prompt or refuses to complete the corrective teaching, staff will ask the child to stop what they are doing and prompt the child to use a self-control strategy by using calm-down time. Children will be expected to follow a simple 4-step calm-down process. The 4 steps to calm down are to sit down, to be quiet, to use a self-control strategy, and to raise your hand when you are ready to work through. This process is designed to provide staff and children a predictable, consistent, and age-appropriate method for children to regain self-control and finish the corrective teaching. If the child becomes disruptive, staff may ask the child to use a self-control strategy in a different area on the unit that is away from others (unit time out).

Follow-up teaching

Once the child is in control of their own behavior, staff will complete follow-up teaching. Follow-up teaching consists of the following 4 steps: test for self-control, set expectations, record negative consequences, and award positive corrections (accepting consequences, practicing relevant skill). As children advance in the program, they are taught and expected to demonstrate more self-control and consistent positive behaviors in order to receive tangible reinforcers. Ultimately, as they demonstrate increasing levels of responsibility, children are transitioned from continuous concrete reinforcement (ie, a motivation card) to more natural general or specific praise.

In the current setting, directors noted that the PEM program was not working as well in the preadolescent unit as it was in the adolescent units. The significantly higher aggression rates in the preadolescent unit was the most evident difference between preadolescent and adolescent groups. It was hypothesized that the Jr PEM program would result in lower rates of physical assaults by youth and decreased use of seclusion and restraint. The Jr PEM program was tested in the preadolescent unit using an ABAB design (A periods were where the PEM model was used, and B periods were where the Jr PEM model was used), and the results are reported here.

METHOD
Participants

This research used information from monthly organizational reports for an RTC in the Midwest for a 32-month period from September 2015 through April 2018. The RTC program has the capacity to serve up to 34 youth, both male and female aged 5 to 18. The population served was divided among three 10- to 12-bed units: unit A comprised girls, generally aged 13 to 18; unit B comprised both girls and boys aged 5 to 12, and unit C comprised boys, generally aged 13 to 18. Youth served on unit B was the target population for the intervention. During this period, the daily census for this unit averaged 10 children in care (standard deviation = 1.2) with a range between 7.4 and 13.4 children. Previous research has shown that typically slightly more than half of these children were boys, were white, had experienced multiple failed placements before admission, and averaged more than 2 psychotropic prescriptions at the time of admission.[1] The program is Medicaid funded, and children must have a *Diagnostic and Statistical Manual of Mental Disorders* (Fourth Edition) diagnosis and be referred by a licensed clinician to be admitted. The most common primary diagnostic classes at admission are behavioral disorders (61%), followed by mood disorders (29%).

All data used in this research came from organizational reports that summarized monthly incident data for unit B over time (no individual-level information was used), and institutional review board review determined this qualified it as exempt from the Common Rule.

Program

Overall, the RTC is a 24-hour lock-secured residential treatment program for children aged 5 to 18 with psychiatric disorders. It is a long-term residential program providing medically directed care for more seriously troubled children who require supervision, safety, and therapy, but not inpatient psychiatric care. Many of the children are admitted to the program following residence in an even more restrictive setting (eg, inpatient hospitalization, juvenile justice detention). Children receive schooling in a special education classroom within the unit. The RTC has a full-time child/adolescent psychiatrist who serves as the Medical Director, 6 therapists (licensed mental health practitioners), and 9 nurses (behavioral health RNs). The program maintains a minimum of a 4:1 child-to-staff ratio during day/evening hours and a minimum of a 6:1 ratio for overnight hours, with behavioral health technicians (BHTs) providing most of the cognitive-behavioral intervention.

Direct-support staff, called BHTs, are hired and assigned to 1 of the 3 units based on preference, skill assessment during new-hire orientation training, and the staff's gender (female staff are permitted to work with youth of both sexes; male staff are generally prohibited from working with adolescent female youth). BHTs are assigned to a specific unit. Providing consistent core staff to a unit's cohort is imperative in developing trusting relationships and familiarity of youths' treatment goals, youths' triggers, and successful interventions. Staffing schedules and assignments are designed to reduce the amount of staff "floating" across units.

Intervention Implementation, Disruption, and Continuance

April 4, 2016 was the date selected for implementation of the Jr PEM model in unit B. In March 2016, all core unit B BHTs and the unit shift manager received an 8-hour training session on the Jr PEM model, including skill practicing on the revised teaching interactions. Likewise, unit B youth also received an orientation of the Jr PEM system, including a review of the new motivation cards and the new motivation schedules and incentives. Role playing was conducted with youth on the revised teaching interactions.

In August 2017, unit assignments required restructuring because of an influx of 12- to 18-year-old female adolescent admissions that fall. To accommodate the high admission rate of these female adolescents, some youth on Jr PEM (unit B) were reassigned to a different unit. Although some female youth who had experienced Jr PEM remained in unit B, all Jr PEM boys were moved to the adolescent boys' unit C. Unit restructuring created several environmental and programmatic challenges and interferences related to the implementation of Jr PEM, including the following: (1) *A breakdown of core staff*. Unit B staff, trained exclusively in Jr PEM, were required to work with female adolescents and attempted to implement both Jr PEM and PEM simultaneously. Likewise, unit C staff were required to work with younger boys on Jr PEM without adequate training or knowledge of that population and model. (2) *A disruption of program components*. Staffing ratios were maintained during this period, but unit program schedules were revised on units B and C in an attempt to accommodate the frequent reinforcement periods built into Jr PEM while also incorporating a schedule that met the needs of the adolescents. Despite best planning, separate program schedules and reinforcement periods proved too complex to consistently implement. As a result, Jr PEM youth were expected to adapt to a program schedule that was geared to adolescents, making it difficult for them to gain access to the privilege/environmental benefits of the Jr PEM system. (3) *A disruption in supervision*. Unit B shift manager, a Jr PEM expert, was required to supervise a unit of new adolescent girls and the unit C shift manager, untrained with Jr PEM, attempted to oversee implementation of the PEM and Jr PEM systems. Summary data for unit B continued to be reported to the program, with unit B not being solely preadolescent. Assault, restraint, and seclusion averages for this period of time were recalculated using only preadolescent data for use in the analysis presented here.

Around the end of December 2017 and beginning of January 2018, all preadolescent youth were reassigned back to unit B and core unit B staff were retrained in the Jr PEM model. Schedule and Jr PEM program were fully restored at that time.

Measures

All data used in this come from critical incident data recorded daily in an instrument called the Treatment Progress Checklist (TPC) and are based on direct observation of behaviors and events. The TPC is a modified version of Chamberlain's Parent Daily Report.[26] The TPC report logs all significant events (eg, property damage, self-destructive behavior, physical assault) that occur at the setting during each of the 3 shifts each day. Each clinically significant recorded incident includes a descriptive narrative of the behavior or event and the selection of at least 1 of 46 codes. Each code has been behaviorally defined so charting is consistent across staff entries. Some incidents may include more than 1 code. Direct-care staff record these events in a TPC (paper form) at the end of each shift for each child (1 form per day, divided into 3 sections, 1 section for each shift). Staff are trained in the use of the TPC during a 2-week preservice course and 1 week of job shadowing a more experienced staff member. TPC data are entered into the organization's clinical database by the overnight direct-care staff at the end of every day.

Assaults were the sum of the following 3 incident codes: physical assault of an adult, physical assault of a peer, and an attempted physical assault. An assault may or may not have resulted in an injury, but involves an intentional aggressive physical contact (eg, biting, choking, kicking, punching, scratching, pushing, jumping on, spitting at, throwing objects at, head-butting). An attempted physical assault is when a child attempts to harm another person through aggressive physical contact but is unsuccessful because the other person moves to avoid the contact.

Seclusions and restraints are single items on the TPC. They are emergency safety interventions and require documentation via a physician's order. Seclusions are the medically authorized use of a safe, secure, locked environment to prevent injury to youth or others. Restraints are a staff member or other adult therapeutically holding a youth to keep him/her from harming self or others. The program uses Safe Crisis Management, a nationally recognized restraint model for personal restraint techniques.

Analysis

The data used in this research follow an ABAB repeated-measures design. The A periods were times when the PEM model was used in the preadolescent unit, and B periods were times when the Jr PEM model was used in preadolescent unit. The authors used R (3.6.1) single-case randomization test,[27] probability, and effect size (standardized mean difference between A and B periods) analyses.

RESULTS

Fig. 1 shows the change in program averages for the dependent measures over time for the ABAB conditions (A = PEM; B = Jr PEM). The PEM and Jr PEM treatment conditions were significantly different (**Table 1**), with assaults decreasing from an average of 132.2 during the PEM months to 64.4 during the Jr PEM months. In other words, during the PEM months, there averaged 1 assault every 2.3 days per preadolescent, whereas during the Jr PEM months there averaged 4.7 days between assaults. The treatment effect size for the Jr PEM program was $d = 1.83$, which indicates that during the Jr PEM condition the children had 96.6% fewer assaults than the average during the PEM condition (Cohen's U3).[28]

Restraints decreased from 45.1 to 16.2, and seclusions decreased from 41.5 to 18.9 during the PEM and Jr. PEM months, respectively. These decreases correspond to restraints per child decreasing from 1 every 6.7 days for the PEM condition to 1 every 18.5 days for the Jr PEM condition, and seclusions per child decreased from 1 every 7.2 days for the PEM condition to 1 every 15.9 days for the Jr PEM condition. The treatment effect size for the Jr PEM program decrease in restraints was $d = 1.80$ and $d = 1.72$ for seclusions, indicating that during the Jr PEM condition, children had 96.4% fewer restraints and 95.7% fewer seclusions than children during the PEM condition.

DISCUSSION

The PEM program was designed many years ago in the context of working with troubled adolescents. When this program was later used in the care of preadolescents, it soon became obvious that it was not as effective for younger children. The shortcomings of the PEM model when used for preadolescents was most obvious in the significantly higher aggression rates for the younger group. Consequently, a

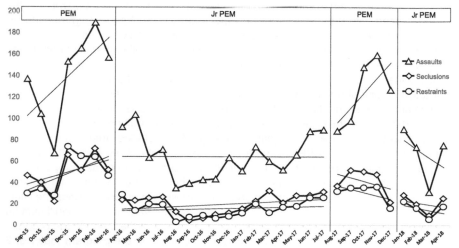

Fig. 1. Frequency of assaults, seclusions, and restraints per month per 10 children.

Table 1 Randomization test statistic, alpha, and effect size for the aggression, seclusion, and restraint			
Dependent Variable	Randomization Test Statistic	P	ES d
Assaults	67.8	.004	1.83
Seclusion	22.1	.024	1.72
Restraint	30.4	.007	1.80

developmentally sensitive adaptation of the PEM program, called the Jr PEM, was designed to address the needs of younger children, reinforce approximations of appropriate behaviors, and address delayed gratification by shortening time to access privileges.

The results support the effectiveness of the Jr PEM program in helping preadolescents decrease their aggressive behaviors and the decreased use of seclusion and restraint within the unit. The effect sizes for the intervention across the dependent measures ranged from 1.72 to 1.83, indicating that this developmentally informed intervention can provide a very robust means to helping behaviorally troubled preadolescents.

Jr PEM is a balance of accountability and patience. There are still behavioral expectations occurring, but within the scope of a young child's maturity and skill level. For instance, the Jr PEM program recognizes that it is age-appropriate for younger children to be impetuous, less skilled, and immature in their emotional and cognitive reactions. Jr PEM, therefore, allows for minor lapses in compliance that can be attributed to normal impulsivity and distractibility. One approach for doing this is incorporating prompts for the appropriate behavior and not expecting immediate compliance, giving the child the opportunity to still earn positive points and praise for degrees of compliance within the prompts. In some instances, when a child is extremely disruptive and/or volatile, Jr PEM enables clinicians to be flexible by directing focus on 1 key problematic behavior (assault, self-injurious behavior, property destruction, and so on) and deliver privileges based on the reduction of that specific behavior. Jr PEM also gives children in-the-moment opportunities to earn privilege time, rather than summarizing how things went at the end of the day, which is the approach used with adolescents in the PEM model. More frequent, immediate rewards and consequences are closer to what happens in family homes.

One lesson learned from the disruption period was that full implementation and fidelity are essential to the success of Jr PEM. For the program to be effective, it must be the sole focus of the interventionists. Partial application, through either distraction or lack of training, was not enough to produce desired outcomes.

There are several limitations to this research. First, the ABAB design was not intentional, and therefore, the transitions between the A and B conditions were not as definitive as it would have been in a planned design. For instance, there was an initial attempt to continue the Jr PEM program with the preadolescents during the second "A" stage (ie, the discontinuation of the Jr PEM program was not as complete as it would have been in an intentional design). Nonetheless, the unintentional reversal period was very helpful in showing a rebound in undesirable outcomes once the intervention was removed or even not the sole focus of the intervention. A second limitation was that the data did not control for the relative difficulty of the youth in the program from month to month (ie, the case-mix). There is a sense in the program that 1 or 2 highly troubled children can radically impact the aggression, seclusion, and restraint rates. This question will have to be answered in future research. Specifically, to what extent do severely troubled youth impact outcome measures? This answer will require using individual, rather than program aggregated, data. Finally, the Jr PEM program has only been used in a single setting, so there is a question as to the degree to which the findings are generalizable. The effectiveness of Jr PEM in other settings and potentially different populations is also something that will have to be tested going forward. The strength of the effect sizes found in this setting, however, is encouraging that the approach underlying the Jr PEM program will also be beneficial elsewhere.

DISCLOSURE

The authors have nothing to disclose.

REFERENCES

1. Huefner JC, Vollmer DG. Characteristics and treatment needs of preadolescent versus adolescent children in an intensive residential treatment program. Residential Treat Child Youth 2014;31(4):301–15.
2. Baker AJL, Archer M, Curtis PA. Age and gender differences in emotional and behavioural problems during the transition to residential treatment: the Odyssey Project. Int J Social Welfare 2005;14:184–94.
3. Grave J, Blissett J. Is cognitive behavior therapy developmentally appropriate for young children? A critical review of the evidence. Clin Psychol Rev 2004;24(4):399–420.
4. Friedberg RD, Wilt LH. Metaphors and stories in cognitive behavioral therapy with children. J Ration Emot Cogn Behav Ther 2010;28(2):100-13.
5. Armelius B-k, Andreassen TH. Cognitive-behavioral treatment for antisocial behavior in youth in residential treatment. Cochrane Libr 2007;(4):1–42.
6. Andrews DA, Bonta J. The psychology of criminal conduct. 4th edition. Newark (NJ): Lexis/Nexis; 2006.
7. Lipsey MW. The primary factors that characterize effective interventions with juvenile offenders: a meta-analytic overview. Victims Offenders 2007;4(2):124–47.
8. Lipsey MW, Howell JC, Kelly MR, et al. Improving the effectiveness of juvenile justice programs: a new perspective on evidence-based practice. Washington, DC: Center for Juvenile Justice Reform; 2010.
9. Duke SG, Scott J, Dean AJ. Use of restrictive interventions in a child and adolescent inpatient unit – predictors of use and effect on patient outcomes. Australas Psychiatry 2014;22(4):360–5.
10. Stewart SL, Baiden P, Theall-Honey L. Factors associated with the use of intrusive measures at a tertiary care facility for children and youth with mental health and developmental disabilities. Int J Ment Health Nurs 2013;22:56–68.
11. Kingery JN, Roblek TL, Suveg C, et al. They're not just "little adults": developmental considerations for implementing cognitive-behavioral therapy with anxious youth. J Cogn Psychotherapy 2006;20(3):263–73.
12. Ollendick TH, Grills AE, King NJ. Applying developmental theory to the assessment and treatment of childhood disorders: does it make a difference? Clin Psychol Psychotherapy 2001;8(5):304–14.
13. Southam-Gerow M, Kendall PC. Cognitive-behaviour therapy with youth: advances, challenges, and future directions. Clin Psychol Psychotherapy 2000;7(5):343–66.
14. Stallard P. Cognitive behaviour therapy with children and young people: a selective review of key issues. Behav Cogn Psychotherapy 2002;30(3):297–309.

15. Garber J, Frankel SA, Herrington CG. Developmental demands of cognitive behavioral therapy for depression in children and adolescents: cognitive, social, and emotional processes. Annu Rev Clin Psychol 2016;12:181–216.
16. Gosch EA, Flannery-Schroeder E, Mauro CF, et al. Principles of cognitive-behavioral therapy for anxiety disorders in children. J Cogn Psychotherapy 2006;20(3):247–62.
17. Jolstead KA, Caldarella P, Hansen B, et al. Implementing positive behavior support in preschools: an exploratory study of CW-FIT Tier 1. J Positive Behav Interventions 2017;19(1):48–60.
18. Friedberg RD, McClure JM. Clinical practice of cognitive therapy with children and adolescents: the nuts and bolts. New York: Guilford; 2002.
19. Sauter FM, Heyne D, Westenberg PM. Cognitive behavior therapy for anxious adolescents: developmental influences on treatment design and delivery. Clin Child Fam Psychol Rev 2009;12(4):310–35.
20. Briggs-Gowan MJ, Godoy L, Heberle A, et al. Assessment of psychopathology in young children. In: Cicchetti D, editor. Developmental psychopathology. Hoboken (NJ): John Wiley & Sons; 2016. p. 1–45.
21. Hong JS, Tillman R, Luby JL. Disruptive behavior in preschool children: distinguishing normal misbehavior from markers of current and later childhood conduct disorder. J Pediatr 2015;166(3):723–30.
22. Wakschlag LS, Briggs-Gowan MJ, Carter AS, et al. A developmental framework for distinguishing disruptive behavior from normative misbehavior in preschool children. J Child Psychol Psychiatry 2007;48(10):976–87.
23. Woodlock D, Juliano N, Ringle JL. Giving hope to troubled adolescents: diverse treatment approach emphasizes self-control skills. Behav Healthc Tomorrow 2002;11(4):8–11.
24. Daly DL, Davis JL. Long-term residential program training manual. Boys Town (NE): Boys Town Press; 2003.
25. O'Brien C, Ringle JL, Larzelere RE. Serving youths by modifying treatment: girls and Boys Town approach uses ongoing outcome measures. Behav Healthc Tomorrow 2001;10:19–21.
26. Chamberlain P, Reid JB. Parent observation and report of child symptoms. Behav Assess 1987;9(1):97–109.
27. Koehler MJ, Levin JR. Regulated randomization: a potentially sharper analytical tool for the multiple-baseline design. Psychol Methods 1998;3(2):206–17.
28. Cohen J. Statistical power analysis for the behavioral sciences. 2nd edition. Hillsdale (NJ): Erlbaum; 1988.

Psychopharmacology of Treating Explosive Behavior

Carrie Vaudreuil, MD[a,b], Abigail Farrell, BS[a], Janet Wozniak, MD[a,b,*]

KEYWORDS

- Psychopharmacology • Pediatric • Explosiveness • Irritability

KEY POINTS

- Pharmacologic management of explosive behavior should be based on the first-line treatment of the primary psychiatric diagnoses of the patient.
- Risperidone has strong evidence for use in the treatment of explosive behavior.
- Divalproex sodium and lithium also have some evidence to support the treatment of explosive behavior.
- Stimulant medications may be helpful in treating explosive behavior in children with attention-deficit/hyperactivity disorder.

INTRODUCTION

Explosive behavior in children poses safety risks and impairs emotional, social, and academic development. Pharmacotherapy may be required despite a limited evidence base. A report by the Agency for Healthcare Research and Quality (AHRQ) summarizes data regarding first-generation antipsychotics (FGAs) and second-generation antipsychotics (SGAs). Explosive behavior was not specifically evaluated, but SGAs were found to probably decrease conduct problems and aggression in children with attention-deficit/hyperactivity disorder (ADHD) and disruptive behavior disorders (DBDs) and to probably decrease irritability in autism spectrum disorder (ASD). Evidence was insufficient to compare medications within the class or to draw conclusions for young children (<8 years old).[1]

Studies addressing explosiveness in youth are limited by lack of distinction of the level of symptoms. Irritability is heterogeneous, and explosive behavior of varying severity cuts across many disorders, such as ADHD, oppositional defiant disorder (ODD), conduct disorder (CD), bipolar disorder (BPD), disruptive mood dysregulation

[a] Clinical and Research Program in Pediatric Psychopharmacology and Adult ADHD, Massachusetts General Hospital, 55 Fruit Street, Warren 705, Boston, MA 02114, USA; [b] Department of Psychiatry, Harvard Medical School, Boston, MA, USA
* Corresponding author. Harvard Medical School, Massachusetts General Hospital, 55 Fruit Street, Warren 705, Boston, MA 02114.
E-mail address: jwozniak@partners.org

Child Adolesc Psychiatric Clin N Am 30 (2021) 537–560
https://doi.org/10.1016/j.chc.2021.04.006
1056-4993/21/© 2021 Elsevier Inc. All rights reserved.

disorder (DMDD), depressive disorders, posttraumatic stress disorder, ASD, anxiety disorders, tic disorders, Tourette syndrome, substance use disorders, learning disabilities, and intellectual disabilities. When physical concerns exist, medical work-up may be indicated.

Two published guidelines regarding the treatment of explosive youth are the Treatment Recommendations for the Use of Antipsychotics for Aggressive Youth (TRAAY)[2,3] and the Treatment of Maladaptive Aggression in Youth: CERT Guidelines.[4,5] In summary:

1. Conduct a thorough initial evaluation, including diagnostic work-up.
2. Initiate treatment based on evidence for first-line psychosocial, therapeutic, and psychopharmacologic management for the identified diagnoses.
3. Assess treatment effects and outcomes. Use standardized symptom and behavior rating scales at regular time points before and during treatment.
4. For chronic aggression, first use psychosocial and educational treatment. Next, use appropriate pharmacologic treatment of primary disorders before prescribing antipsychotics for aggression. If using an atypical antipsychotic, start with an SGA, because they have a safer acute side effect profile than FGAs. Use a conservative dosing strategy: start low, go slowly, routinely assess for side effects and drug interactions, ensure an adequate trial (at least 2 weeks), and avoid using 4 or more medications simultaneously. If no response, try a different SGA. If partial response, consider augmentation with a mood stabilizer. If good response, continue treatment for 6 months and then attempt to taper if tolerated.
5. For acute aggression, perform a risk assessment and refer for emergency evaluation if necessary. Use psychosocial crisis management techniques before medication. If necessary, use pharmacologic management of acute aggression before resorting to physical and mechanical restraints. If as-needed medications are frequently required, readjust the behavioral treatment plan and medication regimen.

These guidelines are general and leave the choice of medication up to the clinician's judgment. This article provides a summary of the evidence base for pharmacotherapy for explosive behavior in youth. The existing literature was reviewed using PubMed, PsycINFO, and Medline and the search algorithm (("psychopharmacology" or "treatment" or "pharmacotherapy" or "pharmacology") and ("explosive behavior" or "explosions" or "rage" or "extreme irritability" or "aggression") and ("child" or "pediatric")). References from identified journal articles were also reviewed. **Table 1** includes a summary of the medications and studies reviewed in this article.

ANTIMANIC AGENTS
Second-Generation Antipsychotics

SGAs are increasingly used to treat aggression in children and adolescents.[6] Although FGAs were primarily used in the 1980s, concerns about side effects and safety of FGAs in children has led clinicians to use SGAs more frequently since their development. Both risperidone and aripiprazole are US Food and Drug Administration (FDA) approved for the treatment of irritability in ASD in children. Risperidone, aripiprazole, olanzapine, quetiapine, lurasidone, paliperidone, and asenapine are FDA approved for use in adolescents and are indicated for the treatment of acute and mixed mania and/or schizophrenia. The use of SGAs to treat disruptive, explosive, or aggressive behavior is off label. SGAs are often associated with side effects, particularly weight gain, type II diabetes, metabolic syndrome, and cardiac rhythm abnormalities.

Table 1
Summary of studies on all medication classes

	Number of Total Studies	Types of Studies	Length of Studies	Review of Data
SGAs				
Risperidone[7–17]	11	6 double-blind, placebo-controlled trials 1 open-label trial 1 longitudinal study 1 naturalistic study 2 meta-analyses	4 wk to 12 mo	All 11 studies show reductions in aggression, irritability, conduct problems, and/or temper outbursts
Aripiprazole[18–27]	10	3 double-blind, placebo-controlled trials 3 open-label trials 1 case series 1 retrospective chart review 1 post hoc analysis 1 review article	6–52 wk	8 studies show efficacy in treating irritability associated with ASD 2 studies show improvements in irritability, aggression, disruptive behaviors, or explosive outbursts 1 study indicates tolerability, although 22% discontinued treatment
Olanzapine[28–31]	4	3 open-label trial 1 case report	2–12 wk	All 4 studies show improvements in aggression or explosive rage 1 study indicates a high discontinuation rate because of side effects
Ziprasidone[32–37]	6	2 case series 4 retrospective chart reviews	6–30 wk	4 studies show beneficial effects on aggression and agitation Compared with other medications, 1 study does not show any beneficial effects and 1 study shows worse outcomes
Quetiapine[38,39]	2	1 open-label trial 1 post hoc analysis	4–8 wk	Both studies show a reduction in aggression 1 study indicates good tolerability
Lurasidone[40]	1	1 double-blind, placebo-controlled trial	6 wk	Found no benefit compared with placebo for irritability in ASD

(continued on next page)

Table 1
(continued)

	Number of Total Studies	Types of Studies	Length of Studies	Review of Data
FGAs[1,41–45] 1 multiple FGAs 1 haloperidol 1 haloperidol and thioridazine 1 molindone and thioridazine 1 thioridazine 1 droperidol	6	2 double-blind, placebo-controlled trials 1 double-blind comparison trial 1 meta-analysis 1 retrospective chart review 1 review article	3–8 wk	1 study found insufficient evidence for conduct problems or irritability in ASD 5 studies indicate efficacy for aggression and CD 1 study notes a greater effect size for haloperidol compared with thioridazine 2 studies note considerable side effects
Lithium[41,48–52]	6	5 double-blind, placebo-controlled trials 1 longitudinal study	2 wk to 10 y	4 studies indicate beneficial effects on aggression or symptoms of CD 2 studies show no beneficial effects in CD or SMD 1 study notes fewer side effects than haloperidol and 1 study notes more side effects than placebo
Antiepileptics				
Divalproex sodium[39,53–58]	7	3 double-blind, placebo-controlled trials 1 double-blind, controlled trial 1 open-label trial 2 post hoc analyses	4–12 wk	6 studies indicate beneficial effects on aggression, irritability, mood lability, or symptoms of CD, alone or as adjunctive treatment 1 study shows efficacy for treatment of impulsivity, but not aggression
Carbamazepine[95,96]	2	1 double-blind, placebo-controlled trial 1 open-label trial	3–6 wk	1 study shows an improvement in aggression and explosiveness 1 study indicates no beneficial effects compared with placebo and more side effects Small N for both studies

Stimulants[12,13,63–71] 4 multiple stimulants 7 methylphenidate	11	6 double-blind, placebo-controlled trials 3 open-label trials 1 naturalistic study 1 meta-analysis	1 d to 6 mo	11 studies show efficacy for aggression, oppositional behaviors, ADHD symptoms, antisocial behaviors, externalizing symptoms, irritability, emotional lability, anger, and/or explosive rage, alone or combined with an SGA or behavior therapy 1 study noted improvement in aggression in less than half (49%) of participants 1 study noted worsened irritability in 19% of participants
Alpha agonists[72–75] 2 clonidine 2 guanfacine	4	2 double-blind, placebo-controlled trials 1 open-label trial 1 case report	6 wk to 18 mo	All 4 studies show improvements in aggression, conduct-related behaviors, oppositional behaviors, or symptoms of ASD, including impulsivity and self-injurious behavior, either alone or combined with a stimulant
Atomoxetine[2,97]	2	2 meta-analyses	6 wk to 9 mo	1 study shows reductions in symptoms of ODD and ADHD 1 study indicates a small effect size for aggression
Antidepressants[43,76–86] 1 multiple antidepressants 1 multiple SSRIs 2 citalopram 2 fluoxetine 1 fluvoxamine 1 nortriptyline 2 desipramine 2 trazodone	12	6 double-blind, placebo-controlled trials 3 open-label trials 2 case reports 1 meta-analysis	1–16 wk	7 studies show improvements in aggression, oppositional symptoms, impulsivity, or OCD, alone or combined with stimulants 1 study noted a small effect size of antidepressants on aggression, with desipramine as the largest 3 studies note no therapeutic benefit on aggression or functional impairment 1 study indicates that some may worsen on trazodone

(continued on next page)

Table 1
(continued)

	Number of Total Studies	Types of Studies	Length of Studies	Review of Data
Antihistamines[98,99] 1 all antihistamines 1 diphenhydramine	2	1 double-blind, placebo-controlled trial 1 retrospective chart review	2 h	1 study notes a high frequency of use for the management of aggressive events 1 study indicates no beneficial effects compared with placebo
Vitamins/minerals[87–94] 2 omega-3 fatty acids 4 EMPower family 2 other vitamins/minerals	8	3 double-blind, placebo-controlled trials 1 single-blind, controlled trial 1 open-label trial 2 case series 1 naturalistic study	8 wk to 6 mo	All 8 studies show improvements in aggression, mood, angry outbursts, irritability, emotional regulation, and/or violent behaviors

Abbreviations: OCD, obsessive-compulsive disorder; SSRI, selective serotonin reuptake inhibitor.

Risperidone

Of the SGAs, risperidone has the most evidence supporting its use as an intervention for children with explosive behavior. In children with CD, risperidone has been shown to be effective at reducing aggressive symptoms compared with placebo.[7] Two meta-analyses have shown that risperidone is effective for reducing aggression and conduct problems in youth with DBDs, but noted a lack of substantial evidence for other SGAs.[8,9]

In children with ADHD and DBDs, risperidone has been shown to reduce aggressive behavior, both alone[10] and in combination with stimulant medications.[11–13]

In a study of 21 children with severe mood dysregulation (SMD), a precursor to DMDD, risperidone was shown to reduce irritability and the frequency of temper outbursts in an 8-week open-label trial.[14]

Risperidone has also been shown to be effective at reducing aggression in children with subaverage cognitive abilities in an inpatient hospital setting[15] and an outpatient setting,[16] and has been effective at reducing aggression in children with ASD.[17] **Table 2** provides a summary of studies on risperidone.

Aripiprazole

Multiple studies have shown the use of aripiprazole to be effective in the treatment of irritability associated with ASD.[18–25] However, fewer studies have evaluated its use for the treatment of aggressive or explosive behavior. Pan and colleagues[26] performed an open-label trial of aripiprazole and methylphenidate in 24 children with ADHD and DMDD. The combination was found to be associated with significant improvement across multiple domains, including irritability, externalizing symptoms, disruptive behaviors, and aggression.[26] A retrospective, observational study of 37 children with Tourette noted improvement in explosive outbursts with aripiprazole. However, 22% of patients discontinued the treatment.[27]

Other second-generation antipsychotics

The data regarding the use of other SGAs for aggression are not robust. Several small, open-label studies have investigated the use of olanzapine for children and adolescents with explosive behavior and aggression and have shown that it may be helpful, although it was associated with significant side effects (weight gain, akathisia, sedation).[28–31]

Several reports noted that intramuscular (IM) ziprasidone used for acute agitation or aggression was effective and well tolerated,[32,33] but 1 study did report oversedation as a side effect.[34] IM ziprasidone was found to be less effective than IM olanzapine[35] and as effective as IM haloperidol plus lorazepam.[36] A small, open-label study of oral ziprasidone to treat ASD or pervasive developmental disorder (PDD) with irritability and aggression found that half of the participants responded to the treatment.[37]

Two small studies investigating the use of quetiapine concluded that it may be effective for the treatment of aggression in children with DBDs.[38,39]

A randomized, double-blind study of lurasidone for moderate to severe irritability in ASD found no benefit compared with placebo.[40]

First-Generation Antipsychotics

Although some FGAs carry FDA approval for the treatment of agitation in children, they have fallen out of favor in recent years because of the risk of side effects and the development of newer agents. Specifically, concerns about sedation, extrapyramidal side effects (EPSs), tardive dyskinesia, and neuroleptic malignant syndrome have been noted.

Table 2
Summary of studies on risperidone

	Study Design	Subjects	Medication Dose	Duration	Main Results
Findling et al,[7] 2000	Double-blind, placebo-controlled trial	20 children aged 5–15 y with CD	Initial dosage: 0.25–0.5 mg/d Final dosage: 0.75–1.5 mg/d	10 wk	Reduced aggressive symptoms compared with placebo
Loy et al,[8] 2017	Meta-analysis	Children aged 5–18 y with DBDs	0.98–1.7 mg/d	4–10 wk	Reduced aggression and conduct problems
Balia et al,[9] 2018	Meta-analysis	Children aged 5–18 y with CD	0.4–4 mg/d	4–10 wk	Reduced aggression and conduct problems
Masi et al,[10] 2017	Open-label trial	20 boys aged 6–16 y with ADHD and ODD	Initial dosage: 0.25 mg/d Final dosage: 0.5–2.5 mg/d	Up to 6 mo	Reduced aggressive behavior
Gadow et al, 2016[11]	Double-blind, placebo-controlled trial with extension	108 children aged 6–12 y with ADHD and DBDs	Not reported	9-wk clinical trial with 12-mo follow-up	Reduced aggressive behavior when combined with stimulants
Aman et al, 2014[12]	Double-blind, placebo-controlled trial	168 children aged 6–12 y with ADHD and DBDs	0.5–3.5 mg/d	9 wk	Reduced aggressive behavior when combined with stimulants
Armenteros et al, 2007[13]	Double-blind, placebo-controlled trial	25 children aged 7–12 y with ADHD and aggression	Initial dosage: 0.5 mg/d Final dosage: 1.08 ± 0.63 mg/d	4 wk	Reduced aggression when combined with stimulants
Krieger et al,[14] 2011	Open-label trial	21 children aged 7–17 y with SMD	Initial dosage: 0.5 mg/d Final dosage: 0.5–3 mg/d	8 wk	Reduced irritability and frequency of temper outbursts

Buitelaar et al,[15] 2001	Double-blind, placebo-controlled trial	38 inpatient children aged 12–18 y with DBDs and subaverage cognitive abilities	Initial dosage: 1mg/d Final dosage: 1.5-4 mg/d	6 wk	Reduced aggression compared with placebo
Snyder et al,[16] 2002	Double-blind, placebo-controlled trial	110 children aged 5–12 y with DBDs and subaverage cognitive abilities	Initial dosage: 0.01 mg/kg/d Final dosage: 0.02–0.06 mg/kg/d	6 wk	Reduced aggressive behavior compared with placebo
Nagaraj et al,[17] 2006	Double-blind, placebo-controlled trial	40 children aged 2–9 y with ASD	Initial dosage: 0.5 mg/d Final dosage: 1 mg/d	6 mo	Reduced symptoms of aggression

The AHRQ report did not find any benefit for FGAs in the treatment of conduct problems or irritability in ASD because of insufficient evidence. FGAs may cause less weight gain and body mass index increase compared with SGAs, but they have a higher risk for EPS symptoms and are equally likely to cause sedation.[1]

Haloperidol was shown to be effective at treating children with CD and aggression, aged 5 to 12 years, but was noted to cause side effects of sedation, drooling, and acute dystonic reaction.[41] Molindone and thioridazine have also been used in children with CD and aggression.[42] A meta-analysis of 3 randomized controlled trials of FGAs (2 haloperidol, 1 thioridazine) found a medium effect size for aggressive behavior, but it was noted that the effect size for haloperidol was large, and the effect size for thioridazine was smaller.[43] A comparison of thioridazine with methylphenidate in 30 children with low intelligence quotient, ADHD, and/or CD found that methylphenidate was superior to thioridazine and thioridazine was superior to placebo based on teacher-rated measure of conduct problems, but there were no improvements on either medication based on parent-report measures.[44]

A chart review of adolescents and young adults who received droperidol for agitation in the emergency department found that 42 out of 68 patients responded to the medication and no significant adverse events were noted.[45]

Lithium

Lithium is a mainstay of treatment of adults with BPD and may also prevent suicide in adults with mood disorders.[46] In children, there remain limited data available about the use of lithium, although studies have shown some benefit in pediatric mania and for the management of aggression in children with CD.[47] Lithium carries an FDA approval for the treatment of mania in adolescents.

In a 10-year longitudinal study of pediatric BPD, Hafeman and colleagues[48] showed that children on lithium displayed less aggression compared with children on other mood-stabilizing medications. However, in children with SMD, which is characterized by chronic irritability and explosive outbursts, lithium was not superior to placebo in a 6-week, double-blind trial.[49]

In the inpatient setting, lithium has been shown to be superior to placebo in the treatment of children with CD and aggression in several double-blind, placebo-controlled studies.[41,50,51] Children on lithium were noted to have more side effects compared with placebo,[51] but 1 study found that lithium caused fewer side effects than haloperidol.[41] A 2-week study investigating the use of lithium in inpatient adolescents with CD and aggression did not find any significant benefit compared with placebo, and noted few responders to treatment overall, perhaps suggesting that a longer trial of lithium is needed to see an effect.[52] **Table 3** provides a summary of studies on lithium.

ANTIEPILEPTIC MEDICATIONS

Antiepileptic drugs (AEDs) are primarily used for the management of seizure disorders or epilepsy. Although various AEDs may be used by clinicians for the treatment of psychiatric disorders, only divalproex sodium carries an FDA indication for the treatment of BPD in adults, and none carry an indication for the treatment of psychiatric disorders in children.

Divalproex Sodium

Divalproex sodium is FDA approved for the treatment of mania and mixed episodes in adults with BPD but does not currently carry an FDA approval for the treatment of psychiatric disorders in children. Divalproex sodium is approved for the treatment of seizure

Table 3
Summary of studies on lithium

	Study Design	Subjects	Medication Dose	Duration	Main Results
Hafeman et al,[48] 2019	Longitudinal study	340 children aged 7–17 y at intake with BPD	Not reported	Up to 10 y	Lower likelihood of displaying aggression compared with other mood stabilizers
Dickstein et al,[49] 2009	Double-blind, placebo-controlled trial	25 children aged 7–17 y with SMD	Initial dosage: 300 mg/d Final dosage: 600 mg/d or therapeutic dose	6 wk	Not superior to placebo for the treatment of SMD
Campbell et al,[41] 1984	Double-blind, placebo-controlled trial	61 inpatient children aged 5–13 y with CD, aggression, and explosiveness	Initial dosage: 250 mg/d Final dosage: 500–2000 mg/d	4 wk	Superior to placebo (to the same degree as haloperidol) in the treatment of behavioral symptoms of CD Associated with fewer side effects than haloperidol
Campbell et al,[50] 1995	Double-blind, placebo-controlled trial	50 inpatient children aged 5–12 y with CD, aggression, and explosiveness	Initial dosage: 600 mg/d Final dosage: 600–2100 mg/d	6 wk	Superior to placebo in the treatment of aggression in CD
Malone et al,[51] 2000	Double-blind, placebo-controlled trial	40 inpatient children aged 10–17 y with CD and aggression	Initial dosage: 600 mg/d Final dosage: 900–2100 mg/d	4 wk	Superior to placebo in the treatment of aggression in CD Associated with more side effects compared with placebo
Rifkin et al,[52] 1997	Double-blind, placebo-controlled trial	33 inpatient children aged 12–17 y with CD and aggression	Therapeutic dose	2 wk	Few responders and no significant benefits compared with placebo

disorders in children aged 10 years and older, and it is noted to carry the risk of hepato-toxicity, with increased risk of fatal hepatotoxicity in children less than 2 years old.

Divalproex sodium has been shown to be effective in the treatment of explosive temper and mood lability in children with ODD or CD.[53,54]

In children aged 6 to 13 years with ADHD and aggression on a stimulant medication, divalproex was shown to be superior to placebo as an adjunctive medication.[55]

In children with BPD and aggression, divalproex was shown to reduce aggression and irritability in children who were hospitalized for a manic or mixed state,[56] and was shown to be as effective as quetiapine in the treatment of impulsivity and reactive aggression.[39] In an open-label study of the offspring of bipolar parents, 24 children with mixed psychiatric diagnoses participated in a 12-week open-label trial of divalproex; 71% showed a reduction in aggression.[57]

In ASD, divalproex was found to be superior to placebo in the treatment of irritability in a 12-week, double-blind controlled trial. However, there were no significant findings with respect to measures of aggression.[58] **Table 4** provides a summary of studies on divalproex.

Carbamazepine

Carbamazepine has limited evidence (see **Table 1**).

STIMULANTS

Psychostimulants are considered the first-line treatment of ADHD. FDA indications for the use of stimulant medications include the use of methylphenidate for adults and children aged 6 years and older and the use of amphetamine salts in adults and children, with some formulations approved as young as age 3 years.

Emotional dysregulation has been shown to be a feature of ADHD in up to 50% of patients.[59] In addition, ADHD is frequently comorbid with other disorders that are associated with explosive behaviors. The treatment of ADHD with psychostimulant medications has been associated with improvement in emotional dysregulation in multiple studies,[60–62] although notably stimulants should be used in caution in children with BPD. Psychostimulants have been shown to be useful in the treatment of children with comorbid ADHD and aggression. A meta-analysis examined the effects of stimulants on aggression in ADHD and found that stimulants were effective for aggression, with moderate to large effect sizes.[63]

There is also some evidence that stimulants are effective at treating ODD/CD symptoms in children with comorbid ADHD.[64–66] In children with SMD and DMDD, stimulants have been shown to be well tolerated and effective at treating externalizing symptoms.[67–69] In children with ADHD and ASD, stimulants have been shown to cause improvements in symptoms of ADHD, as well as aggression and explosive behaviors.[70]

Several studies have also investigated the use of stimulant medications in combination with adjunctive agents for the treatment of aggression and explosive behaviors. Two studies stabilized children with ADHD and aggression on a stimulant medication, and then added risperidone versus placebo. Both studies found that the addition of risperidone led to an additional decrease in aggressive behavior.[12,13] An open-label study in 24 adolescent patients with ADHD and DBD, already stabilized on methylphenidate, found that the addition of quetiapine led to clinically significant improvement in 49%, and 79% of patients on the combination showed minimal aggression after 9 weeks.[71] **Table 5** provides a summary of studies on stimulants.

Table 4
Summary of studies on divalproex sodium

	Study Design	Subjects	Medication Dose	Duration	Main Results
Steiner et al,[53] 2003	Double-blind, controlled trial	71 boys aged 14–18 y with CD	High-dosage condition: 500–1500 mg/d Low-dosage condition: 250 mg/d	7 wk	High-dosage condition was significantly more effective in the treatment of CD
Donovan et al,[54] 2000	Double-blind, placebo-controlled crossover trial	20 children aged 10–18 y with ODD or CD	Final dosage: 750–1500 mg/d	6 wk	Effective in the treatment of explosive temper and mood lability
Blader et al,[55] 2009	Double-blind, placebo-controlled trial	27 children aged 6–13 y with ADHD and ODD or CD with aggressive behavior after stabilization on a stimulant	Initial dosage: 250 mg/d Final dosage: 567 ± 291 mg/d	8 wk	Superior to placebo as an adjunctive medication in the treatment of aggression
Delbello et al,[56] 2004	Post hoc analysis of a double-blind trial	15 children aged 12–18 y with BPD hospitalized for a manic or mixed episode	Initial dosage: 20 mg/kg/d Final dose: therapeutic dose	6 wk	Significantly reduced irritability and aggression
Barzman et al,[39] 2006	Post hoc analysis of a double-blind trial	33 children aged 12–18 y with BPD and DBDs	Initial dosage: 20 mg/kg/d Final dosage: 1172 ± 384 mg/d	4 wk	Effective (to the same degree as quetiapine) for the treatment of impulsivity and reactive aggression
Saxena et al,[57] 2006	Open-label trial	24 offspring aged 6–18 y of bipolar parents with major depression, cyclothymia, ADHD, dysthymia, or ODD	Initial dosage: 125–250 mg/d Final dosage: 375–1,500 mg/d	12 wk	71% of participants with at least a 50% reduction in overt aggression
Hollander et al,[58] 2010	Double-blind, placebo-controlled trial	27 children aged 5–17 y with ASD	Initial dosage: 125–250 mg/d Final dose: therapeutic dose	12 wk	Superior to placebo in the treatment of irritability, but not aggression

Table 5
Summary of studies on stimulants

	Study Design	Subjects	Medication Dose	Duration	Main Results
Connor et al,[63] 2002	Meta-analysis	Children younger than 18 y with ADHD and aggression	7.5–60 mg/d methylphenidate or 10–30.1 mg/d dextroamphetamine or 109.2–181.1 mg/d pemoline	1–42 d	Effective for both covert and overt aggression
Kaplan et al,[64] 1990	Double-blind, placebo-controlled crossover trial	6 children aged 13–16 y with CD, ADHD, and aggression	Initial dosage: 20 mg/d methylphenidate Final dosage: 60 mg/d methylphenidate	3 wk	Reduced aggression
Gadow et al,[65] 2008	Double-blind, placebo-controlled trial	31 children aged 6–12 y with ODD, ADHD, and a tic disorder	0.2, 0.6, and 1 mg/kg/d methylphenidate	2 wk	Improved oppositional and ADHD behaviors
Klein et al,[66] 1997	Double-blind, placebo-controlled trial	84 children aged 6–15 y with CD with or without ADHD	41.3 ± 1.0 mg/d methylphenidate	5 wk	Reduced antisocial behaviors associated with CD
Waxmonsky et al,[67] 2008	Double-blind, placebo-controlled crossover trial	33 children aged 5–12 y with SMD	0.45, 0.9, or 1.8 mg/kg/d methylphenidate	3 wk	Improved externalizing symptoms when combined with behavior modification therapy; well tolerated
Winters et al,[68] 2018	Open-label trial	22 children aged 9–15 y with ADHD and DMDD	Initial dosage: Not reported Final dosage: 61 ± 10.9 mg/d methylphenidate	4 wk	Improved irritability, emotional lability, negative affect, and anger and was well tolerated Irritability worsened in 19% of participants

Baweja et al,[69] 2016	Open-label trial	38 children aged 9.4 ± 1.7 y with ADHD and DMDD	Not reported; therapeutic doses of stimulants	6 wk	Reduced externalizing behaviors and was well tolerated
Santosh et al,[70] 2006	Naturalistic study	52 children aged 11.08 ± 2.63 y with ADHD with and without ASD	Not reported; therapeutic doses of stimulants	1–6 mo	Improvements in symptoms of ADHD, aggression, and explosive rage
Aman et al,[12] 2014	Double-blind, placebo-controlled trial	168 children aged 6–12 y with ADHD and DBDs	18–72 mg/d methylphenidate or comparable alternative	9 wk	Reduced aggressive behavior when combined with risperidone
Armenteros et al,[13] 2007	Double-blind, placebo-controlled trial	25 children aged 7–12 y with ADHD and aggression	Not reported; constant stimulant dose required	4 wk	Reduced aggression when combined with risperidone
Kronenberger et al,[71] 2007	Open-label trial	24 children aged 12–16 y with ADHD and DBDs	Initial dosage: 18 mg/d methylphenidate Final dosage: 54 mg/d methylphenidate	9 wk	Reduced aggression and ADHD symptoms when combined with quetiapine

ALPHA AGONISTS

The alpha agonists include clonidine and guanfacine and are approved by the FDA for the treatment of ADHD in children aged 6 years and older. However, these medications are frequently used off label for the treatment of other psychiatric conditions.

Presently, there is limited evidence on the use of alpha agonists in the treatment of aggression or explosive behavior. An open-label trial of clonidine in aggressive children aged 5 to 15 years noted decreased aggression in 15 out of 17 patients.[72] A study of clonidine versus placebo in 67 children aged 6 to 14 years with ADHD and comorbid CD/ODD who were already taking a stimulant medication found that significantly more children treated with clonidine had improvements in conduct-related behaviors compared with placebo.[73]

A randomized, double-blind, placebo-controlled trial investigating the use of guanfacine extended release (XR) in 217 children aged 6 to 12 years with ADHD and oppositional behaviors found a greater improvement in ADHD symptoms and oppositional behaviors in the guanfacine group compared with placebo.[74] A case report of guanfacine in a child with ASD, impulsivity, and self-injurious behavior noted significant improvement in symptoms using guanfacine XR.[75]

Atomoxetine

Atomoxetine has limited evidence (see **Table 1**).

ANTIDEPRESSANTS

There are several different classes of antidepressants approved for the treatment of children, although none specifically indicated for the treatment of explosive behavior. Several selective serotonin reuptake inhibitors (SSRIs) (escitalopram, fluoxetine, fluvoxamine, and sertraline), duloxetine (a selective norepinephrine reuptake inhibitor), and clomipramine (a tricyclic antidepressant) carry FDA approvals for the treatment of children with obsessive-compulsive disorder (OCD), depression (fluoxetine and escitalopram), and anxiety (duloxetine).

Data regarding the use of antidepressants for aggression are limited. A meta-analysis of 6 randomized controlled trials of antidepressants measuring aggressive behavior showed that the effect size of antidepressants was small. However, the antidepressants included in the meta-analysis were not in the same class (3 bupropion, 2 fluoxetine, 1 desipramine), and not all studied the use of antidepressants for the same condition.[43] In the meta-analysis, desipramine was noted to have the biggest impact on aggressive behavior in a 6-week, randomized controlled trial of children with ADHD.[43,76] Prince and colleagues[77] found improvement in oppositional symptoms with nortriptyline in a 9-week, placebo-controlled discontinuation study of 35 patients with ADHD.

In depression, 1 study noted no therapeutic benefit of fluoxetine on aggression in a randomized controlled trial of 96 youth, despite improvement in depressive symptoms.[43,78] However, in a randomized controlled trial of depressed adolescents randomized to fluoxetine, cognitive behavior therapy (CBT), combination treatment, or placebo for 12 weeks, both the fluoxetine and combination groups had a greater reduction in oppositional symptoms than the placebo and CBT treatment groups, and change in depressive symptoms was observed to be partially responsible for the change in oppositional symptoms.[79]

An open-label study of 19 psychiatrically hospitalized adolescents found no improvement in aggression with the use of SSRIs after a minimum of 5 weeks, and noted some aggressive tendencies seemed to occur more frequently on SSRIs.[80] In contrast, a 6-week, open-label study of citalopram in children with aggression and irritability found a significant improvement in impulsive aggression.[81]

An 8-week study evaluated methylphenidate plus citalopram versus methylphenidate plus placebo in children with ADHD and DMDD, and found that, although a significantly higher proportion of response was found in the citalopram plus methylphenidate group, there were no significant differences in functional impairment at the end of the study.[82] A comparison of desipramine, methylphenidate, and the combination of both in a double-blind, placebo-controlled crossover trial of 16 psychiatrically hospitalized children with DBDs, ADHD, and a mood disorder found that combination treatment improved inattention, hyperactivity, and aggressive behavior compared with placebo.[83]

There is some evidence that trazodone may help treat aggressive behavior, based on a small case report and subsequent open-label study.[84,85] In addition, a case report noted that fluvoxamine successfully treated an 18-year-old with OCD accompanied by aggressive urges.[86]

Children and adolescents taking antidepressant medications should be monitored for suicidal ideation, and many antidepressants specifically carry a black box warning to this effect.

In conclusion, the findings from antidepressants are inconsistent, and benefit is likely related, at least somewhat, to the medication class used and the condition that is being treated.

Antihistamines

Antihistamines have limited evidence (see **Table 1**).

VITAMINS/MINERALS

In addition to more traditional pharmacologic approaches, nutritional supplementation in youth may be appealing because of decreased risk of serious side effects. Several studies provide supporting evidence for various nutritional supplements and micronutrient combinations improving aggression, explosive behavior, irritability, and emotional regulation.

Omega-3 fatty acid supplementation has been shown to improve aggressive behavior in several randomized, double-blind, placebo-controlled trials. In 2 separate trials, supplementation with omega-3 fatty acids led to a reduction in child-reported reactive aggression, with benefits still present after 6 months.[87,88]

A nutritional supplement containing 36 different minerals, vitamins, amino acids, and antioxidants has been studied in children. Two small trials (N = 2, N = 9) of EMPowerplus showed improvements in mood and aggression after 8 to 17 weeks of treatment.[89,90] A retrospective case series found that 44 individuals aged 2 to 28 years with ASD who took EMPower had a greater reduction in irritability compared with 44 similar individuals who chose standard pharmaceutical treatments.[91] A 10-week, randomized, double-blind controlled trial of 93 medication-free children with ADHD treated with EMPowerplus Advanced versus placebo found improvement in emotional regulation and aggression in the EMPowerplus Advanced group.[92]

In addition, various other combinations of micronutrients may be beneficial in the treatment of explosive behaviors. One micronutrient containing a combination of vitamins taken for 16 weeks was effective in improving parent-reported aggressive and violent behaviors in an open-label trial of 31 boys aged 4 to 14 years.[93] Three months of supplementation with omega-3 fatty acids in addition to calcium and 12 vitamins and minerals reduced reactive aggression compared with controls in children aged 11 to 12 years with CD, ODD, or otherwise significant aggression.[94]

SUMMARY

The authors found the most robust evidence for the use of risperidone in the treatment of explosive behavior. The other SGAs had fewer studies supporting their use and no double-blind, placebo-controlled trials. The AHRQ report notes some benefit from SGAs as a class for the treatment of conduct problems in ADHD/DBDs and irritability in ASD. As a class, these medications also cause several side effects; however, the potential benefits of treating children with severe illness and explosive behavior likely outweigh the risks of initiating treatment with an SGA when necessary. There was some evidence supporting the use of divalproex sodium and lithium for the treatment of explosive behavior. Stimulants were shown to be helpful in the treatment of explosive behavior in children with ADHD. Other classes of medications had limited support for their usage. Some natural supplements may be helpful as well, but again the data are limited. Pharmacologic management of explosive behavior should be based on the first-line treatment of the primary psychiatric diagnoses of the patient and should be initiated in combination with appropriate psychosocial interventions.

DISCLOSURE

Dr J. Wozniak receives research support from PCORI and Demarest Lloyd, Jr. Foundation. In the past, Dr J. Wozniak has received research support, consultation fees, or speaker's fees from Eli Lilly, Janssen, Johnson and Johnson, McNeil, Merck/Schering-Plough, the National Institute of Mental Health (NIMH) of the National Institutes of Health (NIH), Pfizer, and Shire. She is the author of the book, *Is Your Child Bipolar*, published May 2008, Bantam Books. Her spouse receives royalties from UpToDate; consultation fees from Advance Medical, FlexPharma, and Merck; and research support from UCB Pharma, Neurometrix, Luitpold, NIMH, and the RLS Foundation. In the past, he has received honoraria, royalties, research support, consultation fees, or speaker's fees from Otsuka, Cambridge University Press, Axon Labs, Boehringer-Ingelheim, Cantor Colburn, Covance, Cephalon, Eli Lilly, GlaxoSmithKline, Impax, Jazz Pharmaceuticals, King, Luitpold, Novartis, Neurogen, Novadel Pharma, Pfizer, Sanofi-Aventis, Sepracor, Sunovion, Takeda, UCB (Schwarz) Pharma, Wyeth, Xenoport, and Zeo. Dr C. Vaudreuil and Ms A. Farrell have nothing to disclose.

REFERENCES

1. Pillay J, Boylan K, Carrey N, et al. In: First- and second-generation antipsychotics in children and young adults: systematic review update. Rockville (MD): Agency for Healthcare Research and Quality, 2017.

2. Pappadopulos E, Macintyre JC Ii, Crismon ML, et al. Treatment recommendations for the use of antipsychotics for aggressive youth (TRAAY). Part II. J Am Acad Child Adolesc Psychiatry 2003;42(2):145–61.

3. Schur SB, Sikich L, Findling RL, et al. Treatment recommendations for the use of antipsychotics for aggressive youth (TRAAY). Part I: a review. J Am Acad Child Adolesc Psychiatry 2003;42(2):132–44.

4. Knapp P, Chait A, Pappadopulos E, et al. Treatment of maladaptive aggression in youth: CERT guidelines I. Engagement, assessment, and management. Pediatrics 2012;129(6):e1562–76.

5. Scotto Rosato N, Correll CU, Pappadopulos E, et al. Treatment of maladaptive aggression in youth: CERT guidelines II. Treatments and ongoing management. Pediatrics 2012;129(6):e1577–86.

6. Pappadopulos E, Jensen PS, Schur SB, et al. "Real world" atypical antipsychotic prescribing practices in public child and adolescent inpatient settings. Schizophr Bull 2002;28(1):111–21.

7. Findling RL, McNamara NK, Branicky LA, et al. A double-blind pilot study of risperidone in the treatment of conduct disorder. J Am Acad Child Adolesc Psychiatry 2000;39(4):509–16.

8. Loy JH, Merry SN, Hetrick SE, et al. Atypical antipsychotics for disruptive behaviour disorders in children and youths. Cochrane Database Syst Rev 2017;8: CD008559.

9. Balia C, Carucci S, Coghill D, et al. The pharmacological treatment of aggression in children and adolescents with conduct disorder. Do callous-unemotional traits modulate the efficacy of medication? Neurosci Biobehav Rev 2018;91:218–38.

10. Masi G, Manfredi A, Nieri G, et al. A naturalistic comparison of methylphenidate and risperidone monotherapy in drug-naive youth with attention-deficit/hyperactivity disorder comorbid with oppositional defiant disorder and aggression. J Clin Psychopharmacol 2017;37(5):590–4.

11. Gadow KD, Brown NV, Arnold LE, et al. Severely aggressive children receiving stimulant medication versus stimulant and risperidone: 12-month follow-up of the TOSCA trial. J Am Acad Child Adolesc Psychiatry 2016;55(6):469–78.

12. Aman MG, Bukstein OG, Gadow KD, et al. What does risperidone add to parent training and stimulant for severe aggression in child attention-deficit/hyperactivity disorder? J Am Acad Child Adolesc Psychiatry 2014;53(1):47–60 e41.

13. Armenteros JL, Lewis JE, Davalos M. Risperidone augmentation for treatment-resistant aggression in attention-deficit/hyperactivity disorder: a placebo-controlled pilot study. J Am Acad Child Adolesc Psychiatry 2007;46(5):558–65.

14. Krieger FV, Pheula GF, Coelho R, et al. An open-label trial of risperidone in children and adolescents with severe mood dysregulation. J Child Adolesc Psychopharmacol 2011;21(3):237–43.

15. Buitelaar J, der Gaag R, Cohen Kettenis P, et al. A randomized controlled trial of risperidone in the treatment of aggression in hospitalized adolescents with subaverage cognitive abilities. J Clin Psychiatry 2001;62(4):239–48.

16. Snyder R, Turgay A, Aman M, et al. Effects of risperidone on conduct and disruptive behavior disorders in children with subaverage IQs. J Am Acad Child Adolesc Psychiatry 2002;41(9):1026–36.

17. Nagaraj R, Singhi P, Malhi P. Risperidone in children with autism: randomized, placebo-controlled, double-blind study. J Child Neurol 2006;21(6):450–5.

18. Marcus RN, Owen R, Kamen L, et al. A placebo-controlled, fixed-dose study of aripiprazole in children and adolescents with irritability associated with autistic disorder. J Am Acad Child Adolesc Psychiatry 2009;48(11):1110–9.

19. Owen R, Sikich L, Marcus RN, et al. Aripiprazole in the treatment of irritability in children and adolescents with autistic disorder. Pediatrics 2009;124(6):1533–40.

20. Findling RL, Mankoski R, Timko K, et al. A randomized controlled trial investigating the safety and efficacy of aripiprazole in the long-term maintenance treatment of pediatric patients with irritability associated with autistic disorder. J Clin Psychiatry 2014;75(1):22–30.

21. Curran MP. Aripiprazole: in the treatment of irritability associated with autistic disorder in pediatric patients. Paediatr Drugs 2011;13(3):197–204.

22. Stigler KA, Posey DJ, McDougle CJ. Aripiprazole for maladaptive behavior in pervasive developmental disorders. J Child Adolesc Psychopharmacol 2004; 14(3):455–63.

23. Aman MG, Kasper W, Manos G, et al. Line-item analysis of the Aberrant Behavior Checklist: results from two studies of aripiprazole in the treatment of irritability associated with autistic disorder. J Child Adolesc Psychopharmacol 2010; 20(5):415–22.

24. Stigler KA, Diener JT, Kohn AE, et al. Aripiprazole in pervasive developmental disorder not otherwise specified and Asperger's disorder: a 14-week, prospective, open-label study. J Child Adolesc Psychopharmacol 2009;19(3):265–74.

25. Jakobsen KD, Bruhn CH, Pagsberg AK, et al. Neurological, metabolic, and psychiatric adverse events in children and adolescents treated with aripiprazole. J Clin Psychopharmacol 2016;36(5):496–9.

26. Pan PY, Fu AT, Yeh CB. Aripiprazole/methylphenidate combination in children and adolescents with disruptive mood dysregulation disorder and attention-deficit/hyperactivity disorder: an open-label study. J Child Adolesc Psychopharmacol 2018;28(10):682–9.

27. Budman C, Coffey BJ, Shechter R, et al. Aripiprazole in children and adolescents with Tourette disorder with and without explosive outbursts. J Child Adolesc Psychopharmacol 2008;18(5):509–15.

28. Krishnamoorthy J, King BH. Open-label olanzapine treatment in five preadolescent children. J Child Adolesc Psychopharmacol 1998;8(2):107–13.

29. Potenza M, Holmes J, Kanes S, et al. Olanzapine treatment of children , adolescents, and adults with pervasive developmental disorders: an open-label pilot study. J Clin Psychopharamcol 1999;19(1):37–44.

30. Horrigan JP, Barnhill LJ, Courvoisie HE. Olanzapine in PDD. J Am Acad Child Adolesc Psychiatry 1997;36(9):1166–7.

31. Holzer B, Lopes V, Lehman R. Combination use of atomoxetine hydrochloride and olanzapine in the treatment of attention-deficit/hyperactivity disorder with comorbid disruptive behavior disorder in children and adolescents 10-18 years of age. J Child Adolesc Psychopharmacol 2013;23(6):415–8.

32. Hazaray E, Ehret J, Posey DJ, et al. Intramuscular ziprasidone for acute agitation in adolescents. J Child Adolesc Psychopharmacol 2004;14(3):464–70.

33. Staller JA. Intramuscular ziprasidone in youth: a retrospective chart review. J Child Adolesc Psychopharmacol 2004;14(4):590–2.

34. Barzman DH, DelBello MP, Forrester JJ, et al. A retrospective chart review of intramuscular ziprasidone for agitation in children and adolescents on psychiatric units: prospective studies are needed. J Child Adolesc Psychopharmacol 2007; 17(4):503–9.

35. Khan SS, Mican LM. A naturalistic evaluation of intramuscular ziprasidone versus intramuscular olanzapine for the management of acute agitation and aggression in children and adolescents. J Child Adolesc Psychopharmacol 2006;16(6): 671–7.

36. Jangro WC, Preval H, Southard R, et al. Conventional intramuscular sedatives versus ziprasidone for severe agitation in adolescents: case-control study. Child Adolesc Psychiatry Ment Health 2009;3(1):9.

37. McDougle CJ, Kem DL, Posey DJ. Case series: use of ziprasidone for maladaptive symptoms in youths with autism. J Am Acad Child Adolesc Psychiatry 2002; 41(8):921–7.

38. Findling RL, Reed MD, O'Riordan MA, et al. Effectiveness, safety, and pharmaco-kinetics of quetiapine in aggressive children with conduct disorder. J Am Acad Child Adolesc Psychiatry 2006;45(7):792–800.
39. Barzman DH, DelBello MP, Adler CM, et al. The efficacy and tolerability of quetia-pine versus divalproex for the treatment of impulsivity and reactive aggression in adolescents with co-occurring bipolar disorder and disruptive behavior disor-der(s). J Child Adolesc Psychopharmacol 2006;16(6):665–70.
40. Loebel A, Brams M, Goldman RS, et al. Lurasidone for the treatment of irritability associated with autistic disorder. J Autism Dev Disord 2016;46(4):1153–63.
41. Campbell M, Small AM, Green WH, et al. Behavioral efficacy of haloperidol and lithium carbonate: a comparison in hospitalized aggressive children with conduct disorder. Arch Gen Psychiatry 1984;41(7):650–6.
42. Greenhill LL, Solomon M, Pleak R, et al. Molindone hydrochloride treatment of hospitalized children with conduct disorder. J Clin Psychiatry 1985;46(8):20–5.
43. Pappadopulos E, Woolston S, Chait A, et al. Pharmacotherapy of aggression in children and adolescents: efficacy and effect size. J Can Acad Child Adolesc Psychiatry 2006;15(1):27–39.
44. Aman MG, Marks RE, Turbott SH, et al. Clinical effects of methylphenidate and thioridazine in intellectually subaverage children. J Am Acad Child Adolesc Psy-chiatry 1991;30(2):246–56.
45. Szwak K, Sacchetti A. Droperidol use in pediatric emergency department pa-tients. Pediatr Emerg Care 2010;26(4):248–50.
46. Cipriani A, Hawton K, Stockton S, et al. Lithium in the prevention of suicide in mood disorders: updated systematic review and meta-analysis. BMJ 2013;346: f3646.
47. Pisano S, Pozzi M, Catone G, et al. Putative mechanisms of action and clinical use of lithium in children and adolescents: a critical review. Curr Neuropharmacol 2019;17(4):318–41.
48. Hafeman DM, Rooks B, Merranko J, et al. Lithium versus other mood-stabilizing medications in a longitudinal study of youth diagnosed with bipolar disorder. J Am Acad Child Adolesc Psychiatry 2019;59(10):1146–55.
49. Dickstein DP, Towbin KE, Van Der Veen JW, et al. Randomized double-blind pla-cebo-controlled trial of lithium in youths with severe mood dysregulation. J Child Adolesc Psychopharmacol 2009;19(1):61–73.
50. Campbell M, Adams P, Small A, et al. Lithium in hospitalized aggressive children with conduct disorder: a double-blind and placebo-controlled study. J Am Acad Child Adoles Psychiatry 1995;34(4):445–53.
51. Malone RP, Delaney MA, Luebbert JF, et al. A double-blind placebo-controlled study of lithium in hospitalized aggressive children and adolescents with conduct disorder. Arch Gen Psychiatry 2000;57(7):649–54.
52. Rifkin A, Karajgi B, Dicker R, et al. Lithium treatment of conduct disorders in ad-olescents. Am J Psychiatry 1997;154(4):554–5.
53. Steiner H, Petersen ML, Saxena K, et al. Divalproex sodium for the treatment of conduct disorder: a randomized controlled clinical trial. J Clin Psychiatry 2003; 64(10):1183–91.
54. Donovan SJ, Stewart JW, Nunes EV, et al. Divalproex treatment for youth with explosive temper and mood lability: a double-blind, placebo-controlled crossover design. Am J Psychiatry 2000;157(5):818–20.
55. Blader JC, Schooler NR, Jensen PS, et al. Adjunctive divalproex versus placebo for children with ADHD and aggression refractory to stimulant monotherapy. Am J Psychiatry 2009;166(12):1392–401.

56. DelBello MP, Adler C, Strakowski SM. Divalproex for the treatment of aggression associated with adolescent mania. J Child Adolesc Psychopharmacol 2004; 14(2):325–8.
57. Saxena K, Howe M, Simeonova D, et al. Divalproex sodium reduces overall aggression in youth at high risk for bipolar disorder. J Child Adolesc Psychopharmacol 2006;16(3):252–9.
58. Hollander E, Chaplin W, Soorya L, et al. Divalproex sodium vs placebo for the treatment of irritability in children and adolescents with autism spectrum disorders. Neuropsychopharmacology 2010;35(4):990–8.
59. Faraone SV, Rostain AL, Blader J, et al. Practitioner Review: emotional dysregulation in attention-deficit/hyperactivity disorder - implications for clinical recognition and intervention. J Child Psychol Psychiatry 2019;60(2):133–50.
60. Suzer Gamli I, Tahiroglu AY. Six months methylphenidate treatment improves emotion dysregulation in adolescents with attention deficit/hyperactivity disorder: a prospective study. Neuropsychiatr Dis Treat 2018;14:1329–37.
61. Kutlu A, Akyol Ardic U, Ercan ES. Effect of methylphenidate on emotional dysregulation in children with attention-deficit/hyperactivity disorder + oppositional defiant disorder/conduct disorder. J Clin Psychopharmacol 2017;37(2):220–5.
62. Childress AC, Arnold V, Adeyi B, et al. The effects of lisdexamfetamine dimesylate on emotional lability in children 6 to 12 years of age with ADHD in a double-blind placebo-controlled trial. J Atten Disord 2014;18(2):123–32.
63. Connor DF, Glatt SJ, Lopez ID, et al. Psychopharmacology and aggression. I: a meta-analysis of stimulant effects on overt/covert aggression-related behaviors in ADHD. J Am Acad Child Adolesc Psychiatry 2002;41(3):253–61.
64. Kaplan SL, Busner J, Kupietz S, et al. Effects of methylphenidate on adolescents with aggressive conduct disorder and ADDH: a preliminary report. J Am Acad Child Adolesc Psychiatry 1990;29(5):719–23.
65. Gadow KD, Nolan EE, Sverd J, et al. Methylphenidate in children with oppositional defiant disorder and both comorbid chronic multiple tic disorder and ADHD. J Child Neurol 2008;23(9):981–90.
66. Klein R, Abikoff H, Klass E, et al. Clinical efficacy of methylphenidate in conduct disorder with and without attention deficit hyperactivity disorder. Arch Gen Psychiatry 1997;54(12):1073–80.
67. Waxmonsky J, Pelham WE, Gnagy E, et al. The efficacy and tolerability of methylphenidate and behavior modification in children with attention-deficit/hyperactivity disorder and severe mood dysregulation. J Child Adolesc Psychopharmacol 2008;18(6):573–88.
68. Winters DE, Fukui S, Leibenluft E, et al. Improvements in irritability with open-label methylphenidate treatment in youth with comorbid attention deficit/hyperactivity disorder and disruptive mood dysregulation disorder. J Child Adolesc Psychopharmacol 2018;28(5):298–305.
69. Baweja R, Belin PJ, Humphrey HH, et al. The effectiveness and tolerability of central nervous system stimulants in school-age children with attention-deficit/hyperactivity disorder and disruptive mood dysregulation disorder across home and school. J Child Adolesc Psychopharmacol 2016;26(2):154–63.
70. Santosh PJ, Baird G, Pityaratstian N, et al. Impact of comorbid autism spectrum disorders on stimulant response in children with attention deficit hyperactivity disorder: a retrospective and prospective effectiveness study. Child Care Health Dev 2006;32(5):575–83.
71. Kronenberger WG, Giauque AL, Lafata DE, et al. Quetiapine addition in methylphenidate treatment-resistant adolescents with comorbid ADHD, conduct/

oppositional-defiant disorder, and aggression: a prospective, open-label study. J Child Adolesc Psychopharmacol 2007;17(3):334–47.

72. Kemph J, DeVane C, Levin G, et al. Treatment of aggressive children with clonidine: results of an open pilot study. J Am Acad Child Adolesc Psychiatry 1993; 32(3):577–81.

73. Hazell PL, Stuart JE. A randomized controlled trial of clonidine added to psychostimulant medication for hyperactive and aggressive children. J Am Acad Child Adolesc Psychiatry 2003;42(8):886–94.

74. Connor DF, Findling RL, Kollins SH, et al. Effects of guanfacine extended release on oppositional symptoms in children aged 6-12 years with attention-deficit hyperactivity disorder and oppositional symptoms: a randomized, double-blind, placebo-controlled trial. CNS Drugs 2010;24(9):755–68.

75. Propper L. Managing disruptive behaviour in autism-spectrum disorder with guanfacine. J Psychiatry Neurosci 2018;43(5):359–60.

76. Biederman J, Baldessarini RJ, Wright V, et al. A double-blind placebo controlled study of desipramine in the treatment of ADD: I. Efficacy. J Am Acad Child Adolesc Psychiatry 1989;28(5):777–84.

77. Prince JB, Wilens TE, Biederman J, et al. A controlled study of nortriptyline in children and adolescents with attention deficit hyperactivity disorder. J Child Adolesc Psychopharmacol 2000;10(3):193–204.

78. Emslie GJ, Rush AJ, Weinberg WA, et al. A double-blind, randomized, placebo-controlled trial of fluoxetine in children and adolescents with depression. Arch Gen Psychiatry 1997;54(11):1031–7.

79. Jacobs RH, Becker-Weidman EG, Reinecke MA, et al. Treating depression and oppositional behavior in adolescents. J Clin Child Adolesc Psychol 2010;39(4): 559–67.

80. Constantino JN, Liberman M, Kincaid M. Effects of serotonin reuptake inhibitors on aggressive behavior in psychiatrically hospitalized adolescents: results of an open trial. J Child Adolesc Psychopharmacol 1997;7(1):31–44.

81. Armenteros JL, Lewis JE. Citalopram treatment for impulsive aggression in children and adolescents: an open pilot study. J Am Acad Child Adolesc Psychiatry 2002;41(5):522–9.

82. Towbin K, Vidal-Ribas P, Brotman MA, et al. A double-blind randomized placebo-controlled trial of citalopram adjunctive to stimulant medication in youth with chronic severe irritability. J Am Acad Child Adolesc Psychiatry 2020;59(3): 350–61.

83. Carlson GA, Rapport MD, Kelly KL, et al. Methylphenidate and desipramine in hospitalized children with comorbid behavior and mood disorders: separate and combined effects on behavior and mood. J Child Adolesc Psychopharmacol 1995;5(3):191–204.

84. Ghaziuddin N, Alessi NE. An open clinical trial of trazodone in aggressive children. J Child Adolesc Psychopharmacol 1992;2(4):291–7.

85. Zubieta JK, Alessi NE. Acute and chronic administration of trazodone in the treatment of disruptive behavior disorders in children. J Clin Psychopharmacol 1992; 12(5):346–51.

86. Poyurovsky M, Halperin E, Enoch D, et al. Fluvoxamine treatment of compulsivity, impulsivity, and aggression. Am J Psychiatry 1995;152(11):1688–9.

87. Raine A, Ang RP, Choy O, et al. Omega-3 (omega-3) and social skills interventions for reactive aggression and childhood externalizing behavior problems: a randomized, stratified, double-blind, placebo-controlled, factorial trial. Psychol Med 2019;49(2):335–44.

88. Raine A, Portnoy J, Liu J, et al. Reduction in behavior problems with omega-3 supplementation in children aged 8-16 years: a randomized, double-blind, placebo-controlled, stratified, parallel-group trial. J Child Psychol Psychiatry 2015; 56(5):509–20.

89. Kaplan BJ, Crawford SG, Gardner B, et al. Treatment of mood lability and explosive rage with minerals and vitamins: two case studies in children. J Child Adolesc Psychopharmacol 2002;12(3):205–19.

90. Kaplan BJ, Fisher JE, Crawford SG, et al. Improved mood and behavior during treatment with a mineral-vitamin supplement: an open-label case series of children. J Child Adolesc Psychopharmacol 2004;14(1):115–22.

91. Mehl-Madrona L, Leung B, Kennedy C, et al. Micronutrients versus standard medication management in autism: a naturalistic case-control study. J Child Adolesc Psychopharmacol 2010;20(2):95–103.

92. Rucklidge JJ, Eggleston MJF, Johnstone JM, et al. Vitamin-mineral treatment improves aggression and emotional regulation in children with ADHD: a fully blinded, randomized, placebo-controlled trial. J Child Psychol Psychiatry 2018; 59(3):232–46.

93. Hambly JL, Francis K, Khan S, et al. Micronutrient therapy for violent and aggressive male youth: an open-label trial. J Child Adolesc Psychopharmacol 2017; 27(9):823–32.

94. Raine A, Cheney RA, Ho R, et al. Nutritional supplementation to reduce child aggression: a randomized, stratified, single-blind, factorial trial. J Child Psychol Psychiatry 2016;57(9):1038–46.

95. Kafantaris V, Campbell M, Padron-Gayol MV, et al. Carbamazepine in hospitalized aggressive conduct disorder children: an open pilot study. Psychopharmacol Bull 1992;28(2):193–9.

96. Cueva J, Overall J, Small A, et al. Carbamazepine in aggressive children with conduct disorder: a double-blind and placebo-controlled study. J Am Acad Child Adoles Psychiatry 1996;35(4):480–90.

97. Biederman J, Spencer TJ, Newcorn JH, et al. Effect of comorbid symptoms of oppositional defiant disorder on responses to atomoxetine in children with ADHD: a meta-analysis of controlled clinical trial data. Psychopharmacology (Berl) 2007;190(1):31–41.

98. Baeza I, Correll CU, Saito E, et al. Frequency, characteristics and management of adolescent inpatient aggression. J Child Adolesc Psychopharmacol 2013;23(4): 271–81.

99. Vitiello B, Hill JL, Elia J, et al. P.r.n. medications in child psychiatric patients: a pilot placebo-controlled study. J Clin Psychiatry 1991;52(12):499–501.

Irritability, Anger, and Aggression in the Context of Pediatric Bipolar Disorder

Luis R. Patino, MD, MSc[a],*, Melissa P. DelBello, MD, MS[b]

KEYWORDS

- Psychopharmacology • Pediatric • Bipolar disorder • Irritability • Aggression

KEY POINTS

- Irritability, anger, and aggression, although not specific for pediatric bipolar disorder (BD), can be a common finding and an important source of distress and impairment in these patients.
- Regardless of intensity and chronicity, irritability, anger, and aggression should not be the sole basis of a diagnosis of pediatric BD.
- Pharmacologic management of irritability, anger, and aggressive behaviors in pediatric BD when in the context of an acute episode should be focused on the first-line treatment of the primary mood episode.
- When irritability, anger, and aggressive behaviors in pediatric BD occur outside of a mood episode, a comprehensive evaluation to determine the patient-specific factors (ie, comorbidities) and environmental context that could be driving these symptoms is necessary before any changes in treatment.

INTRODUCTION

Irritability refers to an increased vulnerability to experiencing anger[1,2] and can be seen in a tonic expression (persistent), a phasic activation (ie, outbursts), or a combination of both.[3] Anger is an emotional state usually elicited by threat or frustration,[4] whereas aggression is only one of many possible behavioral outputs of anger. Conceptually, aggression refers to any definite and observable verbal or motor behavior aimed explicitly or implicitly to cause harm toward any target.[5] Irritability, anger, and aggression are a common cause of referral to child and adolescent psychiatrists.[6]

[a] Department of Psychiatry and Behavioral Neuroscience, Division of Bipolar Disorders Research, University of Cincinnati College of Medicine, 260 Stetson Street, Suite 3200, PO Box 670516, Cincinnati, OH 45219 –0516, USA; [b] Division of Bipolar Disorders Research, Department of Psychiatry and Behavioral Neurosciences, University of Cincinnati College of Medicine, Cincinnati, OH, USA
* Corresponding author.
E-mail address: patinolr@ucmail.uc.edu

Child Adolesc Psychiatric Clin N Am 30 (2021) 561–571
https://doi.org/10.1016/j.chc.2021.04.007
1056-4993/21/© 2021 Elsevier Inc. All rights reserved.

Irritability is a common feature in pediatric bipolar disorder (BD); it can be seen during depressive episodes, manic/hypomanic episodes, and during euthymic periods.[7–9] Youth diagnosed with BD can experience significant distress and impairment related to manifestations of irritability, anger, and aggression.[10] Although there was significant methodological variation across studies on phenomenology, in general, parents of children diagnosed with BD reported higher rates of irritability and aggressive behaviors compared with other diagnostic groups.[8] Compared with clinic children with attention-deficit hyperactivity disorder (ADHD), those with BD had higher rates of verbal and reactive aggression.[11] Furthermore, irritability and aggression seem to be more common in early onset compared with adult-onset BD.[8,12] Finally, high levels of aggression in children and adolescents with BD may be an important predictor of variation in pharmacologic treatment response[13,14] and is also associated with higher risk of depressive relapse.[15]

Over the past 2 decades the diagnostic significance of irritability in pediatric BD has been highly debated.[9,16–18] A publication from The International Society for Bipolar Disorders Task Force report on pediatric BD[19] highlights the now growing consensus that "chronic irritability, regardless of explosiveness or severity, is not sufficient for a diagnosis of BD." Yet, beyond the debate of its diagnostic significance, the clinical importance of irritability, anger, and aggression in youth with BD has been well established. In this review, the authors discuss evaluation and management strategies of irritability, anger, and aggression in youth with BD.

STRATEGIES FOR THE EVALUATION OF IRRITABILITY, ANGER, AND AGGRESSION IN YOUTH WITH BIPOLAR DISORDER

Based on the authors' review of existent literature and their clinical experience, they find the following recommendations useful for the evaluation of irritability, anger, and aggressive behaviors in youth with BD. Although the authors present them in a specific order, aspects of each recommendation pertain to multiple points during treatment and should be tailored to each patient's specific condition and needs.

Conduct a Thorough Evaluation Before Starting/Modifying Treatment

In youth diagnosed with BD, irritability, anger, and aggression may be ubiquitous. Hence, it is crucial to determine the association between irritability, anger, or aggression with either a depressed, manic, or hypomanic episode (either fully active, subthreshold, or partially remitted). Irritability, anger, and aggression associated with a manic/hypomanic episode typically present as a change from the youth's typical/normal behavior and occur concurrently with other manic symptoms (ie, increased energy, elation, grandiosity, rapid thoughts and speech, flight of ideas, and decreased need for sleep). The duration of these symptoms, the change in functioning, and/or level of impairment establishes the distinction between manic and hypomanic episode. Despite controversies regarding mania with irritability and no elation, longitudinal studies have shown that most of the youth with irritable-only manic episodes will eventually report episodes with both irritability and elation or elation only.[15,20,21] During depressive episodes, irritability alongside other symptoms may be more chronically manifested, although a mix of tonic irritability as well as phasic explosive irritability with manifest anger and aggression can also be seen.[22,23]

When explosive irritability, in the context of BD, continues to be a source of distress and impairment during euthymic periods, a comprehensive assessment should also include screening for comorbid conditions. Pediatric BD is a highly comorbid condition,[24] and explosive irritability could be explained by an unaddressed comorbid condition, including anxiety disorders, posttraumatic stress disorder, ADHD, substance use disorders, autism, and other developmental disorders.

A complete assessment should also include the evaluation of developmental, environmental, and contextual factors involved in the patient's expression of mania in general and irritability, anger, and aggression in particular. Parenting styles, school, and neighborhood environment may be exacerbating and perpetuating factors for these symptoms.

Obtaining information from multiple sources (eg, youth and parents) is of paramount importance in child and adolescent psychiatry. However, discrepancies between youth and parental reports are not uncommon.[25] In youth with BD, more than one-third of patients-parent dyads had discordant in the report of history of manic symptoms and episodes.[26,27] Symptom domains that more commonly have youth-parent discordant reports include irritability and aggression.[28] Clinicians should make efforts to clarify discordant reports relating irritability, anger, and aggression between youth and parents or when appropriate obtain information from another source, such as a teacher. Teacher information can be helpful clarifying whether the symptoms of irritability, anger, and aggression are also seen at school; the presence of irritability, anger, and aggression confined to one setting (ie, home) can have different diagnostic implications.[29]

Periodically Reassess the Diagnosis of Bipolar Disorder

Unless the onset of a manic episode is acute, it may be difficult to make a diagnosis. Diagnosing pediatric BD requires changes in mood and behavior that are uncharacteristic of the individual and more extreme than developmentally appropriate, persist long enough to satisfy duration criteria, and have a clear impact on functioning. Under these circumstances, it is important to periodically reassess the diagnosis of BD. Among children and adolescents, irritability, anger, and aggression can be common, and, although they suggest an underlying mental health problem, they are not specific to any one diagnosis. Irritability, anger, and aggression are not proxies for BD and should not be used as the sole basis for a diagnosis of BD. Irritability that waxes and wanes or has episodic changes and is accompanied by changes in energy or sleep suggests a mood disorder. Clinicians should periodically reassess the diagnostic accuracy of the mood disorder, as more information is gathered during follow-up.

Conduct a Risk Assessment and, if Necessary, Consider Referral to Emergency Department and/or Hospitalization

The frequency, intensity, duration, and triggers for the child's aggressive behaviors, regardless of a diagnosis, may predict risk of harm to self or others. If there is imminence of harm, a significant change in mental status, or if the family cannot contain the patient's behavior, specialty or emergency evaluation is indicated. An evaluation of the context, environment, and triggers may also reveal a situation in which a referral to child protective services may be warranted, for example, when the patient's aggression stems from an abusive situation.

Use Validated Clinical Measures to Assess Initial State and Track Treatment Effects and Outcomes

Clinical impressions at a crisis presentation or at a single office visit may not provide full baseline information. Screening and assessment tools can help characterize or quantify irritability, anger, and aggressive behaviors and serve as benchmarks to track treatment progress. Several clinical scales of irritability/anger/aggression have shown robust psychometric characteristics that determine their validity and reliability (see Althoff and colleagues, volume 1). Clinicians will also find it useful to tracking mood symptoms using validated clinical scales (Ref. [30]).

STRATEGIES FOR THE MANAGEMENT OF IRRITABILITY, ANGER, AND AGGRESSION IN YOUTH WITH BIPOLAR DISORDER

Develop an Appropriate Treatment Plan with the Patients and Their Family

Collaboratively establishing specific and realistic goals with the patient and their family increases treatment retention, forms a better therapeutic alliance, and overall leads to improved satisfaction and better outcomes.[31–33] Therapeutic strategies to manage irritability, anger, and aggression in the context of BD should be tailored to patient's needs and current condition. When these symptoms are the result of a relapse or stem from an unsuccessful treatment of a manic or depressive episode, particular attention to adherence and dosing is imperative. Nonadherence can play an important role in continued impairment in BD.[34] In fact, among adolescent patients with BD we have found that over a 1-year posthospitalization follow-up period, 65% reported to be partial or nonadherent to their medications.[35] Moreover, when using electronic pill bottles to track adherence over 6 months, less than a quarter of adolescents with BD meet criteria for adherence (less than 20% missed doses) and self-, parent-, and clinician-reported adherence tended to overestimate the electronic monitoring adherence.[36] An emerging factor associated with nonadherence is weight and weight gain. The authors found that weight gain is the top rated patient-reported barrier to adherence to first-line treatments (ie, second-generation antipsychotics) for youth with BD.[37] For this reason, an open communication among patients, their parents, and their clinicians regarding potential side effects of medications and possible strategies to minimize these side effects is crucial to maximize medication adherence and improve the physical and mental health of this vulnerable population.

Considerations of Pharmacologic Interventions

Although not a systematic review, the authors present some recommendations and an overview of the evidence regarding medication options to treat the irritability, anger, and aggression complex for youth with BD. There are no specific pharmacologic treatments for irritability, anger, and/or aggression in pediatric BD. In fact, there are very few studies specifically addressing the pharmacologic management of irritability, anger, and aggression in the context of BD in pediatric population. Moreover, pharmacologically targeting a mere symptom is an inadequate intervention. Thus, a complete clinical evaluation of youth with irritability, anger, and aggression in the context of BD is important.

Irritability, anger, and aggression in the context of a mood episode

In the presence of an acute mood episode or a partially remitted one, ensuring adherence and optimizing doses are in general a good starting point. It is also important for the clinician to evaluate if the current pharmacologic treatment is adequate for the polarity of the current mood episode. Several medications have been shown to be efficacious and safe to treat acute mood episodes in youth with BD. However, efficacy in the treatment of acute mania does not translate to efficacy in the treatment of bipolar depression, nor does efficacy in adults translate to efficacy in youth.

Based on results from randomized, double-blind, placebo-controlled trials (RCTs), the US Food and Drug Administration (FDA) has approved aripiprazole, asenapine, lithium, olanzapine, quetiapine, and risperidone (http://www.accessdata.fda.gov/scripts/cder/daf/) for mania in youth. In terms of acute mania/mixed episodes, 2 meta-analysis indicate larger effect sizes for second-generation antipsychotics compared with lithium and other mood stabilizers[38,39]; moreover, in a direct head-to-head comparison risperidone outperformed lithium in treating acute mania in patients 6 to 15 years of age.[40] Both oxcarbazepine and divalproex extended release as monotherapy for manic/mixed episodes in youth have well-powered studies failing to show separation from placebo.[41,42]

Meanwhile, for bipolar depression in youth only olanzapine/fluoxetine combination and lurasidone have received FDA approval following positive results from RCTs.[43,44] Quetiapine has been shown to be effective in adults with bipolar depression; however, in youth with bipolar depression, quetiapine has failed to separate from placebo in 2 RCTs.[45,46] Open-label studies of lithium[47] and lamotrigine[48] suggest these agents may be helpful in bipolar depression in youth; however, there are no RCTs confirming these findings.

Irritability, anger, and aggression not related to an acute episode

Given the high rates of comorbidities in pediatric BD, clinicians should carefully review concomitant medications, particularly the use of stimulants and antidepressants. Although treatment of comorbid ADHD in youth with BD with stimulants is generally considered safe and efficacious,[19,49–51] some concerns regarding the effects of stimulants on the course of BD in youth has been brought up in previous research.[52–55] Moreover, stimulants theoretically hold some risk of precipitating mania; but the precise estimates of this risk are lacking, both with and without ongoing mood stabilizer cotreatment.[56] Likewise, antidepressant use has also been associated with inducing manic symptoms in youth with BD[57,58] or at high familial risk for BD[59–61]; yet some longitudinal studies have not seen an increased risk of relapse associated with antidepressant youth.[62] Thus, clinicians should evaluate the potential role of antidepressants and stimulants as destabilizing agents causing irritability, anger, and aggression in the context of either relapsing and/or treatment-resistant manic episodes or maniclike symptoms. Indeed, one study found that discontinuing these medications, at least temporarily, until mood was stabilized was an effective strategy for managing difficult to treat cases of mania in youth with BD.[63] As noted earlier, close follow-up is an absolute essential in teasing apart worsening of ADHD by removing stimulants versus exacerbating mania by continuing them.

After enhancing adherence, optimizing dose of current treatment, removing potential destabilizing concomitant medications, and/or a medication change has been considered, few studies have explored other agents as add-on treatment or as monotherapy for irritability or aggression in youth with BD. Despite divalproex's lack of demonstrated efficacy for the management of acute mania/hypomania or depression in pediatric BD, there are several studies showing this medication might reduce aggressive symptoms. Divalproex in youth with BD was found to reduce aggressive behaviors in 2 retrospective chart reviews[64,65] and in a post-hoc analysis of a randomized, double-blind comparative study of youth with BD and comorbid disruptive behavior disorders.[66] In addition, a 12-week open-label study in youth at high familial risk for BD found treatment with divalproex significantly reduced aggression.[67] However, clinicians should consider potential side effects of divalproex, particularly in girls, before deciding to initiate this medication. Divalproex has been found to increase the risk of developing polycystic ovarian syndrome, infertility, acne, and increase the risk of osteoporosis and obesity in girls.[68] Moreover, a randomized double-blind study found that risperidone outperforms divalproex in reducing aggression in youth with BD,[13] and similar reductions in aggression may be seen with quetiapine.[66]

Even fewer data are available for other pharmacologic options. A retrospective chart review with a small subsample of youth with BD found amantadine to be useful for reducing aggression during hospitalization.[69] There is cross-sectional and transla-tional evidence that deficiency of omega-3 fatty acids is associated with hostility, aggressive behaviors, and impulsivity.[70–74] Despite the absence of systematic studies using omega-3 essential fatty acids to specifically treat aggression in the context of pediatric BD, because of their low side effect and potentially for at least marginal benefit omega-3 essential fatty acid supplementation may be considered an option in milder cases.

Considerations Regarding Psychosocial Interventions

Although in the treatment of pediatric BD pharmacologic agents are the cornerstone of treatment, psychosocial interventions should be included in a comprehensive treat-ment plan to manage irritability, anger, and aggression in the context of pediatric BD. There are several evidence-based psychosocial interventions to manage irritabil-ity, anger, and aggression in youth not specifically designed for BD populations (for a review see:[75–77]). Psychosocial interventions include family-based interventions, patient-oriented techniques (eg, social skills building, conflict-resolution training), parent training (eg, reinforcing positive interactions and improving discipline strate-gies), teacher training (eg, classroom behavioral management strategies), and pro-grams targeting core deficits. Overall, most psychotherapeutic interventions do not distinguish between types of aggression and focus more generally on addressing physical aggression, verbal aggression, or externalizing behaviors. Family-based ap-proaches target aversive patterns of family interactions that may trigger of perpetuate children's disruptive behavior and help parents deliver consistent and effective disci-pline strategies. Psychosocial programs that target core deficits are usually psycho-therapeutic interventions modified to include education and skill building to address issues stemming from anger self-regulation, delay aversion, hostile attribution biases, impulsivity, emotional overarousal, and poor frustration tolerance.[76] A comprehensive evaluation of the behavioral types, context, triggers, and perpetuating factors of the patient's expression of irritability, anger, and aggressive behavior can help select a psychosocial intervention suitable for the patient and family.

Specifically, in youth with BD, there are no unique psychosocial interventions to explicitly target irritability, anger, and aggressive behaviors. However, some psycho-social interventions tailored to youth with BD have reported improvement in these psy-chopathological domains. Specifically, A Child and Family Focused Cognitive Behavioral Therapy designed for patients and families with BD that integrated psycho-education, cognitive behavioral, and interpersonal techniques found that when this intervention is added to pharmacotherapy, youth experienced improvements in measured irritability and aggressive behaviors.[78–80] An adaptation for adolescents of the Family Focused Therapy[81] found that among youth with BD ratings of anger and hostility in families with high levels of expressed emotion can be significantly reduced with this intervention.[82]

SUMMARY

Irritability, anger, and aggression may be common sources of distress and impairment in youth diagnosed with BD. No matter how intense or chronic, these symptoms should not be the sole basis for a diagnosis of BD in children and adolescents. None-theless, disease-specific factors may drive the higher rates of this psychopathological domain for this population, which creates unique management challenges. There is a dire need for more systematic studies addressing these symptoms in youth.

DISCLOSURE

L.R. Patino has received research support from Eli Lilly, Pfizer, Otsuka, Novartis, Lundbeck, Sunovion, AbbVie, and Shire. M.P. DelBello has received research support from Amylin, Eli Lilly, Pfizer, Otsuka, GlaxoSmithKline, Merck, Martek, Novartis, Lundbeck, Pfizer, Sunovion, and Shire and has received consulting/advisory board/honoraria/travel support from Pfizer, Lundbeck, Sunovian, Supernus, and Otsuka.

REFERENCES

1. Brotman MA, Kircanski K, Leibenluft E. Irritability in children and adolescents. Annu Rev Clin Psychol 2017;13:317–41.
2. Buss AH, Durkee A. An inventory for assessing different kinds of hostility. J Consult Psychol 1957;21(4):343–9.
3. Avenevoli S, Blader JC, Leibenluft E. Irritability in youth: an update. J Am Acad Child Adolesc Psychiatry 2015;54(11):881–3.
4. Spielberger CD, Reheiser EC, Sydeman SJ. Measuring the experience, expression, and control of anger. Issues Compr Pediatr Nurs 1995;18(3):207–32.
5. Ramirez JM, Andreu JM. Aggression, and some related psychological constructs (anger, hostility, and impulsivity); some comments from a research project. Neurosci Biobehav Rev 2006;30(3):276–91.
6. Bambauer KZ, Connor DF. Characteristics of aggression in clinically referred children. CNS Spectr 2005;10(9):709–18.
7. Faedda GL, Baldessarini RJ, Glovinsky IP, et al. Pediatric bipolar disorder: phenomenology and course of illness. Bipolar Disord 2004;6(4):305–13.
8. Ryles F, Meyer TD, Adan-Manes J, et al. A systematic review of the frequency and severity of manic symptoms reported in studies that compare phenomenology across children, adolescents and adults with bipolar disorders. Int J Bipolar Disord 2017;5(1):4.
9. Serra G, Uchida M, Battaglia C, et al. Pediatric mania: the controversy between euphoria and irritability. Curr Neuropharmacol 2017;15(3):386–93.
10. Keenan-Miller D, Peris T, Axelson D, et al. Family functioning, social impairment, and symptoms among adolescents with bipolar disorder. J Am Acad Child Adolesc Psychiatry 2012;51(10):1085–94.
11. Doerfler LA, Connor DF, Toscano PF Jr. Aggression, ADHD symptoms, and dysphoria in children and adolescents diagnosed with bipolar disorder and ADHD. J Affect Disord 2011;131(1–3):312–9.
12. Safer DJ, Magno Zito J, Safer AM. Age-grouped differences in bipolar mania. Compr Psychiatry 2012;53(8):1110–7.
13. West AE, Weinstein SM, Celio CI, et al. Co-morbid disruptive behavior disorder and aggression predict functional outcomes and differential response to risperidone versus divalproex in pharmacotherapy for pediatric bipolar disorder. J Child Adolesc Psychopharmacol 2011;21(6):545–53.
14. Masi G, Milone A, Stawinoga A, et al. Efficacy and safety of risperidone and quetiapine in adolescents with bipolar II disorder comorbid with conduct disorder. J Clin Psychopharmacol 2015;35(5):587–90.
15. Hunt JI, Case BG, Birmaher B, et al. Irritability and elation in a large bipolar youth sample: relative symptom severity and clinical outcomes over 4 years. J Clin Psychiatry 2013;74(1):e110–7.
16. Findling RL, Stepanova E, Youngstrom EA, et al. Progress in diagnosis and treatment of bipolar disorder among children and adolescents: an international perspective. Evid Based Ment Health 2018;21(4):177–81.

17. Stringaris A, Baroni A, Haimm C, et al. Pediatric bipolar disorder versus severe mood dysregulation: risk for manic episodes on follow-up. J Am Acad Child Adolesc Psychiatry 2010;49(4):397–405.
18. Stringaris A, Santosh P, Leibenluft E, et al. Youth meeting symptom and impairment criteria for mania-like episodes lasting less than four days: an epidemiological enquiry. J Child Psychol Psychiatry 2010;51(1):31–8.
19. Goldstein BI, Birmaher B, Carlson GA, et al. The International Society for Bipolar Disorders Task Force report on pediatric bipolar disorder: Knowledge to date and directions for future research. Bipolar Disord 2017;19(7):524–43.
20. Birmaher B, Gill MK, Axelson DA, et al. Longitudinal trajectories and associated baseline predictors in youths with bipolar spectrum disorders. Am J Psychiatry 2014;171(9):990–9.
21. Hunt J, Birmaher B, Leonard H, et al. Irritability without elation in a large bipolar youth sample: frequency and clinical description. J Am Acad Child Adolesc Psychiatry 2009;48(7):730–9.
22. Diler RS, Goldstein TR, Hafeman D, et al. Distinguishing bipolar depression from unipolar depression in youth: preliminary findings. J Child Adolesc Psychopharmacol 2017;27(4):310–9.
23. Uchida M, Serra G, Zayas L, et al. Can unipolar and bipolar pediatric major depression be differentiated from each other? A systematic review of cross-sectional studies examining differences in unipolar and bipolar depression. J Affect Disord 2015;176:1–7.
24. Frias A, Palma C, Farriols N. Comorbidity in pediatric bipolar disorder: prevalence, clinical impact, etiology and treatment. J Affect Disord 2015;174:378–89.
25. Cantwell DP, Lewinsohn PM, Rohde P, et al. Correspondence between adolescent report and parent report of psychiatric diagnostic data. J Am Acad Child Adolesc Psychiatry 1997;36(5):610–9.
26. Biederman J, Petty CR, Wilens TE, et al. Examination of concordance between maternal and youth reports in the diagnosis of pediatric bipolar disorder. Bipolar Disord 2009;11(3):298–306.
27. Tillman R, Geller B, Craney JL, et al. Relationship of parent and child informants to prevalence of mania symptoms in children with a prepubertal and early adolescent bipolar disorder phenotype. Am J Psychiatry 2004;161(7):1278–84.
28. Youngstrom E, Meyers O, Youngstrom JK, et al. Diagnostic and measurement issues in the assessment of pediatric bipolar disorder: implications for understanding mood disorder across the life cycle. Dev Psychopathol 2006;18(4):989–1021.
29. Carlson GA, Blader JC. Diagnostic implications of informant disagreement for manic symptoms. J Child Adolesc Psychopharmacol 2011;21(5):399–405.
30. Singh MK. Clinical handbook for the diagnosis and treatment of pediatric mood disorders. Washington, DC: American Psychiatric Association Publishing; 2019.
31. Johnson LN, Wright DW, Ketring SA. The therapeutic alliance in home-based family therapy: is it predictive of outcome? J Marital Fam Ther 2002;28(1):93–102.
32. Kazdin AE, Whitley M, Marciano PL. Child-therapist and parent-therapist alliance and therapeutic change in the treatment of children referred for oppositional, aggressive, and antisocial behavior. J Child Psychol Psychiatry 2006;47(5):436–45.
33. Liddle HA, Jackson-Gilfort A, Marvel FA. An empirically supported and culturally specific engagement and intervention strategy for African American adolescent males. Am J Orthop 2006;76(2):215–25.
34. Cramer JA, Rosenheck R. Compliance with medication regimens for mental and physical disorders. Psychiatr Serv 1998;49(2):196–201.

35. DelBello MP, Adler CM, Whitsel RM, et al. A 12-week single-blind trial of quetiapine for the treatment of mood symptoms in adolescents at high risk for developing bipolar I disorder. J Clin Psychiatry 2007;68(5):789–95.

36. Goldstein TR, Krantz M, Merranko J, et al. Medication adherence among adolescents with bipolar disorder. J Child Adolesc Psychopharmacol 2016;26(10): 864–72.

37. Klein CC, Topalian AG, Starr B, et al. The importance of second-generation antipsychotic-related weight gain and adherence barriers in youth with bipolar disorders: patient, parent, and provider perspectives. J Child Adolesc Psychopharmacol 2020;30(6):376–80.

38. Correll CU, Sheridan EM, DelBello MP. Antipsychotic and mood stabilizer efficacy and tolerability in pediatric and adult patients with bipolar I mania: a comparative analysis of acute, randomized, placebo-controlled trials. Bipolar Disord 2010; 12(2):116–41.

39. Liu HY, Potter MP, Woodworth KY, et al. Pharmacologic treatments for pediatric bipolar disorder: a review and meta-analysis. J Am Acad Child Adolesc Psychiatry 2011;50(8):749–62.e39.

40. Geller B, Luby JL, Joshi P, et al. A randomized controlled trial of risperidone, lithium, or divalproex sodium for initial treatment of bipolar I disorder, manic or mixed phase, in children and adolescents. Arch Gen Psychiatry 2012;69(5): 515–28.

41. Wagner KD, Kowatch RA, Emslie GJ, et al. A double-blind, randomized, placebo-controlled trial of oxcarbazepine in the treatment of bipolar disorder in children and adolescents. Am J Psychiatry 2006;163(7):1179–86.

42. Wagner KD, Redden L, Kowatch RA, et al. A double-blind, randomized, placebo-controlled trial of divalproex extended-release in the treatment of bipolar disorder in children and adolescents. J Am Acad Child Adolesc Psychiatry 2009;48(5): 519–32.

43. DelBello MP, Goldman R, Phillips D, et al. Efficacy and safety of lurasidone in children and adolescents with bipolar i depression: a double-blind, placebo-controlled study. J Am Acad Child Adolesc Psychiatry 2017;56(12):1015–25.

44. Detke HC, DelBello MP, Landry J, et al. Olanzapine/Fluoxetine combination in children and adolescents with bipolar I depression: a randomized, double-blind, placebo-controlled trial. J Am Acad Child Adolesc Psychiatry 2015;54(3): 217–24.

45. DelBello MP, Chang K, Welge JA, et al. A double-blind, placebo-controlled pilot study of quetiapine for depressed adolescents with bipolar disorder. Bipolar Disord 2009;11(5):483–93.

46. Findling RL, Pathak S, Earley WR, et al. Efficacy and safety of extended-release quetiapine fumarate in youth with bipolar depression: an 8 week, double-blind, placebo-controlled trial. J Child Adolesc Psychopharmacol 2014;24(6):325–35.

47. Patel NC, Delbello MP, Bryan HS, et al. Open-label lithium for the treatment of adolescents with bipolar depression. J Am Acad Child Adolesc Psychiatry 2006; 45(3):289–97.

48. Shon SH, Joo Y, Lee JS, et al. Lamotrigine treatment of adolescents with unipolar and bipolar depression: a retrospective chart review. J Child Adolesc Psychopharmacol 2014;24(5):285–7.

49. Findling RL, Short EJ, McNamara NK, et al. Methylphenidate in the treatment of children and adolescents with bipolar disorder and attention-deficit/hyperactivity disorder. J Am Acad Child Adolesc Psychiatry 2007;46(11): 1445–53.

50. Scheffer RE, Kowatch RA, Carmody T, et al. Randomized, placebo-controlled trial of mixed amphetamine salts for symptoms of comorbid ADHD in pediatric bipolar disorder after mood stabilization with divalproex sodium. Am J Psychiatry 2005; 162(1):58–64.

51. Zeni CP, Tramontina S, Ketzer CR, et al. Methylphenidate combined with aripiprazole in children and adolescents with bipolar disorder and attention-deficit/hyperactivity disorder: a randomized crossover trial. J Child Adolesc Psychopharmacol 2009;19(5):553–61.

52. Chang KD, Saxena K, Howe M, et al. Psychotropic medication exposure and age at onset of bipolar disorder in offspring of parents with bipolar disorder. J Child Adolesc Psychopharmacol 2010;20(1):25–32.

53. DelBello MP, Soutullo CA, Hendricks W, et al. Prior stimulant treatment in adolescents with bipolar disorder: association with age at onset. Bipolar Disord 2001; 3(2):53–7.

54. Soutullo CA, DelBello MP, Ochsner JE, et al. Severity of bipolarity in hospitalized manic adolescents with history of stimulant or antidepressant treatment. J Affect Disord 2002;70(3):323–7.

55. Nery FG, Wilson AR, Schneider MR, et al. Medication exposure and predictors of first mood episode in offspring of parents with bipolar disorder: a prospective study. Braz J Psychiatry 2020;42(5):481–8.

56. Goldsmith M, Singh M, Chang K. Antidepressants and psychostimulants in pediatric populations: is there an association with mania? Paediatr Drugs 2011;13(4): 225–43.

57. Biederman J, Mick E, Spencer TJ, et al. Therapeutic dilemmas in the pharmacotherapy of bipolar depression in the young. J Child Adolesc Psychopharmacol 2000;10(3):185–92.

58. Faedda GL, Baldessarini RJ, Glovinsky IP, et al. Treatment-emergent mania in pediatric bipolar disorder: a retrospective case review. J Affect Disord 2004;82(1): 149–58.

59. Baumer FM, Howe M, Gallelli K, et al. A pilot study of antidepressant-induced mania in pediatric bipolar disorder: characteristics, risk factors, and the serotonin transporter gene. Biol Psychiatry 2006;60(9):1005–12.

60. Strawn JR, Adler CM, McNamara RK, et al. Antidepressant tolerability in anxious and depressed youth at high risk for bipolar disorder: a prospective naturalistic treatment study. Bipolar Disord 2014;16(5):523–30.

61. Nery FG, Masifi SL, Strawn JR, et al. Association between poor tolerability of antidepressant treatment and brain functional activation in youth at risk for bipolar disorder. Braz J Psychiatry 2020;43(1):70–4.

62. Geller B, Tillman R, Bolhofner K, et al. Child bipolar I disorder: prospective continuity with adult bipolar I disorder; characteristics of second and third episodes; predictors of 8-year outcome. Arch Gen Psychiatry 2008;65(10):1125–33.

63. Scheffer RE, Tripathi A, Kirkpatrick FG, et al. Guidelines for treatment-resistant mania in children with bipolar disorder. J Psychiatr Pract 2011;17(3):186–93.

64. Barzman DH, McConville BJ, Masterson B, et al. Impulsive aggression with irritability and responsive to divalproex: a pediatric bipolar spectrum disorder phenotype? J Affect Disord 2005;88(3):279–85.

65. MacMillan CM, Korndorfer SR, Rao S, et al. A comparison of divalproex and oxcarbazepine in aggressive youth with bipolar disorder. J Psychiatr Pract 2006; 12(4):214–22.

66. Barzman DH, DelBello MP, Adler CM, et al. The efficacy and tolerability of quetiapine versus divalproex for the treatment of impulsivity and reactive aggression in

adolescents with co-occurring bipolar disorder and disruptive behavior disorder(s). J Child Adolesc Psychopharmacol 2006;16(6):665–70.

67. Saxena K, Chang K, Steiner H. Treatment of aggression with risperidone in children and adolescents with bipolar disorder: a case series. Bipolar Disord 2006; 8(4):405–10.

68. Gotlib D, Ramaswamy R, Kurlander JE, et al. Valproic acid in women and girls of childbearing age. Curr Psychiatry Rep 2017;19(9):58.

69. McGrane IR, Loveland JG, Zaluski HJ. Adjunctive amantadine treatment for aggressive behavior in children: a series of eight cases. J Child Adolesc Psychopharmacol 2016;26(10):935–8.

70. DeMar JC Jr, Ma K, Bell JM, et al. One generation of n-3 polyunsaturated fatty acid deprivation increases depression and aggression test scores in rats. J Lipid Res 2006;47(1):172–80.

71. Gajos JM, Beaver KM. The effect of omega-3 fatty acids on aggression: a meta-analysis. Neurosci Biobehav Rev 2016;69:147–58.

72. Ginty AT, Muldoon MF, Kuan DCH, et al. Omega-3 supplementation and the neural correlates of negative affect and impulsivity: a double-blind, randomized, placebo-controlled trial in midlife adults. Psychosom Med 2017;79(5):549–56.

73. Lotrich FE, Sears B, McNamara RK. Anger induced by interferon-alpha is moderated by ratio of arachidonic acid to omega-3 fatty acids. J Psychosom Res 2013; 75(5):475–83.

74. McNamara RK, Carlson SE. Role of omega-3 fatty acids in brain development and function: potential implications for the pathogenesis and prevention of psychopathology. Prostaglandins Leukot Essent Fatty Acids 2006;75(4–5):329–49.

75. Fossum S, Handegard BH, Martinussen M, et al. Psychosocial interventions for disruptive and aggressive behaviour in children and adolescents: a meta-analysis. Eur Child Adolesc Psychiatry 2008;17(7):438–51.

76. Lee AH, DiGiuseppe R. Anger and aggression treatments: a review of meta-analyses. Curr Opin Psychol 2018;19:65–74.

77. Sukhodolsky DG, Smith SD, McCauley SA, et al. Behavioral interventions for anger, irritability, and aggression in children and adolescents. J Child Adolesc Psychopharmacol 2016;26(1):58–64.

78. Knutsson J, Backstrom B, Daukantaite D, et al. Adolescent and family-focused cognitive-behavioural therapy for paediatric bipolar disorders: a case series. Clin Psychol Psychother 2017;24(3):589–617.

79. Pavuluri MN, Graczyk PA, Henry DB, et al. Child- and family-focused cognitive-behavioral therapy for pediatric bipolar disorder: development and preliminary results. J Am Acad Child Adolesc Psychiatry 2004;43(5):528–37.

80. West AE, Henry DB, Pavuluri MN. Maintenance model of integrated psychosocial treatment in pediatric bipolar disorder: a pilot feasibility study. J Am Acad Child Adolesc Psychiatry 2007;46(2):205–12.

81. Miklowitz DJ, George EL, Axelson DA, et al. Family-focused treatment for adolescents with bipolar disorder. J Affect Disord 2004;82(Suppl 1):S113–28.

82. Millman ZB, Weintraub MJ, Miklowitz DJ. Expressed emotion, emotional distress, and individual and familial history of affective disorder among parents of adolescents with bipolar disorder. Psychiatry Res 2018;270:656–60.

A Review of the Evidence Base for Psychosocial Interventions for the Treatment of Emotion Dysregulation in Children and Adolescents

James G. Waxmonsky, MD[a],*, Raman Baweja, MD, MS[a],
Pevitr S. Bansal, MS[b], Daniel A. Waschbusch, PhD[a]

KEYWORDS

- Emotion dysregulation • Psychosocial treatment • Emotion regulation
- Emotion recognition • Emotion reactivity • Psychotherapy

KEY POINTS

- Emotion dysregulation (ED) is a transdiagnostic factor that meaningfully increases impairment for a wide range of youth with behavioral health disorders.
- Both modified and unmodified versions of currently available evidence-based psychosocial interventions are associated with reduced levels of ED.
- Little is known about how to personalize the psychosocial treatment of youth with ED beyond treating readily identifiable psychiatric comorbidities.
- Future work needs to identify mediational pathways, implement adaptive designs, create stepped care pathways integrating psychosocial and pharmacologic treatment, and test interventions using multimethod assessment batteries in naturalistic settings.

INTRODUCTION

Emotion dysregulation (ED), defined as a failure to modify an emotional state to achieve a goal,[1,2] is a transdiagnostic construct that produces impairment not accounted for by other psychiatric symptoms or by deficits in cognitive or executive function abilities.[3,4] ED is commonly seen in youth with attention-deficit/hyperactivity disorder (ADHD), anxiety, depression, conduct disorder (CD), oppositional defiant disorder (ODD), and autism spectrum disorder (ASD).[5–8] Longitudinal

[a] Department of Psychiatry and Behavioral Health, Penn State College of Medicine, 500 University Dr, Hershey, PA 17033, USA; [b] Department of Psychology in the College of Arts and Sciences at the University of Kentucky, 171 Funkhouser Drive, Lexington, KY, USA
* Corresponding author.
E-mail address: jwaxmonsky@pennstatehealth.psu.edu

Child Adolesc Psychiatric Clin N Am 30 (2021) 573–594
https://doi.org/10.1016/j.chc.2021.04.008
1056-4993/21/© 2021 Elsevier Inc. All rights reserved.

studies show that ED often presents before internalizing disorders.[9–11] Therefore, improvements in ED could reduce current impairments and prevent onset of future internalizing disorders.

ED has been divided into 3 facets: recognition, reactivity, and regulation.[1,2] Recognition requires attending to and appraising emotional stimuli to identify emotions in oneself and others. Deficits in emotion recognition are a common impairment in youth with ASD,[12] with some evidence of impairment in ADHD.[13] It is often measured through laboratory tasks, such as having children identify the type and intensity of emotion in pictures. Reactivity refers to the intensity and duration of an immediate response to a stimulus. It is typically measured using rating scales and direct observation and also evoked response potentials.[14,15] Youth with behavioral disorders show excessive and blunted reactivity,[9] as well as abnormalities in threat and reward processing.[15] In addition, regulation refers to responding to reactivity in an adaptive manner that promotes goal attainment,[1] often to reduce intensity of initial arousal to a stimulus. Effective emotion regulation is thought to require adequate inhibitory control and a capacity for instrumental learning (ie, learning from experience), which are impaired across many psychiatric disorders.[15] It is typically measured using rating scales and direct observation, and more recently using neurophysiologic markers.[16,17]

Challenges in any of these domains can lead to ED and impairments in one can affect the others. For example, difficulty recognizing emotion in others may lead to blunted reactivity, whereas increased reactivity is associated with reduced capacity to regulate emotions.[4,15] Ideally, each area is assessed and used to individualize treatment of ED. Evidence shows emotion regulation is a learned skill that improves with practice,[18] so it is reasonable to assume that psychosocial interventions (PSIs) can reduce ED. Parents are an especially important target for PSIs to reduce ED in children because parents are children's primary models of emotion regulation.[18]

Existing PSIs reliably target each of the ED domains. Parent management training (PMT) improves instrumental learning by clarifying associations between behavior and consequences and by teaching parents optimal responses to the child's excessive reactivity.[15,19] Cognitive behavior therapy (CBT) and dialectical behavior therapy (DBT) address distorted cognitions that impair regulatory efforts and teach skills to regulate excessive emotional reactivity.[20–28] Social information processing interventions address aberrant threat processing and impaired problem-solving skills that overvalue aggression as a means to regulate emotion.[29] Thus, there are several evidence-based PSIs that could potentially benefit youth with ED. Therefore, this article focuses on trials specifically measuring the impact of a PSI on a standardized measure of ED in children or adolescents.

METHODS

MEDLINE was searched for studies in English, published between January 1981 and May 2020, with any of the following keywords: emotional dysregulation, irritability, mood lability, emotion regulation, emotion reactivity, emotion recognition, disruptive mood dysregulation disorder (DMDD), severe mood dysregulation (SMD), ADHD, ODD, CD, ASD, depression, anxiety disorder, bipolar disorder, adolescence, youth, psychotherapy, psychosocial intervention, parent training, CBT, DBT, multimodal treatment, and parent-child interaction therapy (PCIT). References from identified articles were reviewed to ensure that all relevant articles were included. We excluded trials that did not specifically report on changes in ED. Because our focus is on the treatment, we also excluded studies where ED was assessed only through laboratory paradigms with no ratings of change in symptoms or impairment. We also excluded 2 programs meeting all inclusion criteria, multifamily and individual-family psychoeducational psychotherapy, because they are described in detail in a separate article in this issue. Eighteen studies were included in the review.

Studies were organized by intervention modality into 5 categories. The first category was PMT, where either (1) the parent was the sole recipient of the intervention or (2) study staff worked with parent-child dyads supporting parents to modify their children's behavior. The second category was social-emotional training (SET), where study staff (1) directly engaged youth with a focus on identifying and regulating emotions or (2) trained parents to coach their children in regulation strategies. The third category was CBT, where participants were taught strategies to undo unhelpful thinking styles, and behavioral strategies were also taught to parents and/or children. The fourth category was studies that used both SET and PMT. The final category used all 3 components (PMT, CBT, and SET) jointly targeting parents and children. A summary of the reviewed studies can be found in **Table 1**.[19–21,30–37]

RESULTS
Study Demographics

The reviewed studies were published between 2009 and 2020. Ages ranged from 2 to 18 years (mean age, 7.8 years). Approximately two-thirds of youth were male, and 46% were ethnic or racial minorities. The mean number of participants was 104, but there was appreciable variability (median = 75). Nearly a quarter of the studies had fewer than 20 participants.[19,25,34,36] Three larger studies had samples between 229 and 579 subjects, 2 of which were post hoc analyses.[22,24,32]

Inclusion/Exclusion Criteria and Assessment Methods

Multiple measures were used to assess baseline ED severity, often relying on parent report. Three studies explicitly included youth with a DMDD diagnosis.[19,20,34] Others used the related construct of SMD,[38] which includes the 2 core DMDD symptoms plus hyperarousal criteria.[28] The Kiddie Schedule for Affective Disorders and Schizophrenia (KSADS) was most commonly used to assess DMDD/SMD.[39] Other studies enrolled youth with a disruptive behavior disorder[25,27,32] or increased levels of externalizing behavior disorders,[22,26,33] with no specific requirements for ED severity. Waxmonsky and colleagues[28] required increased levels of mood symptoms on the WASH-U KSADS plus a diagnosis of ADHD.[28,40] Work by Luby and coworkers[23,24] focused on the treatment of mood disorders in preschoolers, which did not require a specific ED threshold and used the Preschool Age Psychiatric Assessment (PAPA) to diagnose major depression.[23,24,41] Evans and colleagues[21] used the Child Behavior Checklist (CBCL) to identify minimum levels of ED for inclusion.[21,42] Studies of youth with ASD used the Aberrant Behavior Checklist (ABC), typically using an entry threshold of greater than or equal to 15 on its irritability subscale.[30,31,43] For the 5 studies using the Clinical Global Impressions (CGI) Scale,[44] the mean entry severity score was 4.6 (moderate to markedly ill). Across studies, baseline severity ratings were highest for youth with ASD[30,31] and lowest when trauma was the inclusion criterion.[37]

Therapeutic Targets

There was significant variability across studies in outcomes and measures. Studies requiring a DMDD diagnosis commonly used the CGI to quantify improvement and reported remission rates.[19,20,36] Six studies measured emotion recognition using rating scales and laboratory tasks.[23,24,26,27,34,35] Emotion reactivity was assessed using rating scales, including the ABC,[30,31] the Affective Reactivity Index (ARI),[19,34] items from

Table 1
Summary of the reviewed studies, and their relevant characteristics

Study Investigators, Year, Demographics	Entry Criteria	ED Assessment Method and Other Relevant Measures	Trial Design and Therapy Modality/Format	Medication Procedures	ED Results	Other Findings
PMT						
Aman et al,[30] 2009; N = 124, ages 4–13 y, 75% white	PDDs + aggression, tantrums, self-injury	HSQ, Vineland, Clinical Global Impressions, ABC-I subscale (score ≥ 18) CGI-S: modal entry score of 5 (markedly) ABC irritability subscale: mean entry score of 29.5	24-wk, randomization to med-only vs combined (PT + risperidone) Mean of 10.9 PT sessions The most PT (11 core treatment sessions, 3 optional) concluded at week 16, followed by a face-to-face booster session and 2 follow-up telephone consultations (maximum of 17 sessions), each 60–90 min, delivered individually to families	Risperidone monitored by clinicians 100% on medication (risperidone)	Combined group showed better outcomes on ABC-I (d = 0.48), HSQ, hyperactivity, noncompliance vs medication-only group Added effect of PT + risperidone > than risperidone alone	Mean treatment fidelity = ~95% Effects were significant and large for noncompliance on HSQ, and explosive behavior, and hyperactivity on ABC
Bearss et al,[31] 2015; N = 180, ages 3–7 y, 86% white, 88% boys	Children with DSM-IV-TR diagnosis of autism, PDD-NOS, Asperger Moderate or greater pretreatment behavioral problems on ABC-I and HSQ	ADOS, ADIR; HSQ-ASD and ABC-I (score ≥ 15) CGI-S: modal entry score of (markedly) ABC irritability subscale: mean entry score of 23.8	Randomization 2-groups: • PT (11 sessions, 2 optional sessions, 60–90 min, 1 home visit, 6 parent-child sessions over 16 wk); 1 home visit and 2 telephone boosters between weeks 16 and 24 • PE (12 session, 60–90 min, 1 home visit over 24 wk)	Medication allowed (3% medicated at entry) but could not change	Greater decreases found in PT>PE on the ABC-I and the HSQ ABC-I % reduction posttreatment • PT ~48% vs PE ~32% (standardized ES: 0.62) HSQ % reduction posttreatment • PT 55% vs PE 34% (standardized ES: 0.45)	90% retention at 48-wk for PT Continued improvement on the ABC and HSQ at 48-wk CGI-I scale: 68% for PT vs 40% for PE

Study/Sample	Population	Measures	Design	Medication	Results	Findings
De La Cruz et al,[32] 2015; N = 579 ages 7-10 y, 80% boys, 39% racial/ethnic minority	Youth with ADHD	ADHD diagnosed with DISC-P; Primary outcome 3 DSM ODD items from SNAP Scale: mean entry irritability score of 4.29 (range 0-9)	Examined change in ADHD, ODD symptoms over the 14-mo RCT phase (medication alone, Bmod, Comb, CC) Multimodal treatment	CNS stimulants 3 out of 4 study arms provided medication	Irritability decreased over time: Comb (d = .82) > Beh (d = .42), CC (d = .48) but not medication (d = .63); medication > Beh	Irritability more associated with emotional than conduct problems; Higher ADHD symptoms associated with greater irritability for parent but not teacher ratings; Remission of irritability not seen; irritability treatment effects half as strong as for ADHD; Irritability did not moderate response to ADHD treatments
Rothenberg et al,[33] 2019; N = 86, ages 2-8 y, 69% boys, 78% white	Clinical increases on BASC-2 Externalizing subscale or ECBI intensity score	BASC and ECBI Baseline BASC-2 Externalizing subscale T score: 64.06 Child Emotion Regulation via BASC-2 anger control, Emotion Control, and BRIEF Measured positive parenting using DPICS-III, parent emotion coping using CCNES	PCIT with no modifications to either CDI, and PDI phases Pre-post design	Medication rate not reported	Greater child behavioral improvement ($\beta = -0.65$) during PCIT, and greater parent pretreatment use of positive emotion ($\beta = -0.33$) were both associated with posttreatment reductions in child ED Degree of change in child behavior (but not parenting behaviors) during PCIT mediated the change in ED	Higher baseline levels of ED associated with greater improvements in child behavior; >80% of youth with increased levels of ED normalized by end of treatment

Social-Emotional Training

Stoddard et al,[34] 2016; 3 experiments N = 14 Ages 8-18 y	DMDD	Clinical lifetime diagnosis of DMDD ARI: mean entry score of 7.5 Mean CGI-S (moderate): 3.9	Open clinical trial of Interpretation bias training Active balance-point training 4 sessions	No changes in their medications for at least 2 wk before training and throughout their participation Entry rate not reported	Training was associated with reductions in parent-reported irritability on ARI rating, which persisted 1 and 2 wk after training	Clinician-rated CGI-I scores covering the immediate posttraining period were in the slightly improved range (d = 0.59); In DMDD youth, active training was associated with a shift in balance point toward more happy judgments

(continued on next page)

Table 1
(continued)

Study Investigators, Year, Demographics	Entry Criteria	ED Assessment Method and Other Relevant Measures	Trial Design and Therapy Modality/Format	Medication Procedures	ED Results	Other Findings
Sánchez et al,[35] 2019; N = 64, ages 8–14 y, 81% boys	Youth with ADHD with social/ emotional deteri- oration	Emotional Problems, Emotional Regulation Problems, and Anger Control Problems subtests of the SENA AR subtest of NEPSY II Neuropsychological Battery SENA Anger Management subscale: mean entry T score of 66.5	Single group pre/post 15 groups of 3 to 5 participants 10 sessions: 60 min child only +20 min with parent Multidisciplinary team that includes a neuropediatrician, and psychologists	Entry medication rate not reported	Significant reduction in parent ratings of emotional problems over time [t (63) = 2.63; $P = .01$] and rated emotion regulation [t (63) = 4.11; $P = .00$]	Following the intervention, an improvement in the identification of affect on facial recognition tasks on NEPSY II [t (63) = −3.83; $P = .00$]
CBT						
Johnson et al,[36] 2012; N = 17, ages 7–13 y	ADHD (of any subtype) and ODD	Clinical diagnoses SNAP-IV: median entry score: 20 (range 0–20)	CPS: • Goal is to help parents to understand cognitive factors driving aggression • Steps: define the problem, invite the child to collaboratively solve a problem with therapist focusing on problem- solving skills 6–10 sessions: once a week, 1.5 h Pediatricians/neuropediatri- cians, a clinical psychologist, and a special education teacher	Children had to be unmedicated or on stable psychoactive medications (>6 mo) 6% on medication at baseline	Significant reductions of emotional lability measured using Connors abbreviated form postintervention and at 6-mo follow-up; during the follow-up phase, 8 children were started on CNS stimulants	53% response rate by CGI at postintervention and by 81% at 6-mo follow-up. Reductions in ADHD and ODD scores at postintervention and follow-up

Thornback & Muller,[37] 2015; N = 107, ages 7–12 y, 30.1% boys	Clinically verified trauma experiences	Children's Emotion Management Scales ERC: mean entry lability negativity subscale score: 30.72 (range 15–60)	Randomized to TF-CBT or WL control Average # of sessions were 17.05 TF-CBT Therapists from 9 community site	Stable psychotropic medication regimen 4% were on medication at entry	From preassessment to posttreatment: inhibition and lability/negativity significantly improved on ERC Preassess to 6-mo follow-up: inhibition and dysregulation improved on ERC Pretreatment to posttreatment: lability/negativity on ERC improved	Change in dysregulation and lability best predicted improvement in child-reported posttraumatic stress symptoms at 6-mo follow-up
Kircanski et al., 2018; N = 10, ages 9.3–15.1 y (mean 12.4 y), 6 boys	DSM-5 criteria for DMDD, established via the K-SADS-PL	ARI CGI-S: mean entry score of 4.2 (moderate)	All assigned to active treatment Exposure-based CBT: 12–16 weekly sessions, 60–90 min, manualized Sessions consisted of individual child and parent components as well as joint components	80% children were on medication at entry	Clinician ARI and CGI-S for DMDD scores significantly decreased over time DMDD CGI-I scores significantly lower than score of 5 at posttreatment with no participants worsening	All 10 youth and families attended all sessions, and there were no treatment dropouts
Evans et al,[21] 2020; N = 174 (including 81 with SIMD, ages 7–13 y, 70% boys	Post hoc analysis of just the youth characterized by SIMD drawn from a larger treatment trial	Irritability was measured by averaging 3 CBCL items: (1) tantrums or hot temper, (2) sudden mood changes, and (3) stubborn, sullen, or irritable. Youth with a mean score ≥1.33 on these items, plus evidence of impairment, were identified as SIMD CBCL internalizing, externalizing, and total T scores ranged from 69.5 to 71.2	Cluster randomization design • UC • SMT, 3 standard protocols: Coping Cat for anxiety, PASCET for depression, and Defiant Children for disruptive behavior • MATCH: modular, transdiagnostic, behavioral/cognitive-behavioral intervention	Before treatment, 25% of study youths were taking some psychotropic medication, and, during treatment, 27% of youths used some psychotropic for at least 1 d Medication use was assessed weekly	For youth with SIMD, MATCH and SMT produced faster improvements on parent-reported irritability than UC, with a medium effect size for MATCH (0.60) and a large effect size for SMT (1.02) Among the entire sample, MATCH and SMT equivalently outperformed UC in reducing irritability (ES = 0.49). Irritability did not moderate outcomes	SIMD youths in all conditions showed reductions in DSM diagnoses; only MATCH predicted significantly fewer posttreatment diagnoses (averaging 1.0 fewer; ES = 0.93) Adherence was 93% for SMT, 83% for MATCH, 8% of UC session

(continued on next page)

Table 1
(continued)

Study Investigators, Year, Demographics	Entry Criteria	ED Assessment Method and Other Relevant Measures	Trial Design and Therapy Modality/Format	Medication Procedures	ED Results	Other Findings
Derella et al,[22] 2019; N = 252, ages 6–11 y, 100% boys	Significant behavioral problems: T score >70 on any of the aggressive, rule-breaking, or DSM CD subscales of the CBCL or a T score ≥64 on the overall Externalizing Behavior subscale	Child Symptom Inventory-4: Parent Checklist to measure irritability SCS to measure ER Irritability score was collected using 3 DBDRS items Mean score: 4.6 (range 0–9)	RCT SNAP Program (concurrent parent and child treatment groups weekly for 3 mo followed by individualized therapeutic, academic, or other support services as needed) vs standard services (assistance by project staff to engage in behavioral health services) Data collected at 4 time points over 15 mo	Medication rate not reported	Direct effect of SNAP on irritability did not reach significance (B = −.35, SE = .29, P = .24). SNAP predicted significantly higher ER skills (B = 1.48, SE = .51, P = .004), with small effect size ER skills significantly predictive of reductions in irritability (B = −.07, SE = .03, P = .02)	Adherence to specific SNAP treatment protocols was at least 92% or greater for all treatment groups
Social-Emotional Training/Behavioral therapy						
Luby et al,[23] 2012; N = 54, ages 3–7 y	Meeting criteria for preschool MDD on PAPA	Outcomes = PAPA, PFC-S (preschool depression), functional outcomes (HSQ), emotional recognition (Penn Emotion Differentiation Test) and ER (ERC) Mean ERC negativity lability score: 41.5 (range 15–60)	2-arm RCT: (1) PCIT-ED: 14 sessions in 12 wk, PCIT supplemented with modules to enhance emotional development 3 cores: PCIT, CDI, PDI (2) DEPI (psychoeducation control)	Children taking medications must be on stable doses: no changes 39% were on medication	PCIT-ED showed greater improvements on emotion regulation subscales as rated by parents	29 completed treatment (19 in PCIT-ED, 10 in DEPI) No posttreatment differences on the PAPA MDD, or functional outcomes Maternal depression significantly lower for the PCIT-ED group at posttreatment vs controls Similar patterns found for parenting stress (but only when using intention-to-treat analyses)

Luby et al,[24,62] 2018, 2019; N = 229 (191 completed study), ages 3–7 y	Meeting criteria for preschool MDD	PFC-S, ERC, CBCL ERC negativity lability subscale entry score not reported, CGAS entry score of 42.67	PCIT-ED: 8 sessions for emotion development; 20 sessions total vs WL both lasting 18 wk	Excluded those on antidepressant Use of other medication classes allowed if dose stable but rates not reported	PCIT-ED vs WL controls were less emotionally labile (ES = 1.21) and had higher emotion regulation (ES = 0.69)	All measures (except for CBCL anxiety and externalizing) showed significant improvement using the ED module, with greater improvement in therapy subjects PCIT-ED vs controls were less likely to meet MDD, had lowers scores on MDD outcomes, and less impaired
Chronis-Tuscano et al,[25] 2016; N = 9, ages 3.5–7 y, 5 boys, 7 white	ADHD (+5 ODD, +2 CD)	Posttreatment = CBCL, IRS, ERC Mean entry CBC_ externalizing T score 59.88 ERC negativity lability score: 38.51 IRS overall: 5.50	PCIT-ED, PCIT-Eco integrated into parent and child phases Single-arm pilot	33% were on CNS stimulants	Reliable change on CBCL externalizing problems at posttreatment and follow-up, as well as on the ERC and IRS	Most mothers significantly increased in positive parenting from pretreatment to posttreatment; however, only 1 mother showed reliable change in negative talk

(continued on next page)

Table 1
(continued)

Study Investigators, Year, Demographics	Entry Criteria	ED Assessment Method and Other Relevant Measures	Trial Design and Therapy Modality/Format	Medication Procedures	ED Results	Other Findings
Graziano and Hart,[26] 2016; N = 45, mean age 5.16 y, 76% boys, 84% Hispanic/Latino	Preschool children with EBP EBP T score of 60 or higher on BASC, no history of ASD	C-DISC-IV BASC externalizing; entry parent T score of 66.09 Across all groups: Mean IRS overall entry score of 4.49; entry BASC externalizing parent score of 66.4	RCT, 8 wk, 15 children in 1 of 3 arms: • PMT only (SRPP): ~2 h, traditional PMT in group setting, PCIT CDI skills; 4 optional monthly sessions, parent group discussions • Therapeutic summer camp (STP): daily for 8 h/d; + standard behavioral modification system, PMT and academic curriculum • STP-PreK Enhanced: daily for 8 h/d; all STP aspects plus social-emotional and self-regulation training	No medication	Self-regulation measured via the ER checklist Children in the STP-PreK Enhanced group showed greatest gains across time in emotional knowledge and ER relative to other groups Children in STP-PreK Enhanced continued to show better emotional knowledge and parent-reported ER at the 6-mo follow-up compared with other 2 arms No reliable effects were found for teacher-reported ER or observed ER	STP-PreK Enhanced attended 92% of PT sessions with zero families dropping out. 56% of sessions attended in PMT Children across all 3 intervention groups experienced significant growth in academic achievement ES at the 6-mo follow-up period for children in the STP-PreK Enhanced group (d = 2.22) was significantly larger than children in the STP-PreK group (d = 1.35) or those in the PMT-only group (d = 1.50)
Behavioral therapy/CT/SET						
Webster-Stratton & Reid,[27] 2011 N = 99, age 4-6 y, 75% boys, 27% racial/ ethnic minority	ADHD with or without ODD	Child Symptom Inventory for ADHD and CBCL (≥95% on Attention subscale; no exclusionary criteria besides not meeting ADHD criteria)	Randomized to IY parent and child groups or WL control WL: allowed outside medications and therapy IY: 20 weekly, 2-h sessions, 6	Not at intake At the posttreatment interview, 5 children started	Outcomes: CBCL (significant for aggression and attention), CPRS-R (significant for all domains), ECBI significant for all	By end of study 14% WL and 10% IY added medication Added therapy: 10% WL, 2% IY Overall, improved ER and recognition, ADHD and

	CBCL entry Externalizing T score of 65	families per group with focus on emotional coaching for parents, increasing interpersonal support in family; children groups focused on social and emotional skills; child and parent groups run in parallel	medication in intervention group	domains), DPICS (child deviance and child positive behavior with more effects seen for parent than child behavior), classroom observations (significant effects for social relationships), task to measure social problem-solving skills and emotion recognition (both significant effects); Social Competence Scale for positive social behaviors and ER (significant effects seen on both domains); less effects seen by teacher report; also significant effects for maternal but not paternal parenting behaviors. Dropout 6% WL, 4% IY; mothers attended 18.5/ fathers 17.1. Significant condition × time interactions were observed on parental reports of emotional regulation	ODD symptoms, aggression and social competence with broader effects reported by mothers than fathers. Limited effects at school but was not teacher component. Overall study validated adding the child group to IY, with benefits especially for peer relationships	
Waxmonsky et al,[28] 2016; N = 56, ages 7–12 y, 70% boys, 38% ethnic/racial minority	ADHD plus SMD	DBD-I WASH-U-KSADS parent and child. Needed increased mood symptoms after medication optimization	Randomly assigned to community services or intervention comprised 11,105-min parent and child sessions run in parallel (AIM group)	CNS stimulants that were optimized during study lead-in phase before start	AIM group improved more than time but nonsignificant time × group effects for primary measure of clinician-rated mood severity index that reached significance in	Significant change in ODD (ES = .42) but not ADHD symptoms; >93% completing with mean attendance 9.7 sessions; 90% of parents rated it as	

(continued on next page)

Table 1
(continued)

Study Investigators, Year, Demographics	Entry Criteria	ED Assessment Method and Other Relevant Measures	Trial Design and Therapy Modality/Format	Medication Procedures	ED Results	Other Findings
				of any therapy; doses held stable in therapy phase 100% on medication (CNS stimulant)	those attending 6+ sessions (ES = .53). Parent-rated irritability items (DBDRS) had significant time × group effects (d = .63)	feasible and 83% were satisfied with program
Perepletchikova et al,[20] 2017; N = 43, ages 7–12 y	DMDD Stratified by age and self-harm history	Schedule for Affective Disorders and Schizophrenia for School-Age Children: DMDD modal, CGI-S modal score is 5 (markedly) where average CGAS is 42.65	RCT: DBT-C or TAU TAU not standardized and participants were charged for treatment (through insurance), whereas DBT-C was provided free of charge Divided into child counseling, parent training, and skills training with parents and children; DBT content largely unmodified with addition of parent component being main innovation 32 weekly 90-min sessions, conducted individually with each family; most sessions were joint parent + child Follow-up phase (weeks 33–44): 0–2 booster sessions per month	Were stabilized on medication for 6 wk; no exclusionary medications More in TAU receiving psychiatric medications during study (4 vs 0) 72% were not on any medication at entry	Primary measure of CGI for DMDD response: 90.4% in DBT-C compared with 45.5% in TAU with effect seen by week 16 but not week 8 Remission rates (defined as a CGI-S score no higher than 3): 52.4% for DBT-C and 27.3% for TAU	CGAS at end point: 69.4 for DBT vs 58 for TAU (d = .95) Participants in DBT-C attended 89% (28.5) of sessions compared with 48.6% in TAU (Cohen d: 2.03) but no evidence of dose effects for DBT Dropped out: 36% TAU vs none in DBT-C >90% fidelity for DBT-C Improvements were maintained at 3-mo follow-up (Cohen d: 1.20) with improved CGAS for DBT-C

Abbreviations: ABC, Aberrant Behavior Checklist; ABC-I, Aberrant Behavior Checklist–Irritability subscale; AIM, ADHD medication plus the experimental therapy; AR, affect recognition; ARI, Affective Reactivity Index; ADHD, attention-deficit/hyperactivity disorder; ADIR, Autism Diagnostic Interview–Revised; ADOS, Autism Diagnostic Observation Schedule; ASD, autism spectrum disorder; BASC, Behavior Assessment System for Children; Bmod, behavioral modification; BRIEF, Behavior Rating Inventory of Executive Function Emotional Control subscales; CBCL, Child Behavior Checklist; CC, community care; CCNES, Coping with Children's Negative Emotion; CDI, Child-directed Interaction; C-DISC-IV, Diagnostic Interview Schedule for Children, Computerized Version IV; CGAS, Children's Global Assessment Scale; CGI-S, Clinical Global Impressions Severity; CGI-I, Clinical Global Impressions Improvement; CNS, central nervous system; Comb, combined; CPS, collaborative problem solving; CPRS-R, Conners' Parent Rating Scale–Revised; DBD-I, Disruptive Behavior Disorders Structured Parent Interview; DBT-C, dialectical behavior ther-

Report, Version 3.0; DMDD, disruptive mood dysregulation disorder; DPICS-III, Parent-Child Interaction Coding System-III; DPICS-R, Dyadic Parent-Child Interactive Coding System—Revised; DSM-IV-TR, Diagnostic and Statistical Manual of Mental Disorders [Fourth Edition, Text Revision]; EBP, externalizing behavior problems; ECBI, Eyberg Child Behavior Inventory; ER, emotion regulation; ERC, Emotion Regulation Checklist; ES, effect size; K-SADS-PL, Kiddie Schedule for Affective Disorders and Schizophrenia for School-Age Children—Present and Lifetime Version; HSQ, Home Situations Questionnaire; IRS, Impairment Rating Scale; IY, Incredible Year; MATCH, modular approach to therapy for children with anxiety, depression, trauma, or conduct problems; MDD, major depressive disorder; ODD, oppositional defiant disorder; PAPA, Preschool Age Psychiatric Assessment; PASCET, primary and secondary control enhancement training; PCIT, parent-child interaction therapy; PCIT-ED, Parent-Child Interaction Therapy Emotion Development; PCIT-Eco, PCIT with parent emotion coaching; PDDs, pervasive developmental disorders; PDD-NOS, pervasive developmental disorder–not otherwise specified; PDI, parent-directed interaction; PE, parent education; PFC-S, Preschool Feelings Checklist–Scale; PT, parent training; RCT, randomized controlled trial; SCS, Social Competence Scale–Parent Version; SENA, Spanish Assessment System for Children and Adolescents; SIMD, severe irritability and mood dysregulation; SMD, severe mood dysregulation; SMT, standard manualized treatments; SNAP, Swanson, Nolan, and Pelham; SNAP, Stop Now and Plan; SRPP, School Readiness Parenting Program; TF-CBT, Trauma-focused CBT; TAU, treatment as usual; UC, usual care; WASH-U-KSADS, Washington University in St. Louis Kiddie Schedule for Affective Disorders and Schizophrenia; WL, waiting list.

the CBCL,[21,25,27] the Child Symptom Inventory-4,[22,45] and items from the Disruptive Behavior Disorder Rating Scale (DBDRS).[28,32,46] The ABC was mostly used in studies of ASD and the DBDRS in studies of ADHD. Only 2 studies used the ARI even though it is designed to measure emotional reactivity.[19,34,47] Emotion regulation was measured primarily using the Emotion Regulation Checklist.[23–26,48]

Study Format and Design

Four studies (22%) used PMT only, 2 studies (11%) SET only, 5 studies (28%) CBT only, 4 studies (22%) used SET and PMT, and 3 studies (17%) used PMT, SET, and CBT. Treatment lasted between 6 and 10 weekly sessions in most studies, but ranged from 1 to 32 weeks.[20,30]

Twelve studies used a randomized design with active treatments including combined use of medication and behavioral therapy,[30] combining parent training and/or child-delivered services[20,26,28,32] or enhanced forms of parent-training programs.[23–25] Control comparisons included standardized active treatment,[21,26,30] treatment as usual (TAU) in the community,[20,22,28,32] wait-list conditions,[24,27,37] or a psychoeducation group designed to balance time that study staff spent with parents across the treatment groups.[23,31] Aman and colleagues[30] were unique in that the control arm was only medication (risperidone), whereas active treatment comprised a combination of risperidone and parent training. Three studies were post hoc analyses of randomized controlled trials designed to treat other conditions.[21,22,32,49]

Medication status varied as well. Graziano and Hart[26] did not allow medicated youth into their study, whereas another incorporated a lead-in phase to optimize central nervous system (CNS) stimulant medication before therapy.[28] All participants with ASD were prescribed risperidone.[30] In the Multimodal Treatment Study of Children with ADHD (MTA), 3 of the 4 randomly assigned groups included treatment with CNS stimulants.[32] Collaborative problem solving considers psychoeducation about the role of medication to be an active part of therapy and therefore allowed medication changes during follow-up.[36] Others did not specify the procedures for medication.[33,35]

Treatment Outcomes

Both PMT-only and CBT-only programs were associated with improvements in emotion regulation and reactivity.[19,21,22,36,37] SET was associated with improvements in recognition, regulation, and reactivity.[34,35] Thus, improvements in all 3 domains of ED were observed across different treatment modalities in youth with a wide range of clinical presentations (eg, ADHD, DMDD, depression, autism, trauma).

Additional Clinically Relevant Findings

There was at least an 80% completion rate in active treatment arms across studies.[20–22,26,28,31] For control interventions, rates ranged between 37% and 56%.[20,23,26] When reported, treatment satisfaction rates were high for active treatments[21,23–25,27] versus 50% for control treatments.[20,28] Assessment of global improvement or impairment was limited to 5 studies. Perepletchikova and colleagues[20] observed that youth receiving DBT had significantly better functioning on the Children's Global Assessment Scale (CGAS) at posttreatment and 3-month follow-up compared with youth in the control condition. Chronis-Tuscano and colleagues[25] found that youth experienced reliable change on the Impairment Rating Scale from pretreatment to posttreatment, as did Evans and colleagues[21] on the Brief Impairment Scale[50] and a pair of studies by Luby and colleagues[23,24] that used 2 different measures of impairment.

Follow-up

Follow-up effects were examined in 9 studies. Follow-up periods ranged from a few months to more than 1 year,[20–22,25,26,28,32,36,37] and treatment effects were typically maintained. Graziano and Hart[26] observed that only children in the more intensive summer camp–based treatment arms (vs PMT only) maintained gains in emotion regulation after 6 months.

DISCUSSION

We identified 18 studies examining PSI's capacity to improve aspects of ED. These studies included 3 post hoc analyses, 12 randomized trials, and 3 uncontrolled pilots. All studies reported positive outcomes despite appreciable heterogeneity of samples and variability in treatment modality and design. These results provide a strong preliminary signal supporting PSIs for youth with ED. All 3 ED domains improved, with the strongest evidence for reactivity and regulation. Reduced effects for recognition may be caused by our inclusion criteria requiring assessment of treatment effects outside of the laboratory, where this domain is commonly assessed. However, work by Stoddard and colleagues[34] suggests that emotion recognition is a malleable skill in youth with ED, suggesting that treatments targeting it merit further investigation.

Several approaches were used to identify youth with ED. Outcomes assessments ranged from ad hoc measures using items from existing rating scales to measures specifically designed for ED. There was little quantification of the frequency or severity of temper outbursts or aggressive episodes. This heterogeneity reflects the current lack of consensus on the so-called best practice of assessing ED in youth, although tremendous progress has been made in this area in recent years.

Parents were the primary, and typically sole, informants for measuring ED, which presents methodological challenges because parents are an integral part of all treatments and this may bias their treatment evaluations. Only a few trials accounted for differential contact between parents and study staff in intervention versus control arms.[23,26,31] Treatment efforts for ED would be enhanced if objective measures were available that were psychometrically sound, easy to administer, and sensitive to change. Only a few studies used such measures, which take considerable time and effort to develop and can increase study burden. Other immediately available and useful approaches would be to expand the range of informants (eg, parents, teachers, child) and use observational data and other objective indices that contribute to (1) identifying patients with impairing ED and (2) determining treatment effects, such as the methods used by Graziano and Hart.[26] There are many advantages to multimethod, multi-informant assessments, such as between-informant comparisons, which could shed light on the stability and pervasiveness of ED.[51] Future studies should also measure impairment given that symptomatic reduction may not always translate into reduced impairment.[52]

Most studies used established interventions, and some applied them to ED without any modifications.[30,31,33,36,37] These interventions are effective for comorbidities often seen in youth with ED, including anxiety, depression, ADHD, and ODD.[15,53] This treatment development approach is similar to that followed for psychopharmacology, where most medications used for ED are indicated for another disorder.[30,52,54] There is support for applying existing PSI without modifications to treat ED. PMT has been observed to produce greater improvements in conduct problems in children with ED versus those without ED.[33,55] In some instances, ED effects were equivalent to those in disorders for which the treatments were originally designed,[28,33,36] whereas, in other studies, effects were less.[32] For example, in youth with ASD, treatment effects were much larger for noncompliance, hyperactivity, and aggression than they were for ED.[30] Results across studies may be influenced by trial design issues regarding the use of psychotropics and baseline symptom severity because they have been found to predict treatment effects.[49,56]

Despite these improvements, the need for further refinement and innovation is clear. Youth with ED are more impaired than youth without prominent ED.[2,10,11] These differences often persist after intensive psychosocial and pharmacologic treatment.[32,57] Most studies using modified content to treat ED adapted an existing evidence-based program for another condition. Some modified content for ED to fit a different age range than the original intervention,[20] whereas others added unique content specifically for ED[19,23–26] or integrated multiple evidence-based programs.[21,22,28,35] Most elected to target children and parents either in dyads[23–25,33] or in separate groups.[20,22,28] In children, externalizing problems are often addressed through parent-centered therapies,[58] whereas, for internalizing disorders, treatment centers on the child.[59] Youth with ED often manifest a mix of internalizing and externalizing symptoms,[60,61] so it seems logical to integrate these formats when treating ED. Working together with parents and children allows synchronization of content and creates opportunities for practice of learned skills supported by therapists, which may be particularly important for emotion regulation, because parents are a critical influence for developing these capacities.[5,9]

PCIT has been one of the most commonly adapted programs. In standard PCIT, increasing positive parenting behaviors is not sufficient to produce meaningful ED reductions. Changes in child negative behavior must be seen in session to achieve reduced ED at home.[33] It has been hypothesized that one way to enhance PCIT effects for ED is to add content training parents to be emotion coaches and give them structured opportunities to practice this with their children.[25,33] PCIT with additional emotion regulation sessions has been developed for the treatment of young children with mood disorders.[23,24] It teaches parents to attend to their own emotional reactions to the child's behavior and how to guide their children in recognizing and regulating emotions. In 2 randomized trials of preschoolers with depression, it improved all 3 ED domains, other behavior problems, impairment, and symptoms of depression in children and in parents.[23,24] In a post hoc analysis examining the timing of treatment effects, ED content was associated with changes in mood symptoms, neural response to rewards, and parental emotion coaching efforts that were not seen during standard modules.[62]

For young children with ADHD, ED content is directly integrated into standard PCIT sessions to emphasize the importance of the parent as an emotion coach for youth with challenges with attention and impulse control.[25] Another key modification was creating a sequence of actions for parents. It starts by having parents address their own emotional reactions to their children's behavior, followed by efforts to manage the child's negative behavior to move the child to a calm state, and ends with engaging in emotion coaching with the child only when calm. This model improved levels of ED, ADHD, and impairment in a small open pilot. Similar sequencing of attending to parental emotion, then child behavior, and lastly to child emotion have been observed to be beneficial in other programs.[28]

Whenever evidence-based treatments are modified, there are risks of reducing efficacy either from altering key content or extending duration, which can increase dropout.[58] In the PCIT studies for depression, observed behavioral improvements were comparable with standard PCIT, as were completion and treatment satisfaction ratings.[24] However, reduced effect on conduct problems versus standard PCIT has been observed in other trials when content is added addressing emotion recognition.[63] In the ADHD pilot, there were lower-than-expected reductions in parental negative talk.[25] Whether this was caused by the small sample, a low base rate of negative talk, or by the content modifications was not able to be assessed in the uncontrolled pilot. These observations highlight the value of comparing modified PSIs with standard formats before widespread implementation.

ED is truly a transdiagnostic construct. To paraphrase a classic article by Paul,[64] such heterogeneity argues that it is time to move beyond the simple question of whether treatment works and instead examine which treatments work for whom under what conditions. More finite subtyping of ED is likely needed to successfully match patient to treatment. Evans and colleagues[21] observed quicker rates of response for modular treatments integrating multiple evidence-based interventions than with standardized treatments for both irritable and nonirritable youth, but there has been little other work examining treatment matching in youth with ED.

Adaptive treatment designs are proving to be an important methodological tool that may provide critical information for answering such questions. They are designed to resemble the decisions facing providers more closely in clinical care. Using these designs, it has been found that starting with the most intensive doses of multimodal treatments is unnecessary for many youth with behavioral disorders.[49,65,66] A recent adaptive treatment study found high rates of response to initial treatment with low-dose medication or low-intensity PSIs. For patients needing more care, the sequence of PSI then medication was more efficacious than medication before therapy, in part because of reduced parental attendance for PSIs after ADHD medication was started.[67] Applying these designs to ED could improve knowledge of how to match treatment to patient. Until then, it may be advisable to start with less intensive treatments that are empirically supported for conditions associated with high rates of ED given the wide range of promising PSIs and the low rates of treatment completion often seen with PSI.[68,69]

Several multimodal treatment studies for ADHD and aggression have used sequenced treatments. The typical lead-in phase consists of optimizing CNS stimulant dose plus PMT. Across studies, approximately half of participants do not need additional treatment.[54,70] Given the better tolerability of PSIs and CNS stimulants versus other psychotropic medications used to reduce ED (eg, valproate and atypical antipsychotics),[54,70] it seems reasonable that initial treatments for youth with ED and ADHD should start with optimizing CNS stimulant dose plus a low-intensity evidence-based PSI such as PMT. Waiting to start a PSI until after medication may be less efficacious because medication treatments seem to reduce parental motivation for therapy.[67,68]

Results of this review need to be considered in light of several limitations, most notably the small number of published studies, particularly randomized controlled trials with active comparators. There is a need for additional work testing currently used PSIs under controlled conditions and for developing novel treatments. Next, studies were composed primarily of school-aged boys, although they were moderately ethnically and racially diverse (eg, approximately half of the participants were either black or Hispanic). Future work should aim to recruit diverse samples to strengthen the ability to generalize the findings. Across studies, enrolled participants had a wide range of comorbid disorders. It remains unknown how much ED may differ as a function of psychiatric comorbidity. Moreover, some therapies for ED were originally designed for specific diagnoses or symptom constructs, so it is unclear how efficacious these treatments would be for children with ED not manifesting those conditions. Further, there was limited use of specific measures for the facets of ED. For instance, reactivity was often measured using composite scores from broadband screeners (eg, CBCL) or through change in ODD symptoms. Only 2 studies used a reactivity-specific measure, the ARI. Future work should develop and use measures that better capture the nuances of ED, including methods for reliably coding the severity of observed emotional outbursts. In addition, most studies were conducted in nonnaturalistic office settings that may not generalize to everyday settings (eg, schools, camps). Because optimal emotion regulatory responses are often context dependent, it would be advisable to test interventions in settings where children routinely show ED.

SUMMARY

A variety of existing psychosocial interventions could be efficacious for youth with ED. More studies are needed, particularly those using multimethod batteries of ED and conducting assessments in naturalistic settings. Future work should also focus on identifying mediational pathways and testing treatment sequencing and personalization efforts given the breadth of available treatment options and the heterogeneity of ED. At present, there is the most support for using psychosocial treatments efficacious for psychiatric conditions commonly manifesting ED, such as ADHD or major depression. It seems reasonable to start with less intensive but empirically supported versions of these treatments to promote engagement and uptake while maintaining efficacy. Subsequent treatments can focus on specific residual impairments in order to optimize the functioning of youth with ED.

DISCLOSURE

In the past 3 years, Dr Waxmonsky has received research funding from the National Institutes of Health, Pfizer, and Supernus. The other authors have nothing to disclose.

REFERENCES

1. Gross J, Thompson R. Emotion regulation: conceptual foundations. In: Gross J, editor. Handbook of emotion regulation. New York, NY: Guilford Press; 2007. p. 3–24.
2. Graziano P. ADHD and children's emotion dysregulation: a meta analyses. Clin Psychol Rev 2016;46:106–23.
3. Bunford N, Evans SW, Wymbs F. ADHD and emotion dysregulation among children and adolescents. Clin Child Fam Psychol Rev 2015;18(3):185–217.
4. Berkovits L, Eisenhower A, Blacher J. Emotion regulation in young children with autism spectrum disorders. J Autism Dev Disord 2017;47(1):68–79.
5. Trosper SE, Buzzella BA, Bennett SM, et al. Emotion regulation in youth with emotional disorders: implications for a unified treatment approach. Clin Child Fam Psychol Rev 2009;12(3):234–54.
6. Samson AC, Hardan AY, Podell RW, et al. Emotion regulation in children and adolescents with autism spectrum disorder. Autism Res 2015;8(1):9–18.
7. Shaw P, Stringaris A, Nigg J, et al. Emotion dysregulation in attention deficit hyperactivity disorder. Am J Psychiatry 2014;171(3):276–93.
8. Schoorl J, van Rijn S, de Wied M, et al. Emotion regulation difficulties in boys with oppositional defiant disorder/conduct disorder and the relation with comorbid autism traits and attention deficit traits. PLoS One 2016;11(7):e0159323.
9. Hostinar CE, Cicchetti D. Emotion dysregulation and internalizing spectrum disorders. In: The Oxford Handbook of Emotion Dysregulation. New York, NY. 2018.

10. Copeland WE, Shanahan L, Egger H, et al. Adult diagnostic and functional out-comes of DSM-5 disruptive mood dysregulation disorder. Am J Psychiatry 2014;171(6):668–74.
11. Stringaris A, Cohen P, Pine DS, et al. Adult outcomes of youth irritability: a 20-year prospective community-based study. Am J Psychiatry 2009;166(9):1048–54.
12. Uljarevic M, Hamilton A. Recognition of emotions in autism: a formal meta-anal-ysis. J Autism Dev Disord 2013;43(7):1517–26.
13. Collin L, Bindra J, Raju M, et al. Facial emotion recognition in child psychiatry: a systematic review. Res Dev Disabil 2013;34(5):1505–20.
14. Faraone SV, Rostain AL, Blader J, et al. Practitioner Review: emotional dysregu-lation in attention-deficit/hyperactivity disorder - implications for clinical recogni-tion and intervention. J Child Psychol Psychiatry 2019;60(2):133–50.
15. Brotman MA, Kircanski K, Stringaris A, et al. Irritability in youths: a translational model. Am J Psychiatry 2017;174(6):520–32.
16. Dennis TA, Hajcak G. The late positive potential: a neurophysiological marker for emotion regulation in children. J Child Psychol Psychiatry 2009;50(11):1373–83.
17. Beauchaine TP. Future directions in emotion dysregulation and youth psychopa-thology. J Clin Child Adolesc Psychol 2015;44(5):875–96.
18. Morris AS, Silk JS, Steinberg L, et al. The role of the family context in the devel-opment of emotion regulation. Soc Dev 2007;16(2):361–88.
19. Kircanski K, Clayton ME, Leibenluft E, et al. Psychosocial treatment of irritability in youth. Curr Treat Options Psychiatry 2018;5(1):129–40.
20. Perepletchikova F, Nathanson D, Axelrod SR, et al. Randomized clinical trial of dialectical behavior therapy for preadolescent children with disruptive mood dys-regulation disorder: feasibility and outcomes. J Am Acad Child Adolesc Psychi-atry 2017;56(10):832–40.
21. Evans SC, Weisz JR, Carvalho AC, et al. Effects of standard and modular psycho-therapies in the treatment of youth with severe irritability. J Consult Clin Psychol 2020;88(3):255–68.
22. Derella OJ, Johnston OG, Loeber R, et al. CBT-enhanced emotion regulation as a mechanism of improvement for childhood irritability. J Clin Child Adolesc Psychol 2019;48(sup1):S146–54.
23. Luby J, Lenze S, Tillman R. A novel early intervention for preschool depression: findings from a pilot randomized controlled trial. J Child Psychol Psychiatry 2012;53(3):313–22.
24. Luby JL, Barch DM, Whalen D, et al. A randomized controlled trial of parent-child psychotherapy targeting emotion development for early childhood depression. Am J Psychiatry 2018;175(11):1102–10.
25. Chronis-Tuscano A, Lewis-Morrarty E, Woods K, et al. Parent–child interaction therapy with emotion coaching for preschoolers with attention-deficit/hyperactivity disorder. Cogn Behav Pract 2016;23:62–78.
26. Graziano PA, Hart K. Beyond behavior modification: benefits of social-emotional/self-regulation training for preschoolers with behavior problems. J Sch Psychol 2016;58:91–111.
27. Webster-Stratton CH, Reid MJ, Beauchaine T. Combining parent and child training for young children with ADHD. J Clin Child Adolesc Psychol 2011;40(2):191–203.
28. Waxmonsky JG, Waschbusch DA, Belin P, et al. A randomized clinical trial of an integrative group therapy for children with severe mood dysregulation. J Am Acad Child Adolesc Psychiatry 2016;55(3):196–207.

29. Sukhodolsky DG, Vander Wyk BC, Eilbott JA, et al. Neural mechanisms of cognitive-behavioral therapy for aggression in children and adolescents: design of a randomized controlled trial within the national institute for mental health research domain criteria construct of frustrative non-reward. J Child Adolesc Psychopharmacol 2016;26(1):38–48.

30. Aman MG, McDougle CJ, Scahill L, et al. Medication and parent training in children with pervasive developmental disorders and serious behavior problems: results from a randomized clinical trial. J Am Acad Child Adolesc Psychiatry 2009; 48(12):1143–54.

31. Bearss K, Johnson C, Smith T, et al. Effect of parent training vs parent education on behavioral problems in children with autism spectrum disorder: a randomized clinical trial. JAMA Apr 2015;313(15):1524–33.

32. Fernandez de la Cruz L, Simonoff E, McGough JJ, et al. Treatment of children with attention-deficit/hyperactivity disorder (ADHD) and irritability: results from the multimodal treatment study of children with ADHD (MTA). J Am Acad Child Adolesc Psychiatry 2015;54(1):62–70.e3.

33. Rothenberg WA, Weinstein A, Dandes EA, et al. Improving child emotion regulation: effects of parent–child interaction-therapy and emotion socialization strategies. J Child Fam Stud 2019;28:720–31.

34. Stoddard J, Sharif-Askary B, Harkins EA, et al. An open pilot study of training hostile interpretation bias to treat disruptive mood dysregulation disorder. J Child Adolesc Psychopharmacol 2016;26(1):49–57.

35. Sanchez M, Lavigne R, Romero JF, et al. Emotion regulation in participants diagnosed with attention deficit hyperactivity disorder, before and after an emotion regulation intervention. Front Psychol 2019;10:1092.

36. Johnson M, Ostlund S, Fransson G, et al. Attention-deficit/hyperactivity disorder with oppositional defiant disorder in Swedish children - an open study of collaborative problem solving. Acta Paediatr 2012;101:624–30.

37. Thornback K, Muller RT. Relationships among emotion regulation and symptoms during trauma-focused CBT for school-aged children. Child Abuse Negl 2015;50: 182–92.

38. Leibenluft E. Severe mood dysregulation, irritability, and the diagnostic boundaries of bipolar disorder in youths. Am J Psychiatry 2011;168(2):129–42.

39. Kaufman J, Birmaher B, Brent D, et al. Schedule for affective disorders and Schizophrenia for school-age children-present and Lifetime version (K-SADS-PL): initial reliability and validity data. J Am Acad Child Adolesc Psychiatry 1997;7:980–8.

40. Geller B, Zimerman B, Williams M, et al. Reliability of the Washington University in St. Louis Kiddie Schedule for affective disorders and Schizophrenia (WASH-U-KSADS) mania and rapid cycling sections. J Am Acad Child Adolesc Psychiatry 2001;40(4):450–5.

41. Egger H, Ascher B, Angold A. Preschool age psychiatric assessment (PAPA): version 1.1. Durham, NC: Department of Psychiatry and Behavioral Sciences, Center for Developmental Epidemiology, Duke University Medical Center; 1999.

42. Achenbach TM, Rescorla LA. Manual for ASEBA school-age forms & Profiles. Burlington, VT: University of Vermont Research Center for Children, Youth, an Families; 2001.

43. Aman MG, Singh NN, Stewart AW, et al. The aberrant behavior checklist: a behavior rating scale for the assessment of treatment effects. Am J Ment Defic Mar 1985;89(5):485–91.

44. Guy W. ECDEU Assessment manual for psychopharmacology. Washington DC: US Dept of Health, Education and Welfare; 1976.

45. Gadow KD, Sprafkin J. Childhood symptom inventory-4 screening and norms manual. Stony Brook, NY: Checkmate Plus; 2002.

46. Pelham WE Jr, Gnagy EM, Greenslade KE, et al. Teacher ratings of DSM-III-R symptoms for the disruptive behavior disorders. J Am Acad Child Adolesc Psychiatry 1992;31(2):210–8.

47. Stringaris A, Goodman R, Ferdinando S, et al. The Affective Reactivity Index: a concise irritability scale for clinical and research settings. J Child Psychol Psychiatry 2012;53(11):1109–17.

48. Shields A, Cicchetti D. Emotion regulation among school-age children: the development and validation of a new criterion Q-sort scale. Dev Psychol 1997;33(6): 906–16.

49. The MTA Cooperative Group. A 14-month randomized clinical trial of treatment strategies for attention-deficit/hyperactivity disorder. Multimodal Treatment Study of Children with ADHD. Arch Gen Psychiatry 1999;56(12):1073–86.

50. Bird HR, Canino GJ, Davies M, et al. The Brief Impairment Scale (BIS): a multidimensional scale of functional impairment for children and adolescents. J Am Acad Child Adolesc Psychiatry 2005;44(7):699–707.

51. De Los Reyes A, Augenstein TM, Wang M, et al. The validity of the multi-informant approach to assessing child and adolescent mental health. Psychol Bull 2015; 141(4):858–900.

52. Towbin K, Vidal-Ribas P, Brotman MA, et al. A double-blind randomized placebo-controlled trial of citalopram adjunctive to stimulant medication in youth with chronic severe irritability. J Am Acad Child Adolesc Psychiatry 2020;59(3): 350–61.

53. Mayes SD, Waxmonsky JD, Calhoun SL, et al. Disruptive mood dysregulation disorder symptoms and association with oppositional defiant and other disorders in a general population child sample. J Child Adolesc Psychopharmacol 2016; 26(2):101–6.

54. Blader JC, Pliszka SR, Kafantaris V, et al. Stepped treatment for attention-deficit/hyperactivity disorder and aggressive behavior: a randomized, controlled trial of adjunctive risperidone, divalproex sodium, or placebo after stimulant medication optimization. J Am Acad Child Adolesc Psychiatry 2020;60(2):236–51. https://doi.org/10.1016/j.jaac.2019.12.009.

55. Scott S, O'Connor TG. An experimental test of differential susceptibility to parenting among emotionally-dysregulated children in a randomized controlled trial for oppositional behavior. J Child Psychol Psychiatry 2012;53(11):1184–93.

56. March J, Silva S, Vitiello B, et al. The treatment for adolescents with depression study (TADS): methods and message at 12 weeks. J Am Acad Child Adolesc Psychiatry 2006;45(12):1393–403.

57. Waxmonsky J, Pelham WE, Gnagy E, et al. The efficacy and tolerability of methylphenidate and behavior modification in children with attention-deficit/hyperactivity disorder and severe mood dysregulation. J Child Adolesc Psychopharmacol 2008;18(6):573–88.

58. Kaminski JW, Claussen AH. Evidence base update for psychosocial treatments for disruptive behaviors in children. J Clin Child Adolesc Psychol 2017;46(4): 477–99.

59. Weisz JR, McCarty CA, Valeri SM. Effects of psychotherapy for depression in children and adolescents: a meta-analysis. Psychol Bull 2006;132(1):132–49.

60. Baweja R, Mayes SD, Hameed U, et al. Disruptive mood dysregulation disorder: current insights. Neuropsychiatr Dis Treat 2016;12:2115–24.
61. Roy AK, Klein RG, Angelosante A, et al. Clinical features of young children referred for impairing temper outbursts. J Child Adolesc Psychopharmacol 2013;23(9):588–96.
62. Luby JL, Gilbert K, Whalen D, et al. The differential contribution of the components of parent-child interaction therapy emotion development for treatment of preschool depression. J Am Acad Child Adolesc Psychiatry 2020;59(7):868–79.
63. Salmon K, Dittman C, Sanders M, et al. Does adding an emotion component enhance the Triple P-Positive Parenting Program? J Fam Psychol 2014;28(2): 244–52.
64. Paul GL. Strategy of outcome research in psychotherapy. J Consult Psychol 1967;31(2):109–18.
65. Pelham WE, Burrows-MacLean L, Gnagy EM, et al. A dose-ranging study of behavioral and pharmacological treatment in social settings for children with ADHD. J Abnorm Child Psychol 2014;42(6):1019–31.
66. Sanders MR, Markie-Dadds C, Tully LA, et al. The triple P-positive parenting program: a comparison of enhanced, standard, and self-directed behavioral family intervention for parents of children with early onset conduct problems. J Consult Clin Psychol 2000;68(4):624–40.
67. Pelham WE, Fabiano GA, Waxmonsky JG, et al. Treatment sequencing for childhood ADHD: a multiple-Randomization study of adaptive medication and behavioral interventions. J Clin Child Adolesc Psychol 2016;45(4):396–415.
68. Waxmonsky JG, Baweja R, Liu G, et al. A commercial insurance claims analysis of correlates of behavioral therapy use among children with ADHD. Psychiatr Serv 2019;70(12):1116–22. https://doi.org/10.1176/appi.ps.201800473.
69. Chacko A, Jensen SA, Lowry LS, et al. Engagement in behavioral parent training: review of the Literature and implications for practice. Clin Child Fam Psychol Rev 2016;19(3):204–15.
70. Gadow KD, Arnold LE, Molina BS, et al. Risperidone added to parent training and stimulant medication: effects on attention-deficit/hyperactivity disorder, oppositional defiant disorder, conduct disorder, and peer aggression. J Am Acad Child Adolesc Psychiatry 2014;53(9):948–59.e1.

Preventing Irritability and Temper Outbursts in Youth by Building Resilience

Manpreet K. Singh, MD, MS[a],*, Rebecca Hu, MD[b],
David J. Miklowitz, PhD[c]

KEYWORDS

- Irritability • Temper outbursts • Emotion dysregulation • Resilience • Prevention
- Early intervention

KEY POINTS

- Chronic irritability and temper outbursts are transdiagnostic constructs that can disrupt achievement of typical developmental milestones and result in psychopathology and life-long impairment.
- An evidence base for preventive interventions is limited and more research is needed to determine whether irritability and temper outbursts are disorder-specific or share common neurobiological underpinnings.
- Parent, child, and community-based approaches have empirical support.
- Secondary prevention studies on the relations between changes in family functioning - for example, from family-focused therapy - and changes in the course of high-risk syndromes can help clarify treatment targets and mechanisms.
- Tertiary prevention aims to reduce symptom severity and enhance psychosocial functioning.

INTRODUCTION

Irritability and temper outbursts lead to significant impairment in family and peer relationships as well as academic performance.[1,2] Irritability, which is commonly defined as a tendency to react to stimuli with the experience of negative affective states (eg, an increased proneness to anger) compared with peers at the same developmental level,[3] is observed across multiple psychiatric disorders, and puts youth with one disorder (eg, attention deficit with hyperactivity [ADHD]) at risk for other disorders (eg, depression)[4] and high-risk behaviors like suicidal ideation and self-harming behaviors.[5]

[a] Department of Psychiatry and Behavioral Sciences, Stanford University School of Medicine, 401 Quarry Road, Stanford, CA 94305-5719, USA; [b] University of California, San Francisco School of Medicine, 401 Parnassus Avenue, San Francisco, CA 94143, USA; [c] Department of Psychiatry and Biobehavioral Sciences, UCLA Semel Institute, David Geffen School of Medicine at UCLA, 760 Westwood Plaza Rm A8-256, Los Angeles, CA 90024-1759, USA
* Corresponding author.
E-mail address: mksingh@stanford.edu

Child Adolesc Psychiatric Clin N Am 30 (2021) 595–610
https://doi.org/10.1016/j.chc.2021.04.009
1056-4993/21/© 2021 Elsevier Inc. All rights reserved.

Abbreviations	
ADHD	attention deficit with hyperactivity
DBT	dialectical behavioral therapy
DMDD	disruptive mood dysregulation disorder
FFT-HR	family-focused therapy for youth at high risk for bipolar disorder
ODD	oppositional defiant disorder

Like irritability, temper outbursts are defined as aggressive or nonaggressive behaviors that occur in response to frustration,[6] occur transdiagnostically, and have associated interpersonal and academic impairment. Irritability and temper outbursts are widely accepted examples of dysregulated emotion, although their representation within and beyond mood disorders signal the need for broad-based preventive interventions that should be applicable to a diverse group of youth and across many settings.

The frequency, severity, and intensity of irritability and temper outbursts along with age of onset, persistence and episodicity are key parameters for treatment planning. For example, early onset, persistent, and chronic irritability may suggest a neurodevelopmental or ADHD-like phenotype, whereas a later-onset irritability may be indicative of a mood disorder phenotype.[7] Further, episodic versus chronic and persistent irritability may distinguish adolescents who are at risk for mania versus those who are at risk for depression.[8] With different presentations that portend multifinal outcomes, the developmental context of irritability and temper outbursts have implications for how they are conceptualized, and how and when we treat them.[9]

Irritability and temper outbursts are not only features of multiple disorders and symptom constellations, but they may also be unstable over the course of development, calling into question the usefulness of singular or unifying diagnoses such as the new diagnosis added to the *Diagnostic and Statistical Manual of Mental Disorders,* 5th edition, disruptive mood dysregulation disorder (DMDD), that aimed to distinguish nonepisodic from episodic emotion dysregulation.[10] Despite controversy surrounding the validity of DMDD, evidence points to a clinically significant number of children who are characterized by nonepisodic, chronic, and severe irritability and temper outbursts.[11]

After an initial evaluation of safety considerations and acute stabilization, existing interventions for irritability and temper outbursts are broadly framed around symptom reduction (ie, in frequency and in intensity) and relapse prevention (preventing the undesired behavior from recurring). Importantly, if a behavior can be predicted through early identification and tracking of precursor emotions, behaviors, or triggers, perhaps it can also be prevented. This review summarizes the literature on primary, secondary, and tertiary relapse prevention strategies, with a focus on strategies that promote resilience in youth to prevent the onset and recurrence of irritability and temper outbursts (**Fig. 1**). Although the urgency to treat the frequency and severity of outbursts is self-evident, highlighting interventions in the context of prevention and a resilience framework can enhance our understanding of treatments in terms of causal mechanisms, and illuminate interventions that could be adapted early and transdiagnostically rather than focusing on treating a single disorder. This is principally why more research is needed to guide clinicians on effective treatments to decrease the impact of stress, adversity,[12] and other risk factors, as well as the consequences of common manifestations of emotion dysregulation.

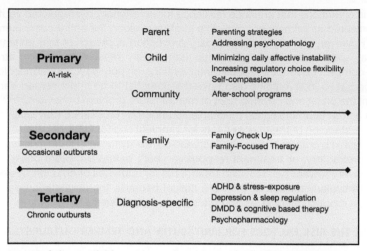

Fig 1. Summary of the available evidence for primary, secondary, and tertiary prevention strategies for irritability and temper outbursts. Primary prevention aims to decrease the risk for disorder onset in susceptible populations through parent, child, or community interventions. Secondary prevention strategies, targeting children with occasional outbursts, are currently predominantly family oriented. Tertiary prevention is diagnosis specific because children with chronic outbursts often are already diagnosed with mental illness. ADHD, attention deficit hyperactivity disorder; DMDD, disruptive mood dysregulation disorder.

WHY IS PROACTIVELY PROMOTING RESILIENCE AN INTRIGUING SOLUTION TO PREVENTING REACTIVE EMOTION DYSREGULATION?

Resilience is a complex process that is defined as the ability of a system to adapt successfully to challenges that threaten the function, viability, or future development of the system.[13] Resilience is dynamic, falls along its own continuum, and can be cultivated with the potential for change across the lifespan to proactively bring about positive outcomes or help avoid or reduce the impact of the negative outcomes of adversity.[14] Resilience has been measured using a variety of scales. The Strength and Difficulties Questonnaire[15] is among the most common metric and evaluates psychopathology risk and resilient factors among youth using emotional, conduct, hyperactive–inattentive, peer, and prosocial factors. The prosocial factor (eg, voluntary actions intended to benefit others) is the single construct of resilience in the Strength and Difficulties Questionnaire, reflecting a key cross-species characteristic that centers on the evolutionarily adaptive drive to be social to promote survival.[16] Several studies have demonstrated a bidirectional inverse relation between prosocial behavior and aggression or delinquency over the course of childhood and adolescence,[17] suggesting the potential for prosociality to be an antidote to various forms of aggression.[18] Thus, resilience, conceptualized in terms of prosociality, could be framed as a preventive intervention, such that skills that encourage prosocial behaviors have the effect of intervening to decrease aggression.

Other studies consistently find that promoting resilience encourages other positive outcomes in the face of adversity by increasing emotion regulation (ability to respond appropriately to situational demands), encouraging life satisfaction, or decreasing depressive symptoms.[19,20] Thus, key factors associated with resilience include prosociality with peers and caregivers, enhancing skills in emotion regulation, and academic engagement.[21]

Novel interventions that enhance resilience for emotionally dysregulated youth could be implemented as primary or adjunctive strategies along the entire continuum of prevention. However, primary and secondary prevention approaches that enhance resilience may yield more enduring effects than tertiary relapse prevention strategies, such as complex psychotherapeutic interventions or poly-psychopharmacology.[22,23] Resilience-based interventions also have the potential to be implemented early in life to prevent the onset and development of myriad future problem behaviors.[24,25] Further, research on the neurobiological mechanisms underlying resilience may open doors to novel understanding of treatment effects for interventions for irritability and temper outbursts. Reliable biomarkers may also increase our ability to identify the most vulnerable, treatment refractory, or treatment responsive youth before symptom onset. Accelerating discovery toward personalized treatments for subtypes of emotion dysregulation that are particularly difficult to treat are critical because the currently available treatments have modest effect sizes and offer nonspecific benefits.[26]

WHAT ARE THE RISK FACTORS FOR IRRITABILITY AND TEMPER OUTBURSTS?

Studies have shown that the risks for irritability and temper outbursts include both environmental and genetic factors. Some known risk factors for irritability include growing up in poverty, homelessness, exposure to violence or abuse, and being the offspring of parents with psychopathology.[19,27–29] When using child self-report measures, twin studies report the heritability of irritability to be around 0.30.[30] Based on parent reports, heritability seems to be higher.[31] Irritability may also be linked to perturbations of the prefrontal cortex that impair emotion regulation.[32] Irritable youth also show abnormalities in neural circuits related to threat and reward processing.[33] Further understanding the neurodevelopmental features of irritability may elucidate novel primary, secondary, and tertiary preventive interventions.[34]

PRIMARY PREVENTION

Primary prevention refers to strategies to prevent disease onset among susceptible populations.[35] Here, we refer to children at risk for developing irritability or temper outbursts as our susceptible population. These sections leverage studies on this at-risk population to highlight targets for interventions that attempt to prevent the development of irritability and temper outbursts. We classify these studies as parent, child, and community focused. **Fig. 2** summarizes the key findings.

Parent-Focused Studies

As discussed elsewhere in this article, resilience is associated with individual intrinsic (eg, problem-solving skills, self-regulation) and relational or prosocial (eg, capacity to form secure attachments) characteristics.[13] The expression and regulation of emotions occur in interpersonal contexts and begin as early as in infancy.[36] Thus, it is not surprising that parenting plays a central role in a child's ability to regulate emotions.

Parental psychopathology has been identified as a risk factor for child internalizing and externalizing behaviors through multiple mechanisms, including increased parenting stress.[37] In their study on mothers with homelessness and problems with substance use disorders, Wu and colleagues[26] found that maternal depressive symptoms and "expressive suppression," defined as the attempt to inhibit emotional expression, were associated with increased parenting stress regarding young children (ages 0–6). In contrast, cognitive reappraisal, or an attempt to reinterpret an emotion-eliciting situation in a way that changes its emotional impact, was associated with decreased parenting stress.[37] Borderline and antisocial personality disorder

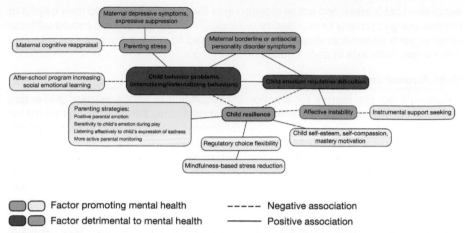

Fig. 2. Summary of the interplay of moderators and targets of primary prevention strategies for irritability and temper outbursts. The main outcome measures are highlighted in the darker color shades (child behavior problems, resilience, emotion regulation difficulties). *Key Terms*: Affective instability, Shifts in emotional intensity over a relatively brief period of time within an individual; Cognitive reappraisal, Reinterpretation of an emotion-eliciting situation in a way that changes its emotional impact; Emotion regulation, Ability to respond appropriately to situational demands and manage the experience and expression of emotions; Expressive suppression, Inhibition of emotional expression; Externalizing behaviors, Actions in the external world, such as aggression, impulsivity, control problems; Instrumental support seeking, Soliciting advice and assistance with planning, decision-making and problem solving; Internalizing behaviors, Characterized by processes within the self, such as anxiety, depression, withdrawal; Mastery motivation, Drive to control and master challenges independently and persistently; Mindfulness-based stress reduction, Developed by Dr. Jon Kabat-Zinn in 1979, an 8-week program teaching mindfulness meditation exercises, initially targeting stress management; Positive parental emotion, Experience of positive emotions by parents; Regulatory choice flexibility, Ability to deploy different emotion regulation strategies based on context; Resilience, Capacity of a system to successfully adapt to threats to its function, viability, or development; Self-compassion, Ability to be kind and nonjudgmental toward the self during stress and failure; Self-esteem, Affectively laden evaluation of one's worth.

symptoms in mothers have been associated with child behavior problems, a relation partially mediated by emotion dysregulation in youth.[29] Maternal irritable depression has also been associated with offspring disruptive behavioral disorders, whereas the remission of maternal depression after 3 months of antidepressant treatment was associated with decreases in psychiatric diagnoses and symptoms in the offspring.[38] Further, the effect of maternal remission on her children may have been mediated by an improvement in maternal symptoms of high anxious distress and irritability.[39] Thus, treating psychopathology and personality pathology among parents should be considered as potential targets for the prevention of psychopathology in children. Dialectical behavior therapy, which targets emotion dysregulation, has been studied extensively as a therapeutic intervention for borderline personality disorder, but its use to improve parenting quality merits evaluation, given that a parent's ability to regulate emotions is critical for effective parenting.[40]

Parental strategies like encouraging positive parental emotion (ie, parents expressing positive emotions toward a child, as measured by the Positive Affect Scale[41]), sensitivity to children's emotions during play, listening effectively to children's expression of sadness, and active monitoring of the child may be particularly helpful to families living in poverty or exposed to violence.[19,28,42] Future studies should address whether such parental strategies can be harnessed to prevent the onset of irritability and temper outbursts in at-risk youth.

Child-Focused Studies

Targeting child risk factors for emotion dysregulation is also a primary prevention strategy. For example, dysregulated temperament[43] may be an early risk factor for mood disorders.[44] Difficult childhood temperaments, with traits like behavioral inhibition, irritability, a high activity level, and poor adaptability are associated with subsequent mood disorders, ADHD, and substance abuse.[45–47] However, these associations have been cross-sectionally determined and merit longitudinal observation to evaluate the predictive validity of early temperament characteristics on developing emotion dysregulation. In 1 longitudinal study, parental temperament of fearfulness moderated the link between childhood fearfulness and their subsequent development of anxiety disorders.[48] This finding may be rooted in either genetics, overprotective parenting practices, or the modeling of avoidant behavior, which could all increase susceptibility to anxiety in children.[48] Thus, intervening on fear-based parenting practices may be a point of intervention in children with temperament vulnerabilities to emotion dysregulation.

Transient mood state changes have also been implicated in persistent emotion dysregulation. A longitudinal study spanning 6 years of adolescence found that day-to-day teen affective instability predicted difficulties in emotion regulation over time, suggesting a process by which mood variability becomes consolidated into enduring patterns of response.[49] Targeting day-to-day affective instability through behavioral or pharmacologic interventions may interrupt the consolidation process that leads to chronic emotion dysregulation. Further, in a national sample of 100 US adolescents, greater trait resilience and support seeking by soliciting advice and assistance with planning, decision-making and problem solving have been associated with lower levels of negative affect instability.[50] An insecure attachment style accounted for the unexpected relation between emotional support seeking and negative affect instability, such that adolescents, and more likely girls, with an insecure–anxious attachment style were more prone to seeking reassurance. It is worth investigating whether interventions that promote instrumental support seeking over emotional support seeking (eg, asking for solutions rather than comfort or validation) are helpful in preventing emotion dysregulation in youth. Indeed, gender differences may moderate the effects of such interventions and should be considered for personalized treatment matching.

Socioemotional functioning and emotion regulation, including self-compassion, self-esteem, and mastery motivation,[25,27,42] may promote resilience against irritability and temper outbursts. In maltreated youth or youth living in poverty, self-esteem[51] plays a protective role against emotional and behavioral problems[52,53] and is associated with greater resilience. Here, resilience was defined as good adaptive functioning and the absence of any significant psychiatric symptomatology based on measures of global functioning (eg, Children's Global Assessment Scale), behavioral disturbance (eg, Child Behavioral Checklist), or depression severity (eg, Childhood Depression Inventory).[24,36] Similarly, in youth experiencing homelessness, higher mastery motivation (the drive to control and master challenges independently and persistently) is associated with better social and emotional functioning.[27]

Self-compassion is a relatively new concept in Western psychology and is the ability to be kind and nonjudgmental toward the self during stress and failure, recognizing that one's suffering is common to the human experience.[54] As such, self-compassion has been theorized to protect against the activation of psychopathological schema after negative affective experiences,[25] that is, a defining feature of irritability. Consequently, interventions that attempt to enhance self-esteem, mastery motivation, and self-compassion may have preventive effects on the onset of irritability. These interventions may benefit both children and parents. For example, in elementary school children, emotion dysregulation has been associated with increased anxiety and decreased prosocial behaviors, and these associations are buffered by maternal agreeableness.[55] Agreeableness is a core trait from the 5-factor model of personality that reflects the degree of expression of empathy, kindness, and consideration toward others.[56] Thus, among children struggling with emotion dysregulation, an early intervention targeting maternal agreeableness or prosociality may decrease a child's risk for irritability and temper outbursts.

Interventions to Promote Emotion Regulation

There are few interventions that encourage emotion regulation skill enhancement. Whether a specific emotion regulation strategy proves adaptive or maladaptive depends on the context in which it is applied. For example, it is adaptive to choose disengagement–distraction for high-intensity emotional stimuli versus engaging–reappraisal for low-intensity stimuli.[57,58] Mindfulness-based practices may increase regulatory choice flexibility through an increased awareness of one's thoughts, sensations, and feelings and decreasing automatic reactivity to emotional experiences. In addition, mindfulness training in the context of family therapy may enhance a family's capacity for emotion regulation.[36] Studies that promote understanding of these and other specific nuances that leverage emotion regulation skills in a family context may lead to additional points of intervention. Outside of the family context, in college students ages 21 to 40 years, Mindfulness-Based Stress Reduction was effective in cultivating "regulatory choice flexibility," or the ability to deploy different emotion regulation strategies based on context to encourage resilience.[59]

Community-level interventions for children at risk for emotional dysregulation are limited.[60] In 1 open trial of an after-school program for urban, middle school African American youth living in poverty, Frazier and colleagues[22] found that encouraging recreational activities that enhance social–emotional learning (ie, problem solving, emotion regulation, effective communication) led to improvements in social skills and decreases in problem behaviors. The specificity of and degree to which such programs lead to long-term changes in problem behaviors in high-risk populations deserves exploration.

SECONDARY PREVENTION

Secondary prevention focuses on addressing subclinical forms of disease as early as possible to prevent progression to full-blown disease states. How can we help youth who have occasional outbursts from developing chronic patterns of emotion dysregulation that will impact their psychosocial functioning or develop into full-blown psychopathology? Lessons can be learned from findings across a number of psychiatric disorders, as well as from interventions developed for specific diagnoses. Indeed, understanding that early alliance in treatment can promote engagement and favorable outcomes underscores the importance of forging a working relationship with a child from intervention outset.[61]

The benefits of early family-based interventions are illustrated by a recent randomized controlled trial assessing the effects of the Family Check Up on dysregulated irritability in early childhood. The Family Check Up, which was designed to improve a child's adjustment by motivating positive behavior support and other family management practices, was composed of a 2-session intervention that was individually tailored to the needs of the family. The sessions typically included an initial contact session, followed by a home-based ecological assessment, and finally a feedback session emphasizing parenting strengths as well as possible areas of change. A total of 8 opportunities for feedback sessions were offered over the 8 years of the study. After feedback sessions each year, families were offered individualized parent training sessions, with 82.8% of families receiving an annual average of less than 3 hours of follow-up intervention services. The authors found intervention effects of Family Check Up on irritability at age 4 years, compared with baseline at age 2, which predicted lower externalizing and internalizing symptoms at 10.5 years of age.[62] Decreases in irritability at age 4 predicted long-term improvements in oppositional defiant disorder (ODD), generalized anxiety, and major depression at 10.5 years of age. These findings confirm that irritability in early childhood is a transdiagnostic risk indicator that can be used to identify children and families in need of intervention, and the Family Check Up may have salutary effects on long-term functional outcomes.[62]

Studies of youth at familial risk for bipolar disorder—who often present with depression, irritability, anxiety, and subthreshold manic states—indicate the benefits of early intervention in delaying progression to full-blown mood disorders. In a pilot randomized controlled trial of 40 high-risk youth, family-focused therapy for youth at high risk for bipolar disorder (FFT-HR), given during 12 sessions over 4 months, was found to hasten time to recovery from depressive symptoms and improve 1-year symptom trajectories compared with a brief educational control. In a more definitive 3-site trial of 127 high-risk youth, FFT-HR was associated with longer time to mood episodes, and specifically, longer well intervals before depressive episodes and lower levels of suicidal ideation and behavior when compared with standard psychoeducation of equal duration.[63–65] Youth who received FFT-HR also showed increased ventrolateral prefrontal and anterior default mode brain network connectivity from baseline to end of treatment compared with youth who received standard psychoeducation, demonstrating improved functional connectivity in emotion regulatory neural networks.[66] That neural plasticity in these networks preceded any observable mood outcome differences between treatment groups raises the intriguing possibility of neurobiological targeting to prevent mood progression. Time to conversion to bipolar I or II disorder over an average of 2 years of follow-up did not differ between FFT-HR and standard psychoeducation. Larger samples and longer follow-up might more definitively confirm the preventative potential of FFT-HR for mania onset or recurrence.[64]

In youth with depressive spectrum disorders and transient manic symptoms, Nadkarni and Fristad[67] found that immediate treatment with multifamily psychoeducation groups was associated with lower rates of conversion to subthreshold and full threshold bipolar spectrum disorders than a waitlist control. Further research is necessary to clarify the relation between changes in family functioning and changes in the course of illness among high-risk youth, who often present with multiple comorbid disorders and myriad subthreshold mood symptoms.

TERTIARY PREVENTION

For youth already struggling with significant and functionally impairing irritability and temper outbursts, tertiary prevention measures aim to reduce symptom severity and enhance psychosocial functioning. These children are commonly diagnosed with psychiatric disorders such as depression, ADHD, autism, DMDD, or other disruptive behavioral disorders (eg, conduct disorder or ODD). Given the variable contexts in which irritability and temper outbursts occur in these youth, the question arises as to whether emotion dysregulation is a manifestation of the same or distinct psychopathologies. Will the same intervention for chronic emotion dysregulation be efficacious across disorders despite differences in underlying etiologies, or should interventions be tailored to a specific disorder? The answers to these questions are not yet clear; therefore, we provide a cursory review of extant literature on tertiary prevention in the context of specific disorders. We focus on depression, ADHD, autism, and DMDD owing to their common association with irritability or temper outbursts, and defer to other articles in this volume for details.

Depression

Worsening irritability while on antidepressant treatment is associated with poorer outcomes and a decreased likelihood of remission.[68] Indeed, youth with depression and a family history of bipolar disorder may be particularly predisposed to antidepressant-related adverse events that include irritability and temper outbursts, underscoring the importance of assessing illness risk factors when weighing treatment benefits against risks.[69] In a study on depressed youth in remission after acute treatment with fluoxetine (12 weeks), higher levels of residual irritability, as well as insomnia were associated with increased odds of depressive relapse.[70] In contrast, higher levels of resilience, and in particular positive affectivity, were related to a lesser occurrence of residual symptoms after remission from depression.[71] Thus, targeting both risk factors for worsening irritability and predictors of residual symptoms early in treatment may decrease relapse rates or clinical worsening.

Attention Deficit Hyperactivity Disorder

Stimulants and behavioral treatment can improve irritability in ADHD.[72,73] However, even with optimally titrated first-line stimulant treatment, a subset of youth have persistent aggressive behavior, indicating disability beyond that of ADHD alone.[74] Indeed, emotion dysregulation is as much a feature of ADHD as of mood disorders.[75] Mood disorders comorbid with ADHD, ODD, or conduct disorder and with high levels of anger or irritability may benefit from risperidone or divalproex sodium augmentation.[74,76] The choice of agents is critical here[77,78]: recent meta-analyses of psychostimulant trials indicate that methylphenidate derivatives (eg, methylphenidate hydrochloride [Ritalin]) may be associated with decreased risk of irritability, whereas amphetamine derivatives (eg, amphetamine/dextroamphetamine [Adderall]) seem to be associated with increased risk of irritability.[77,78]

Aside from pharmacologic approaches, Hartman and colleagues[54] emphasize that assessing stressful conditions in a child's home should be integral to the diagnosis and treatment of ADHD. Specifically, cumulative high-stress exposure, including chronic illnesses in the child or immediate family member(s), academic pressure, problems at home or the neighborhood, unemployment, financial difficulties, having fewer friendships, being bullied, and having enduring conflicts, related strongly to a persistent course of ADHD with worsening irritability, anxiety, and depression.[12] The literature on specific interventions targeting irritability and temper outbursts in children exposed to early life stress or trauma is sparse, but may be benefited by effective treatment of a primary disruptive behavioral disorder.

Autism

Extensive literature has demonstrated the efficacy of pharmacologic treatment for irritability and aggression in autism, which may manifest as temper outbursts and self-injurious behaviors.[79] However, pharmacologic interventions do not address the underlying causes of irritability and temper outbursts in autism. Rather, contextual reasons for irritability in autism should be explored so that an appropriate evidence-based nonpharmacologic intervention can target those reasons. If this search strategy fails or if the magnitude of the irritability needs more urgent treatment, psychopharmacologic intervention may prove helpful. To clarify the stepwise guidelines for youth with autism and temper outbursts, a multidisciplinary workgroup has developed a practice pathway for pediatric primary care providers. This pathway emphasizes assessing contextual risk factors (eg, medical, functional communication challenges, psychosocial stressors, maladaptive reinforcement patterns, co-occurring psychiatric conditions) in each patient.[80] Appropriate treatment is then based on such contextual factors. For instance, irritability or temper outbursts arising from difficulties using functional communication should be followed up with speech and language evaluations, with the inclusion of a communication component in a behavior treatment plan. In contrast, irritability arising from psychosocial stressors, such as poor adjustment to classroom or program characteristics, would warrant communication with the school to address potential changes to the classroom or curriculum. If co-occurring psychiatric disorders are present, treatment with medications may then be considered.

Disruptive Mood Dysregulation Disorder

DMDD is characterized by recurrent temper outbursts in the context of ongoing depressed, anxious, or irritable moods. The current literature has primarily focused on psychopharmacologic treatments for DMDD. Open-label studies of methylphenidate with or without aripiprazole and combined with parent training have shown efficacy in improving irritability and other clinical symptoms (eg, emotional lability, negative affect, and anger) in DMDD and its related precursor severe mood dysregulation.[81,82] Exposure-based cognitive behavioral therapy in which youth with DMDD are exposed to frustrating situations is currently being evaluated. This treatment is theorized to engage cognitive control and top-down regulation of frustration to interrupt symptom reinforcement.[83] How to integrate and personalize pharmacologic and psychosocial treatments beyond treating readily identifiable psychiatric comorbidities is an unmet need in our field.

Given the high rates of comorbid psychopathology associated with DMDD (eg, ODD, ADHD, anxiety disorders),[84] other symptom dimensions often need intervention. One study in children with DMDD (with and without ADHD) found that an association between DMDD and sleep problems is mediated by their shared association with oppositional behaviors.[85] Thus, oppositional behaviors may need targeting before other symptoms such as sleep dysregulation are addressed. Building resilience through teaching emotion regulation skills, classically included in dialectical behavioral therapy (DBT), may decrease the frequency of temper outbursts and associated psychosocial impairments. A pilot randomized controlled trial of 43 children with DMDD (7–12 years old) demonstrated the feasibility and preliminary efficacy of DBT (adapted for preadolescents in 32 weekly 90-minute sessions) compared with a comparison group receiving individual therapy and medication management.[86] Notably, the DBT versus comparison group had higher response rates (90.4% vs 45.5%, respectively). Importantly, the improvements from DBT were achieved without a need to start new psychiatric medications. The efficacy of DBT for decreasing DMDD behaviors should be further tested in randomized controlled trials that include manualized, equally intensive comparison treatments.

SUMMARY

Chronic irritability and temper outbursts—both indicators of emotional dysregulation—are transdiagnostic constructs that can significantly disrupt achievement of typical developmental milestones and result in psychopathology and impairment. An evidence base for early interventions is scarce, but the need to identify at-risk children and intervene early to promote positive neurodevelopmental outcomes cannot be understated. Wakschlag and colleagues,[87] in their translational road map entitled *Mental Health, Earlier*, recommend primary care screening of irritability as a risk factor for lifelong mental health problems, and low intensity interventions to promote self-regulation within an implementation science framework.

More research is needed to determine whether irritability and temper outbursts are disorder specific or share common neurobiological underpinnings. Primary prevention strategies can intervene at the level of the parent (eg, targeting parental mental health and parenting skills), the child (eg, targeting affective instability, self-esteem and self-compassion), and the community (eg, after school programs for at-risk youth to promote socioemotional learning, gun control, and violence prevention programs). Secondary prevention strategies might focus on intervening on family systems and effecting positive changes in the course of high-risk syndromes. Accelerating biomarker discovery and investigating clinically meaningful treatment targets and mechanisms would support the development of novel tertiary prevention strategies to reduce symptom burden and impairment. A research agenda focused on identifying interventions in the context of primary, secondary, and tertiary prevention of chronic irritability and temper outbursts will be essential to promoting resilience and reducing risks of lifelong psychopathology.

DISCLOSURE

Dr M.K. Singh has received research support from Stanford's Maternal Child Health Research Institute and the Department of Psychiatry, National Institute of Mental Health, National Institute on Aging, Johnson and Johnson, Allergan, and the Brain and Behavior Foundation. She is on the advisory board for Sunovion, has been a consultant for X: The moonshot factory (Alphabet Inc), and Limbix, and receives royalties from the American Psychiatric Association Publishing. Dr D.J. Miklowitz has received grant funding from the National Institute of Mental Health (NIMH), the Danny Alberts Foundation, the Attias Family Foundation, the Carl and Roberta Deutsch Foundation, the Kayne Family Foundation, the Jewish Foundation of Los Angeles, AIM for Youth Mental Health, and the Max Gray Fund; and book royalties from Guilford Press and John Wiley and Sons.

REFERENCES

1. Dougherty LR, Smith VC, Bufferd SJ, et al. Disruptive mood dysregulation disorder at the age of 6 years and clinical and functional outcomes 3 years later. Psychol Med 2016;46(5):1103–14.
2. Wesselhoeft R, Stringaris A, Sibbersen C, et al. Dimensions and subtypes of oppositionality and their relation to comorbidity and psychosocial characteristics. Eur Child Adolesc Psychiatry 2019;28(3):351–65.
3. Stringaris A, Vidal-Ribas P, Brotman MA, et al. Practitioner review: definition, recognition, and treatment challenges of irritability in young people. J Child Psychol Psychiatry 2018;59(7):721–39.
4. Eyre O, Riglin L, Leibenluft E, et al. Irritability in ADHD: association with later depression symptoms. Eur Child Adolesc Psychiatry 2019;28(10):1375–84.
5. Benarous X, Consoli A, Cohen D, et al. Suicidal behaviors and irritability in children and adolescents: a systematic review of the nature and mechanisms of the association. Eur Child Adolesc Psychiatry 2019;28(5):667–83.

6. American Psychiatric Association. Diagnostic and statistical manual of mental disorders. 5th edition. Arlington (VA): American Psychiatric Association; 2013.

7. Riglin L, Eyre O, Thapar AK, et al. Identifying novel types of irritability using a developmental genetic approach. Am J Psychiatry 2019;176(8):635–42.

8. Leibenluft E, Cohen P, Gorrindo T, et al. Chronic versus episodic irritability in youth: a community-based, longitudinal study of clinical and diagnostic associations. J Child Adolesc Psychopharmacol 2006;16(4):456–66.

9. Blader JC, Pliszka SR, Kafantaris V, et al. Prevalence and treatment outcomes of persistent negative mood among children with attention-deficit/hyperactivity disorder and aggressive behavior. J Child Adolesc Psychopharmacol 2016;26(2):164–73.

10. Mayes SD, Mathiowetz C, Kokotovich C, et al. Stability of disruptive mood dysregulation disorder symptoms (irritable-angry mood and temper outbursts) throughout childhood and adolescence in a general population sample. J Abnorm Child Psychol 2015;43(8):1543–9.

11. Evans SC, Burke JD, Roberts MC, et al. Irritability in child and adolescent psychopathology: an integrative review for ICD-11. Clin Psychol Rev 2017;53:29–45.

12. Hartman CA, Rommelse N, van der Klugt CL, et al. Stress exposure and the course of ADHD from childhood to young adulthood: comorbid severe emotion dysregulation or mood and anxiety problems. J Clin Med 2019;8(11):1824.

13. Masten AS. Resilience theory and research on children and families: past, present, and promise. J Fam Theory Rev 2018;10(1):12–31.

14. Fergus S, Zimmerman MA. Adolescent resilience: a framework for understanding healthy development in the face of risk. Annu Rev Public Health 2005;26:399–419.

15. Goodman R. Psychometric properties of the strengths and difficulties questionnaire. J Am Acad Child Adolesc Psychiatry 2001;40(11):1337–45.

16. Wilson DS, O'Brien DT, Sesma A. Human prosociality from an evolutionary perspective: variation and correlations at a city-wide scale. Evol Hum Behav 2009;30(3):190–200.

17. Padilla-Walker LM, Memmott-Elison MK, Coyne SM. Associations between prosocial and problem behavior from early to late adolescence. J Youth Adolesc 2018;47(5):961–75.

18. Jung J, Schröder-Abé M. Prosocial behavior as a protective factor against peers' acceptance of aggression in the development of aggressive behavior in childhood and adolescence. J Adolesc 2019;74:146–53.

19. Huang S, Han M, Sun L, et al. Family socioeconomic status and emotional adaptation among rural-to-urban migrant adolescents in China: the moderating roles of adolescent's resilience and parental positive emotion. Int J Psychol 2019;54(5):573–81.

20. Poole JC, Dobson KS, Pusch D. Anxiety among adults with a history of childhood adversity: psychological resilience moderates the indirect effect of emotion dysregulation. J Affect Disord 2017;217:144–52.

21. Gartland D, Riggs E, Muyeen S, et al. What factors are associated with resilient outcomes in children exposed to social adversity? A systematic review. BMJ Open 2019;9(4):e024870.

22. Frazier SL, Dinizulu SM, Rusch D, et al. Building Resilience After School for Early Adolescents in Urban Poverty: Open Trial of Leaders @ Play. Adm Policy Ment Health 2015;42:723–36.

23. Carlson GA, Chua J, Pan K, et al. Behavior modification is associated with reduced psychotropic medication use in children with aggression in inpatient

treatment: a retrospective cohort study. J Am Acad Child Adolesc Psychiatry 2020;59(5):632–41.e4.

24. Schäfer JÖ, Naumann E, Holmes EA, et al. Emotion regulation strategies in depressive and anxiety symptoms in youth: a meta-analytic review. J Youth Adolesc 2017;46(2):261–76.

25. Trompetter HR, de Kleine E, Bohlmeijer ET. Why does positive mental health buffer against psychopathology? An exploratory study on self-compassion as a resilience mechanism and adaptive emotion regulation strategy. Cognit Ther Res 2017;41(3):459–68.

26. Wu Q, Slesnick N, Murnan A, et al. Understanding parenting stress and children's behavior problems among homeless, substance-abusing mothers. Infant Ment Health 2018;39:423–31.

27. Ramakrishnan JL, Masten AS. Mastery motivation and school readiness among young children experiencing homelessness. Am J Orthopsychiatry 2020;90(2): 223–35.

28. Caiozzo CN, Yule K, Grych J. Caregiver behaviors associated with emotion regulation in high-risk preschoolers. J Fam Psychol 2018;32(5):565–74.

29. Kaufman EA, Puzia ME, Mead HK, et al. Children's emotion regulation difficulties mediate the association between maternal borderline and antisocial symptoms and youth behavior problems over 1 year. J Pers Disord 2017;31(2):170–92.

30. Rappaport LM, Carney DM, Brotman MA, et al. A population-based twin study of childhood irritability and internalizing syndromes. J Clin Child Adolesc Psychol 2020;49(4):524–34.

31. Roberson-Nay R, Leibenluft E, Brotman MA, et al. Longitudinal stability of genetic and environmental influences on irritability: from childhood to young adulthood. Am J Psychiatry 2015;172(7):657–64.

32. Blair C, Zelazo PD, Greenberg MT. The measurement of executive function in early childhood. Dev Neuropsychol 2005;28(2):561–71.

33. Leibenluft E. Pediatric irritability: a systems neuroscience approach. Trends Cogn Sci 2017;21(4):277–89.

34. Wakschlag LS, Perlman SB, Blair RJ, et al. The neurodevelopmental basis of early childhood disruptive behavior: irritable and callous phenotypes as exemplars. Am J Psychiatry 2018;175(2):114–30.

35. Kisling LA, Das J M. Prevention strategies. In: StatPearls. StatPearls Publishing; 2020.

36. Brody JL, Scherer DG, Turner CW, et al. A conceptual model and clinical framework for integrating mindfulness into family therapy with adolescents. Fam Process 2018;57(2):510–24.

37. Wu Q, Slesnick N, Murnan A. Understanding parenting stress and children's behavior problems among homeless, substance-abusing mothers. Infant Ment Health J 2018;39(4):423–31.

38. Weissman MM, Pilowsky DJ, Wickramaratne PJ, et al. Remissions in maternal depression and child psychopathology: a STAR*D-child report. JAMA 2006; 295(12):1389–98.

39. Weissman MM, Wickramaratne P, Pilowsky DJ, et al. Treatment of maternal depression in a medication clinical trial and its effect on children. Am J Psychiatry 2015;172(5):450–9.

40. Zalewski M, Lewis JK, Martin CG. Identifying novel applications of dialectical behavior therapy: considering emotion regulation and parenting. Curr Opin Psychol 2018;21:122–6.

41. Watson D, Clark LA, Tellegen A. Development and validation of brief measures of positive and negative affect: the PANAS scales. J Pers Soc Psychol 1988;54(6): 1063–70.

42. Buckner JC, Mezzacappa E, Beardslee WR. Characteristics of resilient youths living in poverty: the role of self-regulatory processes. Dev Psychopathol 2003; 15(1):139–62.

43. West AE, Schenkel LS, Pavuluri MN. Early childhood temperament in pediatric bipolar disorder and attention deficit hyperactivity disorder. J Clin Psychol 2008; 64(4):402–21.

44. Akiskal HS, Hirschfeld RMA, Yerevanian BI. The relationship of personality to affective disorders: a critical review. Arch Gen Psychiatry 1983;40(7):801–10.

45. Biederman J, Hirshfeld-Becker DR, Rosenbaum JF, et al. Further evidence of association between behavioral inhibition and social anxiety in children. Am J Psychiatry 2001;158(10):1673–9.

46. Krueger RF, Hicks BM, Patrick CJ, et al. Etiologic connections among substance dependence, antisocial behavior, and personality: modeling the externalizing spectrum. J Abnorm Psychol 2002;111(3):411–24.

47. Pisecco S, Baker DB, Silva PA, et al. Boys with reading disabilities and/or ADHD: distinctions in early childhood. J Learn Disabil 2001;34(2):98–106.

48. Klein DN, Finsaas MC. The stony brook temperament study: early antecedents and pathways to emotional disorders. Child Dev Perspect 2017;11(4):257–63.

49. Van Lissa CJ, Hawk ST, Koot HM, et al. The cost of empathy: parent-adolescent conflict predicts emotion dysregulation for highly empathic youth. Dev Psychol 2017;53(9):1722–37.

50. Vannucci A, Finan L, Ohannessian CM, et al. Protective factors associated with daily affective reactivity and instability during adolescence. J Youth Adolesc 2019;48(4):771–87.

51. Leary MR, Baumeister RF. The nature and function of self-esteem: sociometer theory. In: Zanna MP, editor. Advances in experimental social psychology, vol. 32. Cambridge (MA): Academic Press; 2000. p. 1–62.

52. Arslan G. Psychological maltreatment, emotional and behavioral problems in adolescents: the mediating role of resilience and self-esteem. Child Abuse Negl 2016;52:200–9.

53. Dang MT. Social connectedness and self-esteem: predictors of resilience in mental health among maltreated homeless youth. Issues Ment Health Nurs 2014;35(3):212–9.

54. Hartman CA, Rommelse N, van der Klugt CL, et al. Stress Exposure and the Course of ADHD from Childhood to Young Adulthood: Comorbid Severe Emotion Dysregulation or Mood and Anxiety Problems. J Clin Med 2019.

55. Hipson WE, Gardiner SL, Coplan RJ, et al. Maternal agreeableness moderates associations between young children's emotion dysregulation and socioemotional functioning at school. J Genet Psychol 2017;178(2):102–7.

56. McCrae RR, Costa PT. Validation of the five-factor model of personality across instruments and observers. J Pers Soc Psychol 1987;52(1):81–90.

57. Schönfelder S, Kanske P, Heissler J, et al. Time course of emotion-related responding during distraction and reappraisal. Soc Cogn Affect Neurosci 2014; 9(9):1310–9.

58. Sheppes G, Scheibe S, Suri G, et al. Emotion regulation choice: a conceptual framework and supporting evidence. J Exp Psychol Gen 2014;143(1):163–81.

59. Alkoby A, Pliskin R, Halperin E, et al. An eight-week mindfulness-based stress reduction (MBSR) workshop increases regulatory choice flexibility. Emotion 2019;19(4):593–604.

60. Biglan A. The nurture effect: how the science of human behavior can improve our lives and our world. Oakland (CA): New Harbinger Publications; 2015. p. xii, 253.

61. Flückiger C, Rubel J, Del Re AC, et al. The reciprocal relationship between alliance and early treatment symptoms: a two-stage individual participant data meta-analysis. J Consult Clin Psychol 2020;88(9):829–43.

62. Smith JD, Wakschlag L, Krogh-Jespersen S, et al. Dysregulated irritability as a window on young children's psychiatric risk: transdiagnostic effects via the family check-up. Dev Psychopathol 2019;31(5):1887–99.

63. Miklowitz DJ, Schneck CD, Singh MK, et al. Early intervention for symptomatic youth at risk for bipolar disorder: a randomized trial of family-focused therapy. J Am Acad Child Adolesc Psychiatry 2013;52(2):121–31.

64. Miklowitz DJ, Schneck CD, Walshaw PD, et al. Effects of family-focused therapy vs enhanced usual care for symptomatic youths at high risk for bipolar disorder: a randomized clinical trial. JAMA Psychiatry 2020;77(5):455–63.

65. Miklowitz DJ, Merranko JA, Weintraub MJ, et al. Effects of family-focused therapy on suicidal ideation and behavior in youth at high risk for bipolar disorder. J Affect Disord 2020;275:14–22.

66. Singh MK, Nimarko AF, Garrett AS, et al. Changes in intrinsic brain connectivity in family-focused therapy versus standard psychoeducation among youths at high risk for bipolar disorder. J Am Acad Child Adolesc Psychiatry 2021;60(4):458–69.

67. Nadkarni RB, Fristad MA. Clinical course of children with a depressive spectrum disorder and transient manic symptoms. Bipolar Disord 2010;12(5):494–503.

68. Jha MK, Minhajuddin A, South C, et al. Worsening anxiety, irritability, insomnia, or panic predicts poorer antidepressant treatment outcomes: clinical utility and validation of the concise associated symptom tracking (CAST) scale. Int J Neuropsychopharmacol 2018;21(4):325–32.

69. Angal S, DelBello M, Zalpuri I, et al. Clinical conundrum: how do you treat youth with depression and a family history of bipolar disorder? Bipolar Disord 2019; 21(4):383–6.

70. Kennard BD, Mayes TL, Chahal Z, et al. Predictors and moderators of relapse in children and adolescents with major depressive disorder. J Clin Psychiatry 2018; 79(2):15m10330.

71. Hoorelbeke K, Van den Bergh N, Wichers M, et al. Between vulnerability and resilience: a network analysis of fluctuations in cognitive risk and protective factors following remission from depression. Behav Res Ther 2019;116:1–9.

72. Fernández de la Cruz L, Simonoff E, McGough JJ, et al. Treatment of children with attention-deficit/hyperactivity disorder (ADHD) and irritability: results from the multimodal treatment study of children with ADHD (MTA). J Am Acad Child Adolesc Psychiatry 2015;54(1):62–70.e3.

73. Galanter CA, Pagar DL, Davies M, et al. ADHD and manic symptoms: diagnostic and treatment implications. Clin Neurosci Res 2005;5(5):283–94.

74. Blader JC, Pliszka SR, Kafantaris V, et al. Stepped treatment for attention-deficit/hyperactivity disorder and aggressive behavior: a randomized, controlled trial of adjunctive risperidone, divalproex sodium, or placebo after stimulant medication optimization. J Am Acad Child Adolesc Psychiatry 2021;60(2):236–51.

75. Marwaha S, He Z, Broome M, et al. How is affective instability defined and measured? A systematic review. Psychol Med 2014;44(9):1793–808.

76. Farmer CA, Brown NV, Gadow KD, et al. Comorbid symptomatology moderates response to risperidone, stimulant, and parent training in children with severe aggression, disruptive behavior disorder, and attention-deficit/hyperactivity disorder. J Child Adolesc Psychopharmacol 2015;25(3):213–24.
77. Pozzi M, Carnovale C, Peeters GGAM, et al. Adverse drug events related to mood and emotion in paediatric patients treated for ADHD: a meta-analysis. J Affect Disord 2018;238:161–78.
78. Stuckelman ZD, Mulqueen JM, Ferracioli-Oda E, et al. Risk of irritability with psychostimulant treatment in children with ADHD: a meta-analysis. J Clin Psychiatry 2017;78(6):e648–55.
79. Fung LK, Mahajan R, Nozzolillo A, et al. Pharmacologic treatment of severe irritability and problem behaviors in autism: a systematic review and meta-analysis. Pediatrics 2016;137(Suppl 2):S124–35.
80. McGuire K, Fung LK, Hagopian L, et al. Irritability and problem behavior in autism spectrum disorder: a practice pathway for pediatric primary care. Pediatrics 2016;137(Suppl 2):S136–48.
81. Winters DE, Fukui S, Leibenluft E, et al. Improvements in irritability with open-label methylphenidate treatment in youth with comorbid attention deficit/hyperactivity disorder and disruptive mood dysregulation disorder. J Child Adolesc Psychopharmacol 2018;28(5):298–305.
82. Pan P-Y, Fu A-T, Yeh C-B. Aripiprazole/methylphenidate combination in children and adolescents with disruptive mood dysregulation disorder and attention-deficit/hyperactivity disorder: an open-label study. J Child Adolesc Psychopharmacol 2018;28(10):682–9.
83. Kircanski K, Craske MG, Averbeck BB, et al. Exposure therapy for pediatric irritability: theory and potential mechanisms. Behav Res Ther 2019;118:141–9.
84. Leibenluft E. Severe mood dysregulation, irritability, and the diagnostic boundaries of bipolar disorder in youths. Am J Psychiatry 2011;168(2):129–42.
85. Waxmonsky JG, Mayes SD, Calhoun SL, et al. The association between disruptive mood dysregulation disorder symptoms and sleep problems in children with and without ADHD. Sleep Med 2017;37:180–6.
86. Perepletchikova F, Nathanson D, Axelrod SR, et al. Randomized clinical trial of dialectical behavior therapy for preadolescent children with disruptive mood dysregulation disorder: feasibility and outcomes. J Am Acad Child Adolesc Psychiatry 2017;56(10):832–40.
87. Wakschlag LS, Roberts MY, Flynn RM, et al. Future directions for early childhood prevention of mental disorders: a road map to mental health, earlier. J Clin Child Adolesc Psychol 2019;48(3):539–54.

Psychoeducational and Skill-building Interventions for Emotion Dysregulation

Taban Salem, PhD[a], Kimberly A. Walters, PhD[b],
Joseph S. Verducci, PhD[c], Mary A. Fristad, PhD[d,e,*]

KEYWORDS

- Psychoeducation • Emotion dysregulation • Depression • Bipolar disorder
- Disruptive behavior • Children • Family therapy • Psychotherapy

KEY POINTS

- Family psychoeducation plus skill building is a class of interventions considered to be well-established for youth with mood disorders/emotion dysregulation.
- Psychoeducational psychotherapy (PEP) is 1 of 3 well-tested examples of family psychoeducation plus skill building.
- PEP is family-based and incorporates psychoeducation and skill building.
- PEP helps reduce rage, mood symptoms, disruptive behavior, and executive functioning deficits.
- PEP may improve functioning and increase appropriate service utilization for years after initial treatment.

Family conflict is a major risk factor for depression and bipolar disorder in children and adolescents; likewise, depressive and manic symptoms in youth can lead to poorer parent-child relationships.[1,2] For example, a 2-year study that examined family functioning and mood symptoms in adolescents with bipolar disorder found longitudinal relationships between youth's depressive symptoms and family cohesion, adaptability, and conflict; furthermore, decreases in parent-child conflict predicted decreases in youth's manic symptoms.[2] Clinical and population-based studies show

[a] Department of Psychology and Neuroscience, Millsaps College, 1701 North State Street, Jackson, MS 39210, USA; [b] Statistics Collaborative, Inc., 1625 Massachusetts Avenue NQ, Suite 600, Washington, DC 20036, USA; [c] Department of Statistics, The Ohio State University, 404 Cockins Hall, 1458 Neil Avenue, Columbus, OH 43210, USA; [d] Department of Psychiatry and Behavioral Health, The Ohio State University Wexner Medical Center, Harding Hospital, Suite 460H, 1670 Upham Drive, Columbus, OH 43210, USA; [e] Nationwide Children's Hospital Behavioral Health Pavilion, 444 Butterfly Gardens Drive #3207, Columbus, OH 43215, USA
* Corresponding author. Nationwide Children's Hospital, Behavioral Health Pavilion, 444 Butterfly Gardens Drive #3207, Columbus, OH 43215, USA.
E-mail address: Mary.Fristad@nationwidechildrens.org

Child Adolesc Psychiatric Clin N Am 30 (2021) 611–622
https://doi.org/10.1016/j.chc.2021.04.010
1056-4993/21/© 2021 Elsevier Inc. All rights reserved.

links between family conflict and suicidal ideation and behavior in youth.[3,4] Additionally, positive parent-child relationships can buffer against the negative impact of peer stress and help to build a child's resilience.[5]

Thus, a family-based approach to intervention for youth with emotion dysregulation is a logical strategy. For the purposes of this article, emotion dysregulation refers to the inability to manage the frequency, intensity, and/or duration of irritable, sad, angry, or fearful emotions. In this context, emotion dysregulation includes but is not limited to symptoms occurring as part of a manic, or depressive or mixed episode, and frequently is accompanied by dysregulated (eg, aggressive or withdrawn) behavior.

Family psychoeducation plus skill building is a class of interventions that is considered well-established for youth with mood disorders.[6] These interventions share 3 common elements: (1) they are family-based; (2) they include psychoeducation on symptoms and their management; and (3) they include skills training for youth and parents. Three examples of this class are family-focused treatment,[7,8] child and family–focused cognitive-behavior therapy,[9,10] and psychoeducational psychotherapy (PEP).[11] These 3 manualized interventions all have been tested in randomized controlled trials (RCTs) with improvements demonstrated both in child and family outcomes. All 3 capitalize on the importance of the family system and incorporate psychoeducation on mood disorders and their treatments tailored to parents and youth, cognitive-behavior–focused skill building to help youth learn to better manage and control their mood symptoms, and strategies for parents to better facilitate school-based interventions, develop specific symptom management techniques, and generate coping strategies for the entire family.

Although each of these 3 interventions has unique aspects, their similarities far exceed their differences. This article focuses on 1 of these 3 interventions, PEP, to illustrate the utility of psychoeducation plus skill building in improving emotion regulation. An overview of PEP is provided, which can be delivered in a multifamily (MF-PEP) group format or to individual families (IF-PEP).[11] Evidence then is presented of PEP's efficacy, including novel findings from secondary analyses of an RCT of MF-PEP showing specific benefits for reducing irritability and aggressive behavior. Results from long-term follow-up of IF-PEP participants are discussed[12], along with possible mechanisms of action that may account for sustained improvements in functioning following PEP for emotion dysregulation.

PSYCHOEDUCATIONAL PSYCHOTHERAPY OVERVIEW

PEP was designed to treat children with bipolar and depressive spectrum disorders—these children often experience severe impairment due to emotion dysregulation, executive functioning deficits, and disruptive behavior.[11] IF-PEP and MF-PEP are similar in their content, structure, and goals (Table 1). IF-PEP includes alternating parent sessions and child sessions, whereas MF-PEP sessions begin and end with children and parents together while the majority of each session is held separately for children and parents (see Table 1). IF-PEP covers certain topics in more detail and allows greater flexibility to modify sessions to meet a family's needs. MF-PEP adheres to a specific schedule, because multiple families' needs are taken into consideration. Although less flexible, MF-PEP has an added benefit of peer support—children with emotion dysregulation and their parents are able to meet other families going through similar struggles.

Every PEP session begins with a check-in regarding the child's/family's past week and a review of take-home projects assigned in the previous session(s). Child sessions begin with parents present so that the therapist can check in with children and parents

Table 1
Psychoeducational psychotherapy session order, attendees, and main topics

Attendees/ Session Number	Session Topics and Goals (Each Session Includes Deep Breathing Practice)
Child session IF-PEP 1 MF-PEP 1	Mood disorders and symptoms • Introduce the child to PEP. • Help the child recognize mood symptoms in general. • Help the child recognize and rate his/her own mood and other symptoms. • Learn the motto (it's not your fault, but it's your challenge). • Set personalized treatment goals.
Parent session IF-PEP 1 MF-PEP 1	Mood disorders and symptoms • Introduce general framework of PEP. • Help parents recognize mood symptoms, especially their child's symptoms. • Give parents hope and motivate them to work hard in PEP. • Learn to chart mood symptoms.
Child session IF-PEP 2 MF-PEP 2	Treatment, including medications • Help the child separate symptoms from self. • Educate the child about treatment, the treatment team, and his/her role on team. • Educate the child about medications.
Parent session IF-PEP 2 MF-PEP 2	Treatment, including medications • Help parents use cost-benefit analysis to make medication decisions. • Overview of medications used to treat mood symptoms—classes, symptom targets, and common side effects.
Child session IF-PEP 3	Healthy habits • Teach the importance of healthy sleeping, eating, and exercise in mood regulation. • Explain how to improve healthy habits. • Help the child select healthy habit priorities to address.
Parent session IF-PEP 3 MF-PEP 3	Mental health services/school services • Give parents an overview of the mental health system, range of mental health professionals, and ways to access different services. • Give parents an overview of educational services for special needs children, who's who in the school system, and ways to build a coalition with the school.
Child session IF-PEP 4 MF-PEP 3	Building a coping tool kit • Help the child identify situations that trigger difficult emotions. • Help the child recognize bodily signals for strong emotions. • Guide the child to developing a list of strategies for coping with feeling mad, sad, or bad.
Parent session IF-PEP 4 MF-PEP 4	Negative family cycles and thinking, feeling, and doing • Increase parents' awareness of how negative family cycles play out in their own family. • Help parents understand how thoughts, feelings, and actions interact in negative cycles and how shifting to more helpful thoughts and actions can improve family functioning.
Child session IF-PEP 5 MF-PEP 4	Thinking, feeling, and doing • Teach the child the difference between helpful and hurtful thoughts,and the ways that thoughts can affect feelings. • Teach the child how to use thoughts and actions to manage difficult feelings.

(*continued on next page*)

Attendees/ Session Number	Session Topics and Goals (Each Session Includes Deep Breathing Practice)
Table 1 *(continued)*	
Parent session IF-PEP 5 MF-PEP 5	Problem solving • Develop parents' problem-solving skills. • Enhance parents' coping skills.
Child session IF-PEP 6 MF-PEP 5	Problem solving • Teach the child the steps of problem solving and ways these can be used to navigate daily challenges.
Parent session IF-PEP 6	Revisiting mental health/school issues and services • See IF-PEP parent session 3.
Child session IF-PEP 7	Revisiting healthy habits • See IF-PEP child session 3.
Parent session IF-PEP 7	School issues (meeting with school personnel) • Improve communication between parents and school personnel. • Develop or enhance school accommodations and/or services.
Child session IF-PEP 8 MF-PEP 6	Nonverbal communication skills • Define "communication" for the child and introduce the 4 steps of the communication cycle. • Increase the child's awareness of his/her own nonverbal communication. • Increase the child's awareness of nonverbal communication in others.
Parent session IF-PEP 8 MF-PEP 6	Improving communication • Improve communication within the family. • Help parents identify hurtful communications and replace these with more helpful communication strategies.
Child session IF-PEP 9 MF-PEP 7	Verbal communication skills • Help the child recognize components of effective verbal communication.
Parent session IF-PEP 9 MF-PEP 7	Symptom and crisis management • Help parents develop strategies to manage mood symptoms and plan for crises. • Help parents develop stress management strategies for themselves. • Prepare for sibling session (IF-PEP). • Plan any additional (in-the-bank) sessions (IF-PEP).
Parent/sibling session IF-PEP 10	Sibling session • Listen to and validate siblings' questions and concerns. • Provide psychoeducation about mood disorders and mood symptoms. • Identify concerns that can be addressed by parents.
Child and parents session IF-PEP 10 MF-PEP 8	Wrap-up/graduation. • Address lingering questions and concerns • Review important PEP lessons.

together. New material is presented via didactics, discussion, handouts, worksheets, and in-session activities. In each session, children practice breathing exercises as an emotion regulation skill, and parents and children are given take-home projects to help them apply newly learned emotion regulation skills to their daily lives. Child sessions end with parents rejoining the child, who is encouraged to share the lesson of the day, the breathing exercise, and project of the week.

Psychoeducation About Mood Disorders and Symptoms

PEP begins by introducing children and parents to the program and providing evidence-based psychoeducation about mood symptoms and disorders. Therapists explain to children that PEP is designed to help them understand how they feel and to develop strategies to manage their challenging feelings. Children are taught to identify and rate the intensity of different feelings and to recognize when feelings become so intense that they enter the "danger zone," where feelings and actions can get out of control. They learn the motto, "it's not your fault, but it's your challenge." The message that they are not to blame for their feelings is both comforting and lays the groundwork for children to develop skills to manage their behavior when they experience intense feelings. Children generate a personal "fix-it list" of problems they would like to work on in PEP.

In a parallel session, parents receive an overview of PEP and information about mood symptoms and disorders. A biopsychosocial framework is utilized, which acknowledges the role of biological factors in developing emotion dysregulation but emphasizes that symptoms can be influenced by environmental stressors, behavioral patterns and habits, and family interactions. This is a counterpart to the children's motto and serves to reduce stigma, blame, and guilt surrounding childhood emotion dysregulation, while also empowering and motivating families to make positive changes and to seek appropriate services and supports. Parents are taught how to keep a mood record of their child's mood symptoms, and they begin the ongoing project of creating and updating parent and family fix-it lists, which are revisited periodically throughout PEP to evaluate progress.

Psychoeducation About Treatment, Including Medications

Children complete a "symptom-self" exercise, in which they first list their positive characteristics then list their mood and comorbid symptoms, as a means to externalize their symptoms, rather than thinking of them as their own personal characteristics. Treatment is described as a way to put their symptoms literally behind them while they let the "real me" show. Treatment modalities, including therapy, school-based support, and medication, are discussed. In their session, parents receive an overview of types of treatment, in particular medication, with an emphasis on how to use cost-benefit analysis to make decisions about medication, monitor treatment response, and communicate effectively with the treatment team to optimize pharmacotherapy.

Building Healthy Habits

PEP addresses the importance of sleep hygiene, healthy eating habits, and regular exercise in promoting mood stability and healthy coping. Therapists describe what healthy habits look like in each domain and then children pick which of these habits to improve upon. Parents are included in problem-solving the pragmatic steps needed to improve healthy habits during initial check-ins and session reviews, but psychoeducation in this domain is focused on children to increase their buy-in and prevent parent-child conflict around making changes.

Psychoeducation About Mental Health and School-based Services

Parents learn about possible components of their child's mental health and school-based treatment teams. PEP also provides parents with a review of various types of school-based services, steps for building a coalition with the school, seeking specific services, and strategies to improve communication and problem solving between parents and school personnel. In addition to decreasing frustration for parents, developing more appropriate school-based services is anticipated to aid the child in successfully engaging in emotion regulation strategies learned in therapy.

Building a Coping Tool Kit

Children are guided to identify triggers that lead to feeling anxious, irritable, angry, or sad. They list physical sensations that accompany "mad," "sad," and "bad" feelings as well as the actions they tend to take when they feel negative emotions. Therapists coach children to evaluate actions by asking: (1) "Does it hurt me?" (2) "Does it hurt someone or something else?" and (3) "Does it get anyone in trouble?" Children work with their therapist to compile tool kits and coping strategies that can be utilized under a variety of circumstances. Between sessions, children and their parents assemble these tool kits with tangible objects (eg, coloring pages and a bottle of bubble bath) and representational objects (eg, photos and phone numbers) to help them cope with negative emotions.

Negative Family Cycles and Thinking, Feeling, and Doing

Parents learn about the typical negative family cycle that occurs when families are dealing with a child's emotion dysregulation: the child becomes upset, the family tries various strategies to change the child's mood/behavior, but those strategies often are ineffective, which causes an escalation of negative emotion in both the child and other family members and often leads to parental conflict. Psychoeducation helps parents understand how a child's emotion dysregulation places stress on families (ie, through unpredictability, failure to meet family expectations and responsibilities, social failures, dangerous or violent outbursts, and disengagement or withdrawal). They learn about the role of thoughts in negative cycles and ways of breaking negative cycles by thinking and doing things differently—using positive strategies—not necessarily by doing more. In the corresponding child session, the cognitive component of cognitive-behavior treatment is added to the prior session's foundation in behavioral intervention. Children learn that actively choosing different actions and thoughts can change their feelings.

Problem Solving

The theme of breaking negative family cycles is carried forward through the next session, which focuses on teaching parents problem-solving and basic coping skills. Standard problem-solving steps are taught, with an emphasis on who in the family should be involved with generating, testing, and evaluating possible solutions. In a parallel session, children learn to problem solve using the steps, stop, think, plan, do, and check.

Improving Communication Through Nonverbal and Verbal Communication Skills

Communication is addressed in 1-parent and 1-child sessions. For children, fundamentals of effective communication are made explicit, because children with mood disorders are prone to misreading nonverbal cues[13] as well as to using indirect, masked, inflammatory, or otherwise unclear language to convey their thoughts and feelings. Children practice conveying varying emotions as well as clear, direct communication both in session and at home with parents. Parents are coached similarly to recognize and replace "hurtful" with "helpful" communication, thereby turning negative communication cycles into positive cycles.

Symptom and Crisis Management

The symptom and crisis management session helps parents develop strategies to manage specific mood symptoms (eg, identifying early and later stages of a manic episode, creating a safety plan, and responding to suicidal threats), acknowledge the needs of all family members, and manage their own stress. If families in IF-PEP wish to have a sibling session, they can plan for it during this session (ie, establish goals, determine who will attend, and determine how to prepare the children for the session).

Sibling Involvement

Siblings of children with emotion dysregulation experience stress due to the direct effects of their sibling's symptoms and behaviors as well as indirect effects on family relationships, such as reduced time and attention that parents have to devote to other children in the household. Thus, IF-PEP includes a session focused on siblings, with goals of helping parents learn about and validate siblings' concerns, providing siblings with psychoeducation about mood disorders, ensuring siblings' safety during crises, and increasing support for siblings' needs.

EFFICACY OF MULTIFAMILY–PSYCHOEDUCATIONAL PSYCHOTHERAPY

Two RCTs of MF-PEP as an adjunct to usual care have been conducted for children aged 8 to 12 with depressive or bipolar spectrum disorders, a pilot study followed by the main study. In the pilot RCT, 35 children and their parents were assigned to either immediate MF-PEP (IMM) or a 6-month waitlist control (WLC) condition, with all participants also receiving treatment as usual (TAU).[14–16] In comparison to WLC, MF-PEP significantly increased parental knowledge about mood disorders and treatments, increased children's perceptions of social support from both parents and peers, and increased appropriate utilization of mental health and school-based services.

In the main RCT (clinicaltrials.gov NCT00050557), 165 children and their parents were randomized to IMM or a 12-month WLC, with assessments at baseline (T1) and again at 6 months (T2), 12 months (T3), and 18 (T4) months.[17,18] Families randomized to the IMM condition participated in MF-PEP in the first 6 months of the study (ie, between T1 and T2), whereas MF-PEP took place between 12 (T3) and 18 (T4) months for those in the WLC condition. Detailed study procedures, including the Consort diagram, are described elsewhere.[18] Children assigned to IMM showed significantly greater decreases in mood symptoms over a 1-year follow-up period than did children assigned to WLC.[18] Moreover, children with greater baseline functional impairment, higher levels of stress, and more historical exposure to traumatic events (which are not directly addressed in PEP but nonetheless moderated response) benefitted the most from MF-PEP.[19] MF-PEP also produced small to medium reductions in disruptive behaviors; parents of children in the IMM condition endorsed significantly fewer symptoms of attention-deficit/hyperactivity disorder (ADHD), oppositional defiant disorder (ODD), and overall disruptive behavior at 12-month follow-up than they had at baseline.[17]

Parents of youth with mood disorders commonly complain of "rage" episodes, which they typically describe as intensely irritable behavior accompanied by aggressive behavior. To address this, the authors derived a Rage Index including 2 items, 1 behavioral (disruptive-aggressive) and 1 affective (irritability), from the Young Mania Rating Scale,[20] and conducted a secondary analysis of this outcome for the main MF-PEP RCT.[18] Rage Index scores can range from 0 to 16. Using the intent-to-treat

(ITT) sample, the authors compared the Rage Index in IMM and WLC groups using a linear mixed effects (LME) model with a random intercept by participant. Basic fixed effects in the LME model were treatment group, continuous time from randomization, and group × time interaction; an indicator for T4 and a group × T4 interaction were included to allow for treatment effect in the WLC group and attenuation of effect in the IMM group. The model also included the number of diagnoses experienced by the primary informant parent, reported on the Psychiatric Diagnostic Interview,[21] as a fixed surrogate effect for the likelihood of a child remaining in the study. To test the hypothesis that rage decreases more rapidly over a 1-year period when immediate psychoeducation is provided, a χ^2 with 1 degree of freedom was derived from the ratio between likelihoods for models with and without the group × time interaction term.

As a supplementary analysis, the Rage Index was modeled in the T3 completers subsample, that is, those participants who remained in the study at least for the 12-month interview.[18] Of the ITT cohort ($N = 165$), 43 were lost to follow-up during the first year, leaving 122 participants (ie, T3 completers) who completed baseline (T1), 6 month (T2), and 12 month (T3) interviews. Of the T3 completers, 113 participated in MF-PEP at some point during the study. Treatment participation was defined as attendance at 6 or more of the 8 group sessions. An additional 13 families were lost to the final assessment.

In both the ITT sample (**Fig. 1**A) and the T3 completers subsample (see **Fig. 1**B), the mean evolution of rage for the IMM group showed a sustained decrease over time with rate attenuation after T3. For the WLC group, rage maintained a more or less steady value until T3 and then showed a marked decrease (that is, after receiving MF-PEP). The drop in rage seen in the full sample at T2 was not seen in the T3 completers ubset. This feature is related to WLC families with generally lower overall mood symptoms dropping out after T2 and before T3.

In constructing the LME model based on observed trends in rage, it was clear there was a time trend in both treatment groups that changed after T3. To evaluate the treatment effect on rage, likelihoods of the final LME model and a model excluding the group × time interaction were compared. In the ITT analysis, the difference in slopes was estimated as 1.36 U per 6 months ($\chi^2 = 8.84$; $df = 1$; $P = .0030$). In the T3 T3 completers subsample, the treatment effect on rage was estimated as a difference of 1.18 U per 6 months between treatment groups ($\chi^2 = 5.89$; $df = 1$; $P = .0152$). These novel findings represent strong evidence that MF-PEP has a beneficial effect on rage in addition to previously published evidence showing other benefits.

EFFICACY OF INDIVIDUAL–PSYCHOEDUCATIONAL PSYCHOTHERAPY

Three pilot RCTs have tested IF-PEP's impact on children's mood and behavior. A pilot RCT compared IF-PEP plus TAU to WLC plus TAU in 20 children ages 8 to 11 with

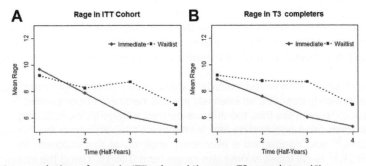

Fig. 1. Mean evolution of rage in ITT cohort (*A*) versus T3 completers (*B*).

bipolar spectrum disorders and their parents.[6] As compared with WLC, IF-PEP yielded significant improvements in mood symptom severity and family climate (assessed using a measure of expressed emotion), and these improvements persisted at 12-month follow-up.[6]

In a pair of 2 × 2 RCTs, 1 trial of 72 youth with major depression, dysthymia, or depression not otherwise specified and the other trial of 23 youth with bipolar disorder not otherwise specified or cyclothymia, participants were assigned to a 12-week course of either IF-PEP paired with omega-3 supplementation or placebo or of active monitoring paired with omega-3 or placebo in a 1:1:1:1 distribution.[22,23] Participants received 7 assessments and a daily vitamin-mineral supplement; families received referrals as requested or needed, payment for assessments, free parking, and child care at appointments. Families assigned to 1 of the 2 PEP conditions (PEP + omega-3 or PEP + placebo) attended two 45-minute to 50-minute sessions per week.

Among youth with bipolar disorder not otherwise specified or cyclothymia, PEP significantly outperformed active monitoring in reducing depressive symptoms occurring in the context of a mood episode and overall yielded medium to large effects on depressive symptoms.[22] Moreover, combined therapy (PEP + omega-3) significantly outperformed either monotherapy condition for the reduction of depressive symptoms.

Among youth with depression, 77% of those randomized to combined therapy (PEP + omega-3) achieved remission over the 12-week follow-up.[23] Youth with more endogenous forms of depression (ie, those depressed despite few environmental stressors) showed greater improvement in response to active treatments (PEP and omega-3) than to placebo, and among youth whose mothers had a history of depression, those who received PEP plus placebo showed significantly greater reduction in depressive symptoms than those in the active monitoring plus placebo condition. These findings suggest that the psychoeducation and skill-building exercises provided through PEP may be especially important especially to achieving improvements in emotion dysregulation among children with family histories of depression and who experience more endogenous forms of emotion dysregulation that emerge despite minimal psychosocial stress.

The combination of PEP and omega-3 supplementation also significantly outperformed placebo in reducing comorbid disruptive behavior (assessed dimensionally as average rating per item on subscales assessing symptoms associated with ADHD and ODD) among depressed youth over the 12-week follow-up period.[24] Specifically, combined treatment yielded large reductions in the severity of hyperactivity/impulsivity and overall behavior problems and reductions in the frequency of disruptive behaviors.

PEP in combination with omega-3 supplements improved executive functioning relative to placebo in the combined bipolar spectrum and depressive disorder samples.[25] Parents completed the Behavior Rating Inventory of Executive Functioning, which measures of their children's functioning in the domains of behavioral regulation (composed of inhibition, shift, and emotional control) and metacognition (composed of initiation, working memory, planning, organization of materials, and monitoring).[26] A global executive functioning composite also was computed by combined scores across domains. Youth across randomization conditions showed deficits in executive functioning at baseline. Following intervention, youth who received a combination of PEP and omega-3 supplements showed significantly greater improvements in global executive functioning and behavioral regulation compared with those who received placebo and active monitoring. Gains in behavioral regulation following the combined PEP and omega-3 treatments were especially robust, indicating that this combined intervention may be helpful particularly for improving inhibitory control, cognitive flexibility, and emotional regulation skills among youth with symptoms of emotion dysregulation.[25]

In a long-term naturalistic follow-up, participants from the original 2 ×2 RCTs assessing benefits of IF-PEP, omega-3 supplementation, or their combination were recontacted 2 years to 5 years after study participation (Fristad et al., under review, 2020). Across intervention conditions, youth continued to report lower mood symptom severity and better executive functioning and overall functioning than they had at RCT baseline. Although depressive symptoms had increased significantly in comparison to the end of the initial RCT, manic symptoms had not. Of those who returned for long-term follow-up, 58% either continued or commenced psychotherapy following RCT participation. Those who had been assigned to IF-PEP conditions during the RCT were significantly more likely than those assigned to active monitoring to seek psychotherapy post-RCT (71% compared with 41%, respectively). Moreover, the 58% who commenced or continued psychotherapy post-RCT had decreased depressive symptom severity at long-term follow-up compared with those who did not. Thus, receiving PEP in the context of the RCT increased subsequent utilization of psychosocial treatments, which in turn led to longer-term improvements in mood symptoms.

When asked to evaluate subjective impact of the RCT, 84% of parents reported that their child's symptoms decreased during the acute trial and 82% reported that at least some symptom improvement was maintained in subsequent years. Regarding specific symptoms, 50% of parents reported long-term improvements in their child's ability to cope with stress, 47% each reported long-term reductions in irritability and dysphoria. Furthermore, 87% of parents reported improvements in family functioning during the acute trial; 74% of parents believed those improvements persisted afterward. Regarding specific improvements, 63% reported long-term increases in feelings of hope, and 58% reported long-term improvements in family communication. Among youth, 82% reported their symptoms decreased during the acute trial and 68% reported that symptom improvement was maintained afterward. Regarding long-term improvements in specific symptoms, 62% of youth reported feeling less annoyed/mad, 59% felt calmer, and 56% reported feeling better about themselves. In addition, 79% of youth reported improvements in family functioning during the acute trial; 68% believed those improvements persisted afterward.

Among parents assigned to active treatment conditions (IF-PEP and/or omega-3), the top reason reported for improvement in their child's symptoms was "My child learned new skills" (76%), and top reasons for improvement in family functioning included "My understanding of my child improved" (71%), "My family learned new skills" (71%), and "I learned new ways to interact with my child" (67%). Among youth assigned to active treatment conditions, top reasons reported for improvement in their own symptoms included "I learned new skills" (84%) and "I learned new ways to talk and behave with my parents" (79%), and top reasons reported for improvements in family functioning were "I learned new ways to talk and behave with my parents" (93%), "My family learned new skills" (73%), and "I learned more about myself" (67%).

SUMMARY

PEP is an example of the class of well-established interventions, family psychoeducation plus skill building for youth with mood disorders who experience considerable emotion dysregulation. The novel findings presented in this article support the efficacy of MF-PEP for reducing irritability and aggressive/disruptive behavior, whereas the summarized prior findings show benefits of MF-PEP for overall mood symptom severity[18] and disruptive behavior.[17] IF-PEP, especially when combined with omega-3 supplementation, also has been shown to reduce mood symptoms,[23] disruptive behavior,[24] and executive functioning deficits.[25] Specific components of PEP may be beneficial especially for children with greater functional impairment[19] and those with family histories of mood disorders.[23] Long-term follow-up indicates that most families have a positive experience with PEP and many report improvements in youth functioning, overall family functioning, and appropriate service utilization even 2 years to 5 years after initial treatment (Fristad et al., under review, 2020). These findings suggest that once equipped with a better understanding of emotion dysregulation and skills to manage their feelings and behavior, children are able to implement coping strategies. Concurrently, parents play a valuable role in their child's treatment, both by recognizing and changing maladaptive family interaction patterns and by encouraging and helping their child with their new emotion regulation skills.

DISCLOSURE

This research was supported by National Institute of Mental Health (RO1 MH61512-01A1, R34 MH090148, and R34 MH085875), the Ohio Department of Mental Health, and the Ohio State University Foundation David Family Funds and Fristad Research Funds. Dr M.A. Fristad receives royalties from Guilford Press, American Psychiatric Press, and Child & Family Psychological Services, and receives research support from Janssen.

REFERENCES

1. Branje SJT, Hale WW III, Frijns T, et al. Longitudinal associations between perceived parent-child relationship quality and depressive symptoms in adolescence. J Abnorm Child Psychol 2010;38(6):751–63.
2. Sullivan AE, Judd CM, Axelson DA, et al. Family functioning and the course of adolescent bipolar disorder. Behav Ther 2012;43(4):837–47.
3. DeVille DC, Whalen D, Breslin FJ, et al. Prevalence and family-related factors associated with suicidal ideation, suicide attempts, and self-injury in children aged 9 to 10 years. JAMA Netw Open 2020;3(2):e1920956.
4. Sewall CJR, Goldstein TR, Salk RH, et al. Interpersonal relationships and suicidal ideation in youth with bipolar disorder. Arch Suicide Res 2020;24(2):236–50.
5. Hazel NA, Oppenheimer CW, Technow JR, et al. Parent relationship quality buffers against the effect of peer stressors on depressive symptoms from middle childhood to adolescence. Dev Psychol 2014;50(8):2115–23.
6. Fristad MA. Psychoeducational treatment for school-aged children with bipolar disorder. Dev Psychopathol 2006;18(4):1289–306.
7. Miklowitz DJ, Chung B. Family-focused therapy for bipolar disorder: reflections on 30 years of research. Fam Process 2016;55(3):483–99.
8. Miklowitz DJ, Schneck CD, Walshaw PD, et al. Effects of family-focused therapy vs enhanced usual care for symptomatic youths at high risk for bipolar disorder: a randomized clinical trial. JAMA Psychiatry 2020;77(5):455–63.
9. Pavuluri MN, Graczyk PA, Henry DB, et al. Child- and family-focused cognitive-behavioral therapy for pediatric bipolar disorder: development and preliminary results. J Am Acad Child Adolesc Psychiatry 2004;43(5):528–37.
10. West AE, Weinstein SM, Peters AT, et al. Child- and family-focused cognitive-behavioral therapy for pediatric bipolar disorder: a randomized clinical trial. J Am Acad Child Adolesc Psychiatry 2014;53(11):1168–78.

11. Fristad MA, Arnold JSG, Leffler JM. Psychotherapy for children with bipolar and depressive disorders. New York: Guilford Press; 2011.
12. Fristad, M.A., Roley-Roberts, M.E.*, Black, S.R.*, & Arnold, L.E. (2021). Moody kids years later: Long-term outcomes of youth from the Omega-3 and Therapy Studies (OATS). J Affective Disorders, 281: 24-52.
13. Deveney CM, Brotman MA, Decker AM, et al. Affective prosody labeling in youths with bipolar disorder or severe mood dysregulation. J Child Psychol Psychiatry 2012;53(3):262–70.
14. Fristad MA, Gavazzi SM, Soldano KW. Multi-family psychoeducation groups for childhood mood disorders: a program description and preliminary efficacy data. Contemporary Family Therapy: An International Journal 1998;20(3): 385–402.
15. Fristad MA, Goldberg-Arnold JS, Gavazzi SM. Multifamily psychoeducation groups (MFPG) for families of children with bipolar disorder. Bipolar Disord 2002;4(4):254–62.
16. Fristad MA, Goldberg-Arnold JS, Gavazzi SM. Multi-family psychoeducation groups in the treatment of children with mood disorders. J Marital Fam Ther 2003;29(4):491–504.
17. Boylan K, MacPherson HA, Fristad MA. Examination of disruptive behavior outcomes and moderation in a randomized psychotherapy trial for mood disorders. J Am Acad Child Adolesc Psychiatry 2013;52(7):699–708.
18. Fristad MA, Verducci JS, Walters K, et al. Impact of multifamily psychoeducational psychotherapy in treating children aged 8 to 12 years with mood disorders. Arch Gen Psychiatry 2009;66(9):1013–20.
19. MacPherson HA, Algorta GP, Mendenhall AN, et al. Predictors and moderators in the randomized trial of multifamily psychoeducational psychotherapy for childhood mood disorders. J Clin Child Adolesc Psychol 2014;43(3):459–72.
20. Young RC, Biggs JT, Ziegler VE, et al. A rating scale for mania: reliability, validity and sensitivity. Br J Psychiatry 1978;133:429–35.
21. Othmer E, Penick EC, Powell BJ, et al. Psychiatric diagnostic interview–revised (pdi-r): administration booklet and manual. Los Angeles (CA): Western Psychological Services; 1989.
22. Fristad MA, Young AS, Vesco AT, et al. A randomized controlled trial of individual family psychoeducational psychotherapy and omega-3 fatty acids in youth with subsyndromal bipolar disorder. J Child Adolesc Psychopharmacol 2015;25(10): 764–74.
23. Fristad MA, Vesco AT, Young AS, et al. Pilot randomized controlled trial of omega-3 and individual–family psychoeducational psychotherapy for children and adolescents with depression. J Clin Child Adolesc Psychol 2019;48(Suppl 1): S105–18.
24. Young AS, Arnold LE, Wolfson HL, et al. Psychoeducational psychotherapy and omega-3 supplementation improve co-occurring behavioral problems in youth with depression: results from a pilot RCT. J Abnorm Child Psychol 2017;45(5): 1025–37.
25. Vesco AT, Young AS, Arnold LE, et al. Omega-3 supplementation associated with improved parent-rated executive function in youth with mood disorders: secondary analyses of the omega 3 and therapy (OATS) trials. J Child Psychol Psychiatry 2018;59(6):628–36.
26. Baron IS. Behavior rating inventory of executive function. Child Neuropsychol 2000;6(3):235–8.

A Modular, Transdiagnostic Approach to Treating Severe Irritability in Children and Adolescents

Spencer C. Evans, PhD[a,b,*], Lauren Santucci, PhD[b,c]

KEYWORDS

- Irritability • Mood dysregulation • Oppositional • Behavioral parent training (BPT)
- Cognitive-behavioral therapy (CBT) • Modular • Transdiagnostic
- Children and adolescents

KEY POINTS

- Severe irritability often occurs in youth externalizing and internalizing problems, for which behavioral parent training and cognitive-behavioral therapy are recommended treatments.
- MATCH is a modular intervention for delivering evidence-based behavioral parent training/cognitive-behavioral treatment strategies to youth with anxiety, depression, trauma, and/or conduct problems.
- MATCH may be effective in the treatment of severely irritable youth, with strengths including its flexible, transdiagnostic, and personalized format.
- We offer strategies for personalized treatment of youth irritability with MATCH, emphasizing behavioral parent training as the first-line approach and cognitive-behavioral treatment elements as complementary or alternative approaches.

Research has demonstrated the clinical and developmental importance of irritability in children and adolescents (herein "youth").[1–4] Conceptualized as an increased proneness to anger, irritability is a common emotional experience with various manifestations moderated by development. In its most severe forms, irritability crosses into psychopathology. Chronic and developmentally inappropriate irritability (eg, severe temper outbursts, persistent angry/irritable mood) can be significantly impairing and warrant clinical attention. Evidence to guide care for severe irritability in youths is limited, although research in this area is rapidly advancing. The best available

[a] Department of Psychology, University of Miami, 5665 Ponce de Leon Boulevard, Coral Gables, FL, 33146, USA; [b] Department of Psychology, Harvard University, 33 Kirkland Street, Cambridge, MA, 02138, USA; [c] McLean Hospital School Consultation Service, Cambridge, MA, USA
* Corresponding author.
E-mail address: sevans@miami.edu

Child Adolesc Psychiatric Clin N Am 30 (2021) 623–636
https://doi.org/10.1016/j.chc.2021.04.011
1056-4993/21/© 2021 Elsevier Inc. All rights reserved.

Abbreviations	
BPT	Behavioral parent training
CBT	Cognitive-behavioral therapy
EST	Empirically supported treatment

evidence supports using behavioral parent training (BPT) with a primary caregiver (herein "parent") and/or cognitive-behavioral therapy (CBT) with the youth directly.[3,5,6] Beyond these general recommendations, specific guidance concerning which techniques to use, how, when, and with whom is lacking.

This article aims to provide clinicians with practical information for treating severe irritability in youth. In doing so, we focus on the Modular Approach to Therapy with Children with Anxiety, Depression, Trauma, and Conduct Problems (MATCH)[7] as one transdiagnostic intervention that can be used to personalize BPT/CBT for irritability and related problems. Although we focus on MATCH, we acknowledge other youth psychotherapies that similarly adopt modular transdiagnostic frameworks and derive from BPT/CBT research and theory. Notable examples include FIRST (Feeling Calm, Increasing Motivation, Repairing Thoughts, Solving Problems, Trying the Opposite)[8]; the Unified Protocol for Children and Adolescents[9] (UP-C/A), and its recent extension to irritability/anger[10]; Brief Intervention Strategy for School Clinicians (BRISC)[11]; and Common Elements Treatment Approach for Youth (CETA-Y).[12] A cursory review of these programs reveals many common "active ingredients" targeting changes in thoughts, behaviors, and parenting practices. What is novel about MATCH and these other examples is that they present evidence-based techniques in a modular format for personalized transdiagnostic treatment of youth emotional and behavioral problems, including severe irritability.

WHY TRANSDIAGNOSTIC?

Irritability is usefully conceptualized as a transdiagnostic phenomenon for several reasons. First, irritability is a central feature in more than a dozen diagnostic categories (eg, oppositional defiant disorder, depression, anxiety disorder, post-traumatic stress disorder, borderline personality disorder) and an associated feature of many more (eg, autism spectrum disorder, attention-deficit/hyperactivity disorder, conduct disorder). Thus, the mere occurrence of irritability as part of the presentation entails numerous differential diagnostic considerations to clarify the nature of the problem.[3] Second, when the presentation is clearly defined by severe, chronic irritability (eg, disruptive mood dysregulation disorder or oppositional defiant disorder with chronic irritability/ anger), this is typically accompanied by 2 to 3 other diagnoses such as attention-deficit/hyperactivity disorder, depression, anxiety, and conduct disorder.[1] Given so many potential treatment targets, a transdiagnostic framework can help the clinician to identify and prioritize co-occurring problems. Third, although severe irritability largely falls in the externalizing spectrum (eg, as a dimension of oppositional defiant disorder[1,13] or by comorbidity[14,15]), irritable youth are also at increased risk for depression, anxiety, suicidality, and other social, behavioral, and functional problems.[1,2,4] So, even in the rare case of a youth with severe irritability but no co-occurring disorders, it remains important to consider internalizing and externalizing problems as potential developmental precursors and outcomes. Finally, although these considerations are specifically relevant for severe irritability, they also generalize to other emotional and behavioral conditions common among treatment-referred youth. This factor underscores the practical usefulness of transdiagnostic approaches for both broad and targeted applications.

OVERVIEW OF A MODULAR APPROACH TO YOUTH COGNITIVE BEHAVIORAL THERAPY AND BEHAVIORAL PARENT TRAINING

MATCH[7] is a modular, transdiagnostic, evidence-based youth psychotherapy. Rather than offering yet another new treatment, MATCH offers a menu of treatment techniques ("practice elements," in MATCH terminology) from empirically supported treatments (ESTs) for anxiety,[16] depression[17] and trauma (all CBT-based) and conduct[18] (BPT). These 4 areas, or "protocols," collectively house 33 brief "modules," each describing a CBT/BPT practice element and how to deliver it. **Fig. 1** illustrates this framework with 17 irritability-relevant modules (eg, Praise, Practicing, and Problem-Solving) from 3 protocols (Conduct, Anxiety, and Depression, respectively). Although this wide array of elements offers intuitive appeal for transdiagnostic flexibility (eg, praise could help with depression, or problem solving with anxiety), MATCH should not be used as an a-la-carte menu of treatment strategies; this practice would dilute its effectiveness. To promote personalization while retaining EST fidelity, MATCH guides clinicians to first select which of the 4 MATCH protocols best captures the core problem. From there, MATCH provides further personalization and decision-making guidance (discussed elsewhere in this article).

MATCH was designed to address common barriers faced by clinicians trying to implement ESTs in everyday settings. Many ESTs were developed for 1 problem or disorder, but in community clinics comorbidity is the norm. Moreover, there is often

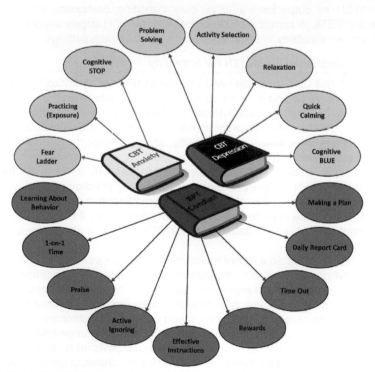

Fig. 1. Selected irritability-relevant modules illustrating the structure of MATCH.

heterogeneity, with the same problem presenting differently across patients, and flux, with problems changing over treatment. To address comorbidity, MATCH was designed for the most common youth mental health concerns (internalizing, externalizing, trauma), covering approximately 75% of outpatient youth mental health referrals. Fluctuations in problems during treatment can be managed via flowchart recommendations, such as addressing sources of treatment "interference" (eg, low motivation) using targeted practice elements (eg, rewards), or shifting to a new protocol (eg, from BPT to CBT-depression) if new problems arise or become primary. For clinics and clinicians, learning MATCH is simpler than learning 4 distinct interventions, and the flexible delivery of MATCH mirrors the way ESTs are administered in the real world.

Effectiveness of MATCH

Evidence for MATCH's effectiveness generally falls into 2 buckets. The first bucket consists of decades of youth psychotherapy research[19–21] demonstrating the efficacy and effectiveness of the ESTs[16–18] from which MATCH is derived. The second and more direct bucket includes trials of MATCH. In the initial randomized effectiveness trial,[22,23] 174 treatment-referred youths ages 7 to 13 years were assigned randomly to receive either standard manualized treatments[16–18] (CBT-Depression, CBT-Anxiety, BPT-Conduct), a modular version of them (MATCH), or usual care. MATCH consistently outperformed usual care and was equally or more effective than the standard treatments in decreasing internalizing, externalizing, total, and top problems, as well as number of diagnoses, over various measurement schedules.[22,23] Moreover, clinicians tended to prefer MATCH, suggesting it showed an optimal balance between responsiveness and effectiveness.[24] More recently, Chorpita and colleagues[25] again found MATCH to outperform a usual care condition composed of community-implemented EBTs. In sum, the evidence base for MATCH largely supports its effectiveness and acceptability in community youth mental health settings.

Preliminary Effectiveness of MATCH for Irritability

As noted, BPT and CBT are considered first-line treatments for irritability, but there is limited guidance regarding how to administer these techniques.[3,5,6] MATCH was designed to provide such guidance. Potential challenges in working with severely irritable youths include heterogeneity, comorbidity, difficult differential assessment, problems shifting over time, and variability across perspectives and settings.[1,3] MATCH was designed with these considerations in mind. Common comorbidities of irritability include anxiety and depression.[1,4] MATCH offers some of the best-supported techniques for these problems (eg, exposure ["practicing"], behavioral activation ["activity selection"]; **Fig. 1**), organized in a modular transdiagnostic framework rather than in separate disorder-specific interventions. Thus, if BPT/CBT techniques are appropriate for severely irritable youth, MATCH could be an appropriate vehicle for delivering them.

This reasoning prompted a recent reanalysis[26] of the original MATCH effectiveness data[22,23] to investigate its effects on severe irritability. Using empirically based cutoffs, the authors[26] identified a subsample of 81 youths with high irritability and impairment who had been randomly and evenly distributed across conditions at baseline. Severely irritable youths who received MATCH improved faster on all outcomes—especially by youth report—than those in other conditions, with medium to large effect sizes. From before to after the treatment, all 3 conditions showed significant reductions in youths' total number of mental health diagnoses (derived via structured diagnostic interviews); however, only MATCH significantly outperformed usual care on this metric, predicting

1.0 fewer diagnoses than usual care after treatment. Finally, MATCH's original effectiveness results[22,23] were not moderated by baseline irritability. In sum, BPT/CBT techniques were effective in reducing irritability in community-referred youths generally and, among severely irritability youth specifically, these effects were most pronounced when delivered via MATCH.

Clinical Application of MATCH to Youth Irritability

Although it is possible that various irritability-specific CBT/BPT techniques could be compiled into a new modular program targeting irritability, such an approach would be limited because it does not build on decades of research on the understanding and treatment of youth psychopathology. The clinical science of irritability is in its infancy, whereas the evidence base for treating other youth emotional and behavioral problems is much farther along. The modular approach draws from a comprehensive distillation of EST techniques for specific problems.[19,20,27] To develop an irritability-specific adaptation of MATCH or a MATCH-like treatment for irritability, it would need to be integrated into this framework and pass a certain threshold of empirical support. In our view, the evidence base for youth irritability treatment is not yet mature enough for this method. Rather, a more feasible and efficient approach is to take EST elements—already well-established and usefully arranged in MATCH—and apply them to irritability as it manifests across the landscape of youth psychopathology. From an evidence-based practice perspective,[28,29] there is never any single approach that is optimally effective for all clinicians with all patients with a given commonality. Nowhere does there exist an evidence base of randomized trials involving you and your patient to guide your clinical decision-making. Instead, best practice exists at the intersection of patient characteristics, clinician expertise, and the best available evidence.

So, where does the best available evidence lead? Generally, some form of BPT, such as MATCH-Conduct, is indicated. Although irritability does occur in anxiety, depression, and other disorders, most manifestations of severe irritability (eg, losing temper, angry/aggressive outbursts) are, by definition, disruptive behaviors. Thus, most presentations predominantly characterized by severe irritability fit this pattern and should probably receive the indicated treatment, BPT.[30–32] For example, in the MATCH irritability reanalysis,[26] 57% of the youths with severe irritability were identified by experts as being appropriate for MATCH-Conduct/BPT as a first-line treatment, as compared with anxiety (26%) and depression (17%). Finally, irritable, angry, and aggressive youths are not always the most motivated psychotherapy participants, but parents tend to be the ones bringing them to treatment and could serve as the agents of change in a youth's social environment.

Behavioral Parent Training (Conduct Protocol)

Evidence for BPT has accumulated over more than 50 years. Dating back to the work of Constance Hanf, Gerald Patterson, and others from the 1960s on,[30,33] various BPT programs have been developed, which—despite variations across settings, populations, and decades—contain essentially the same core intervention components. Thus, meta-analytic and systematic reviews[21,30–32] supporting BPT's effectiveness have broad generalizability. One example of a BPT protocol is Barkley's[18] Defiant Children, which was designed for general youth and family therapy settings and served as the basis for the Conduct protocol in MATCH.

The key premise in BPT is that child behavior problems are maintained by an interplay among child factors, parent factors, parent–child interactions, and other stressors. Treatment involves working with the parent to reverse dysfunctional interactional patterns that have emerged in their relationship, such as coercive cycles. It is up to the parent, working with the therapist as a coach, to enact behavior changes that might reverse those patterns. In MATCH, BPT (ie, the Conduct protocol) begins with engagement building (Engaging Parents) and psychoeducation (Learning About Behavior), followed by 2 major treatment phases. First comes child-directed activities, including special play time between parent and child (One-on-One Time). Positive reinforcement techniques promote behavior change through the skillful application of positive attention (Praise, Rewards). Parental attention is also selectively withdrawn (Active Ignoring) for minor misbehavior. Collectively, these techniques strengthen the parent–child relationship and make the parent's attention even more valuable to the child.

With this foundation in place, BPT shifts to the next phase: parent-directed activities. Core elements include training in giving effective directives (Instructions), a well-specified Time-Out protocol, and Making a Plan for managing behavior on the go. If needed, there is a Daily Report Card for problem behaviors at school. The goal of this second phase is to teach parents to be more consistent, clear, and effective in their requests and consequences, and for children to learn to comply with those requests more often and more quickly. The ultimate goal for the child is to modify their behavior to be more adaptive, understanding the links to the consequences in their environment. Last, treatment gains are reviewed and consolidated (Looking Ahead), with additional support later, if needed (Booster).

These 12 MATCH BPT modules are listed in **Table 1** along with special considerations for severely irritable youth. Importantly, this BPT protocol it is not a fixed, linear, session-by-session sequence, nor does every module need to be given (eg, Daily Report Card is only given when applicable to behavior problems at school). Rather, these elements are organized via flexible flowcharts that help clinicians personalize treatment. **Fig. 2** presents our conceptualization of modular BPT/CBT treatment for youth irritability, embedded in a MATCH-style flowchart framework. As shown, effective treatment must first begin with an accurate assessment to identify the problem(s) to be addressed. Irritability symptoms could reflect an underlying problem of anxiety, depression, or trauma—in which case, the corresponding MATCH protocol would be indicated. Alternatively, the assessment could reveal some other problem (eg, bipolar disorder) for which MATCH is not appropriate as a standalone treatment. But, in general, BPT is likely to be an important part of intervention, often as the first-line treatment.

When following the standard BPT sequence in MATCH, personalization questions arise (see **Fig. 2**, diamonds): Is the family able to proceed with BPT? If there is interference, what is the problem? The flowchart suggests which modules might help with different types of interference. For example, if an irritable-depressed mood is interfering with the parents' ability to engage the youth, the clinician might administer Problem Solving and/or Activity Selection to help improve mood first, and then resume with BPT. If there is a preference/possibility for individual youth-focused work, it may be possible for 2 clinicians to work together, or for 1 clinician to have separate parent and youth appointments regularly or on alternating weeks. It might be doubly beneficial for a youth to work through an anger exposure hierarchy[5] (Fear Ladder and Practicing) while their parent is acquiring positive parenting skills through BPT. However, this kind of dual approach is not standard and might be advisable only in certain circumstances (eg, if there is a basic level of engagement from all parties).

In delivering BPT for severely irritable youth, clinicians should recognize that reward processes are likely to be influential and motivating, but may come with more difficulty learning and changing behaviors, as compared with nonirritable youth[2] (see **Table 1**).

Table 1
BPT techniques and considerations for severe irritability

Module	Goal	Considerations for Severe Irritability
Engaging parents	Establish relationship and treatment plan	BPT involves working with parents to implement techniques themselves, with the clinician occupying a "coach" role. With older youth and/or severely irritable mood, greater involvement from the youth may be warranted, but the parent BPT sequence is still essential. Building rapport and setting expectations at the outset is key.
Learning about behavior	Help parent to understand the factors that may maintain youth misbehavior	Psychoeducation centers on how child and parent factors, consequences, and stressors affect the youth's irritable moods or aggressive outbursts. It may be helpful to normalize strong emotions commonly experienced by children and parents alike, but noting developmental differences (eg, tantrums vs moodiness). This can help parents realize that disruptive behaviors could reflect frustration and dysregulation, not just "acting out."
One-on-one time	Increase positive parent–child interactions, strengthen bond	Parents may have come to know youths' chronic irritability as aversive. Positive interactions, as in one-on-one time, are key to reversing this cycle. It is important to ensure parents can differentiate minor misbehavior vs aggressive outbursts, and how to respond differently to each (active ignoring vs end one-on-one time).
Praise	Teach parents to give child praise effectively	Emphasize the need for frequent labeled praise for good or "just okay" behavior. Praise is especially effective when it is immediate, specific, enthusiastic, and incremental. Attend to the "positive opposites" of target problems when possible (eg, praising putting 1 toy away [positive opposite] rather than criticizing leaving a mess of toys [target problem]). The power of attention may be less apparent for irritable mood, but it is still there; ask parent, "Do these difficulties occur more or less often when others are around?"
Active ignoring	Teach parents to remove attention from minor misbehavior to avoid inadvertently reinforcing it	Even in severely irritable youth, some behaviors are attention-seeking in nature and minor enough to be be actively ignored (aggression being an exception). Extinction bursts can be more severe with irritable youths, as they may take longer to learn from ignoring. Initially, parents should select behaviors they are willing and able to ignore (failing to do so can backfire). Most effective with praise and one-on-one time already in place.

(continued on next page)

Table 1
(continued)

Module	Goal	Considerations for Severe Irritability
Giving effective instructions	Teach parents to give instructions effectively	Common triggers of irritable behaviors include unexpected and unclear demands; effective instructions can reverse this. Parents and youth may be more successful when instructions are first given for trivial tasks before working up to more challenging requests. Extra practice may be needed with irritable youths, and youth preparation can be helpful.
Rewards	Help parent use rewards to increase positive behaviors	Irritable youths are responsive to rewards but may take longer to change behavior. With parents, involve youth in identifying range of potential rewards. Use easy criteria to ensure some success. Consider rewarding skill use and more socially appropriate expressions of emotion (eg, as verbalizing feeling angry).
Time-out	Help parent to decrease target behaviors by briefly removing reinforcement	Willful disobedience and aggression are good candidate behaviors for time-out. Use clinical judgment regarding its fit for the clinical presentation, youth age, and parent willingness. For older youths, consider framing as a "cool-down" (or similar), issue-able by youth or parent. Time-out may be inappropriate for severe aggression; safety is paramount.
Making a plan	Plan ahead to prevent and address behavior problems	Tantrums are often more likely to occur in public settings (eg, the supermarket), where parents often feel less equipped to manage them. Developing a plan for "high-risk" situations helps with maintaining and generalizing skills and gains.
Daily report card	Linking school behavior to home rewards	Applicable if the target mood and behavior problems occur at school. The teacher's perspective on the youth's problems may differ from parents. Prioritize a small, manageable set of problems that are impairing at school.
Looking ahead	Review, plan, and conclude BPT	Irritable/aggressive behaviors can recur or persist over time. As treatment ends, review skills, progress, and plan ahead for high-risk situations.
Booster session	Follow-up support after BPT	If irritable behavior problems do recur, acute challenges arise, or skills fade, call upon this session to review and consolidate skills.

Note. BPT Adapted from Chorpita and Weisz[7] (Copyright 2009, Practicewise). Table developed for this article.

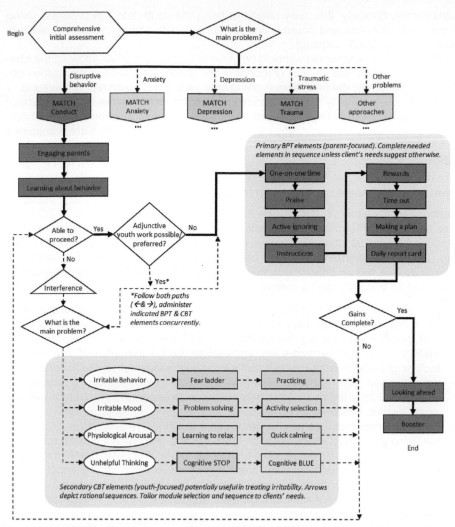

Fig. 2. MATCH-style flowchart conceptualizing youth irritability treatment in a modular framework. Bold: standard MATCH-conduct sequence; Dashed: alternative and adjunctive approaches potentially helpful for irritability when standard parent-focused treatment alone is not optimal; Ellipses: alternative approaches not presented here. (*Adapted from* Chorpita and Weisz[7] (Copyright 2009, PracticeWise). Figure developed for this article.)

Thus, personalizing for irritability could include allowing for more time and practice. Families are likely aware that certain circumstances can trigger angry, aggressive outbursts, and these patterns should be identified early in treatment. Later, when parent-directed strategies (eg, Instructions, Time-Out) are introduced, it is advisable to start small and work up to the more upsetting circumstances.[5] For example, if homework is a daily struggle leading to severe outbursts, the parent might start with more trivial and easily followed instructions (eg, please pass the salt) and later work up to homework directives after some initial success has been achieved. This graded approach may help to increase the parent's confidence so they feel better able to implement skills consistently. Similarly, it is likely helpful to bring the youth into this process, giving them advance notice and possibly equipping them with emotion regulation skills to help cope (eg, Quick Calming).

Finally, regular assessments should be given to monitor progress, allowing the clinician to see whether the youth is responding and make treatment personalization decisions accordingly. We recommend giving brief parent and youth report measures of current problem severity. First, idiographic measures, such as the Top Problems,[34] help to monitor the problems identified by families as their biggest concerns for treatment. Second, various nomothetic measures can be used to obtain a quick snapshot of severity in specific domains such as internalizing and externalizing problems,[35] irritability,[36] or anger.[37]

Tips, Tricks, and Tweaks in Using MATCH for Irritability

Although BPT is generally the first-line treatment, many CBT elements in MATCH may also be helpful for teaching youths skills to manage their irritability and anger directly. This work could be done as a complementary or alternative strategy to BPT (see **Fig. 2**). We highlight elements that, based on evidence and experience, might be beneficial. Still, we emphasize that these applications of MATCH were not explicitly designed for irritability, and therefore should be used with careful clinical judgment.

1. Cognitive-Behavioral Psychoeducation (Learning About [Behavior, Depression, Anxiety]). Potentially helpful psychoeducation elements include: (a) the 3-component CBT model of thoughts (eg, "he meant to do that"), feelings (eg, irritability, anger, somatic arousal), and behaviors (eg, aggression); (b) the metaphor of developing a toolbox of skills, to have the right tool for different situations; (c) the importance of practicing new skills (eg, graded exposure to irritability triggers, mood-enhancing activities); and (d) a feelings thermometer to measure anger and irritability in general, when irritated, and when using skills.
2. Calming Techniques (Learning to Relax, Quick Calming). Techniques, such as deep breathing with visual imagery (Quick Calming) and progressive muscle relaxation (Learning to Relax) can help youths to manage strong emotions. Given that youths with irritability may have difficulty tolerating frustration and inhibiting impulsive actions, learning to recognize the physiologic cues of irritability and using self-calming in these moments can put a space between impulse and action. The clinician might teach the youth calming strategies to use on a regular basis (eg, before bed) to help regulate physiologic arousal at baseline and when emotions escalate.
3. Problem Solving. Irritable youths may respond to challenging situations in ways that make their problems worse. This module teaches a systematic approach to identifying the problem, generating possible solutions, evaluating them, picking one to try, evaluating its success, and trying alternatives if needed. Problem solving involves exploring a full range of possible solutions—including maladaptive ones—that may seem to be viable to the youth to foster objective evaluation. For example, a child who is asked to stop playing videogames might hit their caregiver as an immediate solution. In this case, the problem would be the strong unpleasant emotion the child feels. Hitting would be one possible solution; other solutions could include self-calming, verbally expressing frustration, refusing to comply, and requesting more time.
4. Behavioral Activation (Activity Selection). Considering that irritability is often part of youth depression, behavioral activation may be advisable for irritable/depressed mood. When youths feel sad or depressed, they may withdraw from activities they used to enjoy, which can exacerbate the problem. Behavioral activation

reverses this cycle by promoting engagement in enjoyable and meaningful activities that can be positively reinforcing (eg, an activity that is fun, involves social interaction, provides a sense of accomplishment, or helps someone else). It is important to convey that instead of waiting to feel less irritable or angry before doing something, youths should start doing something to feel better. It can be helpful to allow them to "fake it 'til you make it," because this skill can have a cumulative rather than an immediate effect.

5. Addressing Unhelpful Thoughts (Cognitive STOP, Cognitive BLUE). Youths with irritability may perceive ambiguous situations as threatening or hostile, and then act according to these assumptions. Through cognitive restructuring, youths can learn to identify biased interpretations, evaluate the evidence for and against them, and develop more realistic or helpful interpretations. For example, when asked to put their phone away in class, a student might think, "this is unfair, the teacher is targeting me." In turn, this could lead to the behavior of storming out of class, resulting in disciplinary action. By gathering evidence via Socratic questioning (What's the evidence the teacher is targeting you? Have they ever asked other students to put away their phones?), the clinician might help the student to arrive at the more likely or helpful alternative thought—for example, "The teacher does not allow phones in class"—leading to more adaptive behavior.

6. Graded Exposure (Fear Ladder, Practicing). In anxiety treatment, exposure involves a gradual, step-by-step approach to entering anxiety-provoking situations. Doing so allows the youth to learn that the aversive outcome does not occur or is not as bad as anticipated and that they can handle their strong emotions by staying in the situation rather than avoiding it. Irritability exposure treatment[5] follows the same model but with anger-provoking (not anxiety-provoking) situations. Youths are asked to tolerate strong feelings of anger without acting on them in unhelpful or disruptive ways. First, the clinician helps the youth to identify triggering situations and rate, on a 0 to 10 feelings thermometer, how hard it would be to tolerate emotions rather than act (Fear Ladder, reframed as an anger ladder or similar). Before starting exposure, consider teaching the youth coping strategies (eg, Cognitive STOP) or alternative responses rehearsed outside of the triggering moment.

Here, we have summarized 6 core anxiety/depression CBT strategies relevant to youth irritability. Of course, attention should be given to rapport-building and goal setting at the outset (Getting Acquainted, etc) and to maintaining gains and preventing relapse at the end (eg, Plans for Coping, Wrap Up, Maintenance). Because the youth will continue to experience irritability after treatment ends, it is important to review the need for continued practice, discuss difficulties that might arise, identify what skills could be most helpful, and emphasize persistence in the face of challenges.

SUMMARY AND CAVEATS

Decades of youth psychotherapy research have yielded core techniques that are effective for irritability-related problems in youth. These techniques include BPT for disruptive behavior and CBT for anxiety, depression, and traumatic stress. Rather than developing yet another treatment, MATCH put these effective strategies into a format that clinicians can readily apply to youths presenting with comorbid, heterogeneous, and shifting problems. We have adopted this same philosophy in presenting MATCH as a viable treatment for severe irritability. In addition to the direct and indirect evidence for MATCH, recent evidence suggests that MATCH—in its standard format, without adaptations for irritability—was more effective than usual care and linear ESTs in the treatment of youth with severe irritability. For this and the other reasons presented in this article, we view MATCH as a potentially ideal first-line treatment recommendation for clinically referred youths with severe irritability.

However, this viewpoint must be accompanied by an important caveat: MATCH has not been developed, adapted, or tested specifically as a treatment for youths referred for severe irritability. The recommendations presented in this article are based on the available evidence and our experience as clinicians and trainers, but further research is clearly needed. Several other modular programs[8–12] were noted that could offer similar promise. Additionally, irritability-specific programs (some in this volume) are beginning to show evidence for effectiveness from dialectical behavior therapy,[38] interpersonal psychotherapy,[39] and behavioral/cognitive-behavioral approaches.[5,6,40,41] Such interventions may eventually be known as gold-standard EBTs for youth with severe irritability. Unfortunately, this kind of progress often takes years. In the meantime, MATCH can be used broadly today, with evidence of benefits for addressing irritability and related problems in youth.

ACKNOWLEDGMENTS

The authors thank John Weisz for his mentorship, expertise, and early contributions to many of the ideas presented in this article. This article is not intended to serve as a substitute for or adaptation of the MATCH protocol,[7] to which we refer all interested readers, especially those interested in clinical applications.

DISCLOSURE

The authors have nothing to disclose.

REFERENCES

1. Evans SC, Burke JD, Roberts MC, et al. Irritability in child and adolescent psychopathology: an integrative review for ICD-11. Clin Psychol Rev 2017;53:29–45.
2. Brotman MA, Kircanski K, Leibenluft E. Irritability in children and adolescents. Annu Rev Clin Psychol 2017;13(1):317–41.
3. Stringaris A, Vidal-Ribas P, Brotman MA, et al. Practitioner review: definition, recognition, and treatment challenges of irritability in young people. Journal of Child Psychology and Psychiatry 2018;59(7):721–39.
4. Vidal-Ribas P, Brotman MA, Valdivieso I, et al. The status of irritability in psychiatry: a conceptual and quantitative review. J Am Acad Child Adolesc Psychiatry 2016;55(7):556–70.
5. Kircanski K, Clayton ME, Leibenluft E, et al. Psychosocial treatment of irritability in youth. Curr Treat Options Psychiatry 2018;5(1):129–40.
6. Sukhodolsky DG, Smith SD, McCauley SA, et al. Behavioral interventions for anger, irritability, and aggression in children and adolescents. J Child Adolesc Psychopharmacol 2016;26(1):58–64.
7. Chorpita BF, Weisz JR. MATCH-ADTC: modular approach to therapy for children with anxiety, depression, trauma, or conduct problems. Satellite Beach (FL): PracticeWise; 2009.
8. Weisz JR, Bearman SK. Principle-guided psychotherapy for children and adolescents: the FIRST treatment program for behavioral and emotional problems. New York: Guilford Press; 2019.
9. Ehrenreich-May J, Kennedy SM, Sherman JA, et al. Unified protocols for transdiagnostic treatment of emotional disorders in children and adolescents: therapist guide. New York: Oxford University Press; 2017.

10. Hawks JL, Kennedy SM, Holzman JBW, et al. Development and application of an Innovative transdiagnostic treatment approach for Pediatric irritability. Behav Ther 2020;51(2):334–49.

11. Bruns EJ, Pullmann MD, Nicodimos S, et al. Pilot test of an engagement, triage, and brief intervention strategy for school mental health. Sch Ment Health 2019; 11(1):148–62.

12. Murray LK, Hall BJ, Dorsey S, et al. An evaluation of a common elements treatment approach for youth in Somali refugee camps. Glob Ment Health 2018;5:e16.

13. Burke JD, Boylan K, Rowe R, et al. Identifying the Irritability Dimension of ODD: application of a modified bifactor model across five large community samples of children. J Abnorm Psychol 2014;123(4):841–51.

14. Freeman AJ, Youngstrom EA, Youngstrom JK, et al. Disruptive mood dysregulation disorder in a community mental health clinic: prevalence, comorbidity and correlates. J Child Adolesc Psychopharmacol 2016;26(2):123–30.

15. Copeland WE, Angold A, Costello EJ, et al. Prevalence, comorbidity, and correlates of DSM-5 proposed disruptive mood dysregulation disorder. Am J Psychiatry 2013;170(2):173–9.

16. Kendall PC, Hedtke KA. Cognitive-behavioral therapy for anxious children: therapist manual. Ardmore (PA): Workbook Publishing; 2006.

17. Weisz JR, Southam-Gerow MA, Gordis EB, et al. Primary and secondary control enhancement training for youth depression: applying the deployment-focused model of treatment development and testing. In: Weisz JR, Kazdin AE, editors. Evidence-based psychotherapies for children and adolescents. New York: The Guilford Press; 2003. p. 165–82.

18. Barkley RA. Defiant children: a clinician's manual for assessment and parent training. New York: Guilford press; 2013.

19. Okamura KH, Orimoto TE, Nakamura BJ, et al. A history of child and adolescent treatment through a distillation lens: looking back to move forward. J Behav Health Serv Res 2020;47(1):70–85.

20. Chorpita BF, Daleiden EL. Mapping evidence-based treatments for children and adolescents: application of the distillation and matching model to 615 treatments from 322 randomized trials. J Consult Clin Psychol 2009;77(3):566–79.

21. Weisz JR, Kuppens S, Ng MY, et al. What five decades of research tells us about the effects of youth psychological therapy: a multilevel meta-analysis and implications for science and practice. Am Psychol 2017;72(2):79–117.

22. Weisz JR, Chorpita BF, Palinkas LA, et al. Testing standard and modular designs for psychotherapy treating depression, anxiety, and conduct problems in youth: a randomized effectiveness trial. Arch Gen Psychiatry 2012;69(3):274–82.

23. Chorpita BF, Weisz JR, Daleiden EL, et al. Long-term outcomes for the Child STEPs randomized effectiveness trial: a comparison of modular and standard treatment designs with usual care. J Consult Clin Psychol 2013;81(6):999–1009.

24. Chorpita BF, Park A, Tsai K, et al. Balancing effectiveness with responsiveness: therapist satisfaction across different treatment designs in the Child STEPs randomized effectiveness trial. J Consult Clin Psychol 2015;83(4):709–18.

25. Chorpita BF, Daleiden EL, Park AL, et al. Child STEPs in California: a cluster randomized effectiveness trial comparing modular treatment with community implemented treatment for youth with anxiety, depression, conduct problems, or traumatic stress. J Consult Clin Psychol 2017;85(1):13–25.

26. Evans SC, Weisz JR, Carvalho AC, et al. Effects of standard and modular psychotherapies in the treatment of youth with severe irritability. J Consult Clin Psychol 2020;88(3):255–68.

27. Chorpita BF, Daleiden EL, Weisz JR. Modularity in the design and application of therapeutic interventions. Appl Prev Psychol 2005;11(3):141–56.
28. APA Presidential Task Force on Evidence-Based Practice. Evidence-based practice in psychology. Am Psychol 2006;61(4):271–85.
29. Sackett DL. Evidence-based medicine. Semin Perinatol 1997;21(1):3–5.
30. Kaminski JW, Claussen AH. Evidence base update for psychosocial treatments for disruptive behaviors in children. J Clin Child Adolesc Psychol 2017;46(4): 477–99.
31. McCart MR, Sheidow AJ. Evidence-based psychosocial treatments for adolescents with disruptive behavior. J Clin Child Adolesc Psychol 2016;45(5):529–63.
32. Michelson D, Davenport C, Dretzke J, et al. Do evidence-based interventions work when tested in the "real world?" a systematic review and meta-analysis of parent management training for the treatment of child disruptive behavior. Clin Child Fam Psychol Rev 2013;16(1):18–34.
33. Reitman D, McMahon RJ. Constance "Connie" Hanf (1917–2002): the mentor and the model. Cogn Behav Pract 2013;20(1):106–16.
34. Weisz JR, Chorpita BF, Frye A, et al. Youth top problems: using idiographic, consumer-guided assessment to identify treatment needs and to track change during psychotherapy. J Consult Clin Psychol 2011;79(3):369–80.
35. Weisz JR, Vaughn-Coaxum RA, Evans SC, et al. Efficient monitoring of treatment response during youth psychotherapy: the Behavior and Feelings Survey. J Clin Child Adolesc Psychol 2019;49(6):737–51.
36. Stringaris A, Goodman R, Ferdinando S, et al. The Affective Reactivity Index: a concise irritability scale for clinical and research settings. J Child Psychol Psychiatry 2012;53(11):1109–17.
37. Irwin DE, Stucky BD, Langer MM, et al. PROMIS Pediatric Anger Scale: an item response theory analysis. Qual Life Res 2012;21(4):697–706.
38. Perepletchikova F, Nathanson D, Axelrod SR, et al. Randomized clinical trial of dialectical behavior therapy for preadolescent children with disruptive mood dysregulation disorder: feasibility and outcomes. J Am Acad Child Adolesc Psychiatry 2017;56(10):832–40.
39. Miller L, Hlastala SA, Mufson L, et al. Interpersonal psychotherapy for mood and behavior dysregulation: pilot randomized trial. Depress Anxiety 2018;35(6): 574–82.
40. Waxmonsky JG, Waschbusch DA, Belin P, et al. A randomized clinical trial of an integrative group therapy for children with severe mood dysregulation. J Am Acad Child Adolesc Psychiatry 2016;55(3):196–207.
41. Derella OJ, Burke JD, Romano-Verthelyi AM, et al. Feasibility and acceptability of a brief cognitive-behavioral group intervention for chronic irritability in youth. Clin Child Psychol Psychiatry 2020;25(4):778–89.

Future

The Irritable and Oppositional Dimensions of Oppositional Defiant Disorder

Integral Factors in the Explanation of Affective and Behavioral Psychopathology

Jeffrey D. Burke, PhD*, Oliver G. Johnston, MS, Emilie J. Butler, BA

KEYWORDS

- Oppositional defiant disorder • Chronic irritability • Internalizing disorders
- Antisocial behavior

KEY POINTS

- Chronic irritability is a distinct dimension of symptoms of ODD identified by often being touchy or angry, and often losing temper.
- Chronic irritability and oppositional behavior are distinct but inseparable dimensions of oppositional defiant disorder.
- Whereas chronic irritability is a strong marker for the risk of later depression, anxiety, and suicidality, oppositional behavior is associated with disruptive and aggressive behavior.
- The dimensions of irritability and oppositionality are identifiable in preschool and can continue into adulthood, exerting influence on associated psychopathology and impairment over the life course.

The introduction of disruptive mood dysregulation disorder (DMDD) in the Diagnostic and Statistical Manual (DSM)-5[1] was justified, in part, by an assertion that there was no diagnostic category that reflected the experience of frequent temper outbursts along with persistent anger and irritability. A substantial literature base alternatively suggests that these symptoms are reliable indicators of chronic irritability as a dimension of oppositional defiant disorder (ODD), a diagnostic category that was introduced in the DSM-III-R.[2] The evidence also suggests that the chronic irritability dimension of ODD may predispose toward future depression and anxiety[3,4] and suicidality.[5] A failure to be aware of the evidence base for ODD, including its symptom dimensions,

The authors have no conflicts of interest and no funding sources to report.
Department of Psychological Sciences, University of Connecticut, 406 Babbidge Road, Storrs, CT 06269, USA
* Corresponding author.
E-mail address: jeffrey.burke@uconn.edu

Child Adolesc Psychiatric Clin N Am 30 (2021) 637–647
https://doi.org/10.1016/j.chc.2021.04.012
1056-4993/21/© 2021 Elsevier Inc. All rights reserved.

childpsych.theclinics.com

course into adulthood, and associations with behavioral and affective psychopathology, clouds and confuses efforts to describe the onset and course of chronic irritability. It also risks continued delays in developing interventions for individuals with chronic irritability.

As evidence has emerged regarding DMDD, other challenges arise that are more than a choice between equivalent competing nosologic labels. These challenges are particularly germane to accurately identifying individuals at risk and predicting outcomes associated with presentations of chronic irritability through the lifespan. This is because DMDD appropriated only one of two symptom dimensions from ODD. It selectively features the chronic irritability dimension (losing temper, being touchy, and being angry) while omitting the oppositional behavioral dimension (being defiant, arguing, blaming, annoying others, and being spiteful). The behavioral dimension of ODD is not an inconsequential remainder. Instead, it is an inseparable[6,7] if still distinguishable, dimension that provides important predictive information about risks for future psychopathology. Here, we provide a brief review of the origins of these two disorders.

THE HISTORY OF OPPOSITIONAL DEFIANT DISORDER

The clinical characterization of oppositionality predates the introduction of "oppositional disorder" in the DSM-III.[8] Levy[9] described "oppositional syndrome" as a dimension of rebellious and hostile negativism evident, in somewhat different forms, from childhood to adulthood. A proposed classification of childhood disorders[10] suggested "oppositional personality disorder." This disorder was intended to represent the expression of aggression through passive forms of negativism and stubbornness, including indicators of disobedience, provocative behavior, quarreling, and teasing. Oppositional disorder in the DSM-III similarly described the condition as representing passive aggression, including an indication that passive aggressive personality disorder in adulthood was a likely outcome.

Revisions in the DSM-III-R[2] brought ODD largely into the form it has had to the present date. References to passive aggression were removed, and items indicating chronic anger and touchiness were introduced. Factor analyses have consistently supported the distinction of ODD from other psychiatric diagnoses.[11] In particular, in a two-dimensional structure identified by factor analysis of ODD and conduct disorder (CD) symptoms, ODD symptoms were largely distinguished from CD in a quadrant of "overt nondestructive" symptoms.[12] Thus, from early inceptions to the present, ODD has been characterized by behaviors that are noxious and negativistic, but are not aggressive. Even the symptom of "often loses temper" fell outside of the "aggression" quadrant of ODD and CD behaviors, along with most of the remaining symptoms of ODD, including those related to often being angry and touchy. The role of those symptoms (temper, touchy, and angry) in distinguishing pathways to affective outcomes nevertheless remained unclear for several decades. This may, in part, be because ODD was regarded and categorized as a behavioral disorder that was hierarchically subsumed under CD. In fact, a diagnostic prohibition against assigning a diagnosis of ODD if criteria for CD were met existed up until DSM-5.[1] Because there were no affectively oriented symptoms in CD, the hierarchical framework and prohibition against identifying ODD in the context of CD arguably obscured the importance of chronic irritability and its link to affective disorders.

THE HISTORY OF DISRUPTIVE MOOD DYSREGULATION DISORDER

In response to the question of whether chronic irritability had the same long-term outcomes as episodic irritability, and to describe phenotypes of mania in a range from narrow to broad, Leibenluft and colleagues[13] described a construct called severe mood and behavioral dysregulation. This construct was intended to represent a broad band phenotype of juvenile mania, identified by angry or sad mood, hyperarousal, and reactivity to negative stimuli, including extended tantrums and rages. It did not include a requirement that children experienced circumscribed episodes. Subsequent studies of severe mood dysregulation (SMD)[14] operationalized the construct using chronic irritability from ODD, along with dysphoric mood, symptoms of restlessness, distractibility and hyperactivity from attention-deficit/hyperactivity disorder (ADHD), symptoms of mania (ie, racing thoughts or flight of ideas), and insomnia.[14] The construct of SMD was found not to be particularly predictive of bipolar disorder, but instead was associated with ODD, CD, and ADHD along with depression and anxiety.[14]

Although evidence for SMD was used to support the inclusion of DMDD in the DSM-5,[1] most of the indicators of SMD (ie, restlessness, distractibility, intrusiveness, hyperactivity, racing thoughts, and sadness) were removed as symptoms. What was retained was frequent outbursts along with chronic anger and irritability. These are the symptoms of the chronic irritability dimension of ODD, with the exception that DMDD specifies severe temper outbursts (behavioral or verbal) in contrast to the specification of often losing temper in ODD. Consequently, similar individuals are identified when applying DMDD symptoms and ODD symptoms.[3,15–20] It has also been asserted that DMDD represents a more severe presentation of irritability than ODD, which could theoretically be true given the ways in which temper outbursts are defined as previously. Nevertheless, there is little empirical support for this possibility. Rather, Wiggins and colleagues[20] demonstrated that an empirically derived index of early childhood irritability was specifically associated with the ODD chronic irritability dimension rather than the oppositional behavioral dimension, and found near unity in groups identified by ODD and by DMDD.

There is also little precedent for splitting one diagnosis into two or more distinct and novel diagnostic categories based solely on gradations of severity in the absence of any advantage to doing so. For example, more intense characterization of severe temper outbursts in DMDD, with verbal rages or physical aggression, might imply that when asked about often losing temper, more severe manifestations of temper loss can occur alongside more benign forms of temper loss. Instead of categorizing them as different disorders, a more detailed description of outbursts may help to clarify differences between children who experience chronic irritability but stifle or bottle up any overt response and those who manifest varying levels of intensity of outward behavior. Importantly, the chronic irritability characterized in ODD is not separable from oppositional behavior, and oppositional behavior is particularly relevant to describing a course of overt behavior in the form of CD. The overlap between ODD and DMDD suggests that it may be a mistake to identify and treat DMDD without also assessing for and treating oppositional behavior.

OPPOSITIONAL DEFIANT DISORDER ACROSS DEVELOPMENT

ODD symptoms generally emerge in childhood and are distinguished in children as young as preschool age.[21] There is evidence that ODD symptoms are stable from preschool into early school years.[22–24] Oppositional defiant symptoms and preschool behavior problems as young as age 3 predict later ODD symptoms.[25,26] The presence of even a few symptoms of ODD at age 4 predicts an ODD diagnosis later in childhood.[27] There is also high stability of ODD symptoms from childhood into later adolescence.[22]

Efforts to understand the comorbidity between behavioral and affective disorders, and in particular the strong role of ODD in the prediction to depression and anxiety,[28,29] led to the identification of symptom dimensions within ODD.[30–32] A large literature has developed that makes clear that the structure of ODD is best represented as including dimensions of chronic irritability and oppositional behavior (see Ref.[3] for a review). More recent work has shown that this dimensional structure also holds among adults.[33,34] Of particular relevance for this review, tests of the structure of ODD have consistently failed to find support for a complete dissolution of ODD into separate categories of chronic irritability independent from oppositional behavior[6,7] and instead have supported a structure with correlated subfactors of chronic irritability and oppositional behavior.[35]

SYMPTOM DIMENSIONS AND THE RISK FOR AFFECTIVE AND BEHAVIORAL PSYCHOPATHOLOGY

The relevance of distinguishing between the dimensions of ODD at all is largely in their distinct prediction to affective versus behavioral outcomes. Evidence on this point exists from childhood through young adulthood. The dimensional structure within ODD, including chronic irritability and behavioral subdimensions, has been observed among preschool children.[36] A large study of children from age 3 to 6 found three trajectories of irritability symptoms: (1) high-persistent (31.9%), (2) decreasing (34.9%), and (3) increasing (33.2%).[37,38] Stable trajectories of low-, medium-, and high-severity chronic irritability have also been demonstrated from middle childhood to adolescence in a community sample of girls.[39] In some contrast, Riglin and colleagues,[40–44] using an English population sample of children older than ages 7 to 15, examined trajectories of the chronic irritability dimension of ODD. They found trajectories of irritability over that age range that included low (81.2% of the sample), decreasing (5.6%), increasing (5.5%), late childhood limited (5.2%), and high-persistent (2.4%). In general, chronic irritability shows levels of stability similar to other psychopathology, such as anxiety and depression.[45]

Evidence demonstrates that the distinct dimensions of ODD symptoms show consistent differential comorbid and predictive associations with internalizing psychopathology, even when identified in early or middle childhood.[46,47] As with older samples, the chronic irritability dimension is reliably associated with mood and anxiety symptoms, whereas the behavioral dimension is associated with hyperactivity and conduct problems. In the Riglin and colleagues[40] study, the high-persistent and increasing trajectories were associated with depression, whereas the others were not. However, they did not find a strong link between irritability and generalized anxiety disorder. It should be noted that the study failed to account for the behavioral dimension of ODD symptoms, which might have influenced the associations between trajectories of irritability and comorbid psychopathology.

WHAT HAPPENS TO THE BEHAVIORAL SYMPTOMS OF OPPOSITIONAL DEFIANT DISORDER?

The identification of the chronic irritability dimension of ODD and its role in affective psychopathology has generated substantial interest and focus. Garnering less interest has been the behavioral symptom dimensions of ODD. Despite being initially conceptualized as passive aggression, the remaining symptoms of ODD actually play an important role in predicting future antisocial outcomes (eg, CD, aggression, delinquency, antisocial personality feature). The oppositional behavior symptoms are associated with externalizing disorders, particularly ADHD and CD. However, only a minority of those with ODD develop CD.[48] Nevertheless, the oppositional behavior symptoms may be particularly important in explaining which children with ODD are at risk for developing CD. Furthermore, a set of relevant dimensions for understanding ODD and CD proposed by Wakschlag and colleagues[49,50] included irritability, noncompliance, callousness, and aggression. In regards to trajectories of antisocial outcomes, the evidence suggests that CD plays a greater predictive or explanatory role than ODD. ODD, for example, does not predict antisocial personality disorder over the effects of CD.[48] However, it is possible that ODD has not been sufficiently tested in the context of other dimensions of symptoms.

For example, little attention has been given to the relationship between callous and unemotional features (CU) and ODD. CU includes such characteristics as being callous, lacking remorse or guilt, and having a shallow or deficient affect. CU distinguishes a subgroup of children at risk for more severe and persistent antisocial behavior.[51-53] CU comorbid with CD provides one explanation for the course and severity of antisocial behavioral problems.[51] Yet, unlike the DSM-5, the International Classification of Diseases-11 includes limited prosocial emotions as a specification for CD and ODD.[54] This is consistent with evidence that elevated CU may precede the onset of CD,[52] and may predict antisocial behavior even in the absence of CD. Although most of the literature on the topic does not distinguish ODD from CD, a few studies have. Kumsta and colleagues[55] showed CU to be significantly associated with ODD but not CD. Findings from an unpublished study (Burke and coworkers) suggest that CU was most commonly associated with ODD (91.9%), compared with CD (44.1%) or ADHD (67.1%). When CU was applied as a specifier, ODD + CU was predictive of CD, whereas ODD without CU was not.

Taking together the evidence from longitudinal studies, structural modeling, and behavior genetic studies, chronic irritability seems to have unique associations with internalizing psychopathology, but it also remains linked to externalizing behavior via its connections with the behavioral dimension of ODD. Furthermore, when comorbid with elevated CU, ODD may be associated with the development of antisocial personality disorder. It may be that by more clearly measuring multiple dimensions related to irritability, oppositionality, CU, and aggression would clarify how explosive outbursts are characterized. Consistent with this possibility, Liu and colleagues,[56] using data from a sample of youth with ADHD, tested the structure of ODD symptoms along with items measuring mood swings, "explosive and unpredictable behavior," "cries often and easily," and "demands must be met immediately." These latter items formed a dimension that the authors labeled emotional lability. The authors found that, consistent with all models of chronic irritability in ODD, the symptoms of often being touchy and often being angry formed a separate factor. However, often losing temper loaded with the remainder of the behavioral symptoms on an oppositionality factor. Often losing temper has been found to load with the behavioral dimension in about one-quarter of the studies of ODD dimensionality,[3,57] so it is not without precedent that data by Liu and colleagues[56] provide evidence for such a structure.

OPPOSITIONAL DEFIANT DISORDER IN ADULTHOOD

Childhood and adolescent ODD have been shown to predict mental health disorders[58,59] or impairment[7] in adulthood. But little evidence has accrued to describe ODD specifically in adulthood. In a clinic sample of adults, 28.7% met criteria for ODD,[60] which is within the range estimated for child clinical samples.[61] Retrospective reports of adults find that ODD symptoms persisted into adulthood for 30% reporting a childhood or adolescent history.[62-65]

Using prospective repeated measurement from adolescence into young adulthood in the Victoria Healthy Youth Survey, a stable pattern of persisting ODD symptoms was observed in young men, and a curvilinear pattern for young women, increasing in late adolescence and decreasing in young adulthood, although levels were overall comparable between men and women.[66] Among college-aged men and women, Johnston and colleagues[67] found that approximately 3% to 4% showed criterion level symptom counts for ODD, consistent with prevalence estimates for children.[68] Together, these studies suggest that ODD persists into adulthood.

Irritability and Behavioral Subdimensions of Oppositional Defiant Disorder in Adulthood

ODD symptom dimensions have been examined in adult samples. In a large community sample of youth followed up into young adulthood, Leadbeater and Homel[69] found that the irritability dimension characterized by ODD symptoms of often being irritable, easily annoyed, and angry/resentful persisted into adulthood for men and women, whereas the behavioral symptoms gradually decreased, particularly for women. This study also noted concurrent relations between irritability and internalizing symptoms with some evidence of reciprocal interactions over time during specific developmental periods. This evidence of ODD irritability in youth being associated with ODD irritability and internalizing symptoms in adulthood has also been observed in samples of youth with tic disorders.[70]

In addition to this longitudinal evidence supporting the construct validity of these subdimensions in adults, more recent research has examined the structure of ODD dimensions and their concurrent associations with personality traits and comorbid psychopathology. Using two samples of community adults, Gomez and Stavropoulos[33] found support for a three-factor model of ODD symptoms with two behavioral dimensions (oppositional and antagonistic) and one negative affect subdimension marked by symptoms of often being touchy, angry, and/or spiteful, an index of ODD irritability that has also been supported in certain samples of youth.[30,48] For adults, the oppositional behavior dimension was associated only with aggression and the antagonistic dimension was associated with social potency and harm avoidance, whereas the irritability dimension was found to be associated with Tellegen's multidimensional personality model traits of stress reaction and aggression indicating a greater propensity toward negative mood states and interpersonal transgressions.[33]

Echoing these findings, Johnston and colleagues[34] found support for a two-factor structure of ODD symptoms in a college student sample with an irritability dimension indexed by symptoms of often being touchy, angry, and losing temper and a behavioral dimension indexed by remaining ODD symptoms. Irritability was uniquely associated with anxiety, depression, and the DSM-5 pathological personality traits of negative affectivity and detachment.[34] The behavioral dimension was associated with ADHD, and with personality factors of disinhibition and antagonism. Although the associations with internalizing psychopathology and negative affectivity are similar to the findings of Gomez and Stavropoulos[33] with the trait of stress reaction, it is notable that there was not an association with traits that reflected aggression, but rather an association suggesting a withdrawal from or avoidance of others (ie, detachment). It is possible that these differences are influenced by the presence or absence of spitefulness as an index for irritability. For example, the aggression personality trait that was associated with Gomez and Stavropoulos[33] negative affect dimension (touchy, angry, spiteful) is conceptually similar to the DSM-5 pathology personality trait of antagonism, which was uniquely associated with Johnston & colleagues[34] behavioral dimension of ODD, which includes spitefulness. Regardless of the "true" structure of irritability in adulthood, these findings underscore the importance of considering the behavioral symptoms of ODD in examining the structure and associated characteristics of irritability in adult populations.

The emerging nascent literature on ODD in adulthood finds factor structures, prevalence rates, and differential associations with associated psychopathology and personality dimensions that are in accord with evidence from child and adolescent datasets. Additional work is needed that more explicitly tests CU traits and other constructs and dimensions associated with antisocial behavior to clarify those relationships. However, if consistent results emerge, it seems that the related but distinct ODD dimensions of irritability and oppositional behavior remain present in adulthood and generally speaking have differential associations with internalizing and externalizing psychopathology. It may be that elevations on associated other factors (eg, CU) further clarify which individuals will show more severe antisocial behavior, and which individuals are particularly at risk for depression, anxiety, and suicidality.

SUMMARY

Chronic irritability and oppositional behavior are two dimensions among the symptoms of ODD, and evidence strongly concludes that they should not be considered separately. In reiterating the irritability dimension and omitting the behavioral dimension of ODD, DMDD fails to account for crucial prognostic and diagnostic information regarding antisocial behavioral outcomes. DMDD also obscures a substantial literature base that involves the irritability dimension of ODD, despite evidence that the two conditions are essentially the same. The structure of ODD and the constituent elements of the dimensions are largely consistent from preschool age through adulthood, and across the life span, differential associations with internalizing and externalizing psychopathology are consistently observed in the main. Future work on irritability must account for oppositional behavior, and must expand the evidence regarding ODD and its dimensions further into adulthood.

REFERENCES

1. American Psychiatric Association. Diagnostic and statistical manual of mental disorders (DSM-5®). Arlington, VA: Author; 2013.
2. American Psychiatric Association. Diagnostic and statistical manual of mental disorders (DSM III-R). Arlington (VA): Author; 1987.
3. Evans SC, Burke JD, Roberts MC, et al. Irritability in child and adolescent psychopathology: an integrative review for ICD-11. Clin Psychol Rev 2017;53:29–45.
4. Evans SC, Pederson CA, Fite PJ, et al. Teacher-reported irritable and defiant dimensions of oppositional defiant disorder: social, behavioral, and academic correlates. Sch Ment Health 2016;8(2):292–304.
5. Aebi M, Barra S, Bessler C, et al. Oppositional defiant disorder dimensions and subtypes among detained male adolescent offenders. J Child Psychol Psychiatry 2016;57(6):729–36.
6. Burke JD, Boylan K, Rowe R, et al. Identifying the irritability dimension of ODD: application of a modified bifactor model across five large community samples of children. J Abnormal Psychol 2014;123(4):841.
7. Burke JD, Rowe R, Boylan K. Functional outcomes of child and adolescent ODD in young adult men. J Child Psychol Psychiatry 2014;55:264–72.
8. American Psychiatric Association. Diagnostic and statistical manual of mental disorders. 3rd edition. Arlington, VA: Author; 1980.

9. Levy DM. Oppositional syndromes and oppositional behavior. In: Hoch PH, Zubin J, editors. Psychopathology of childhood. Oxford, England: Grune & Stratton; 1955. p. 204–26.

10. Group for the Advancement of Psychiatry. Psychopathological disorders in childhood group for the advancement of psychiatry psychopathological disorders of childhood: theoretical considerations and a proposed classification (No. 62). New York: Group for the Advancement of Psychiatry; 1966.

11. Hartman CA, Hox J, Mellenbergh GJ, et al. DSM-IV internal construct validity: when a taxonomy meets data. J Child Psychol Psychiatry 2001;42(6):817–36.

12. Frick PJ, Lahey BB, Loeber R, et al. Oppositional defiant disorder and conduct disorder: a meta-analytic review of factor analyses and cross-validation in a clinic sample. Clin Psychol Rev 1993;13(4):319–40.

13. Leibenluft E, Charney DS, Towbin KE, et al. Defining clinical phenotypes of juvenile mania. Am J Psychiatry 2003;160(3):430–7.

14. Brotman MA, Schmajuk M, Rich BA, et al. Prevalence, clinical correlates, and longitudinal course of severe mood dysregulation in children. Biol Psychiatry 2006; 60(9):991–7.

15. Mayes SD, Waxmonsky JD, Calhoun SL. Disruptive mood dysregulation disorder symptoms and association with oppositional defiant and other disorders in a general population child sample. J Child Adolesc Psychopharmacol 2016;26:101–16.

16. Malhi GS, Byrow Y, Fritz K, et al. Does irritability determine mood depending on age? Aust N Z J Psychiatry 2017;51(3):215–6.

17. Merjonen P, Pulkki-Råback L, Puttonen S, et al. Anger is associated with subclinical atherosclerosis in low SES but not in higher SES men and women. The Cardiovascular Risk in Young Finns Study. J Behav Med 2008;31(1):35–44.

18. Mikolajewski AJ, Taylor J, Iacono WG. Oppositional defiant disorder dimensions: genetic influences and risk for later psychopathology. J Child Psychol Psychiatry 2017;58(6):702–10.

19. Mulraney MA, Melvin GA, Tonge BJ. Psychometric properties of the affective reactivity index in Australian adults and adolescents. Psychol Assess 2014; 26(1):148–55.

20. Wiggins JL, Briggs-Gowan MJ, Brotman MA, et al. Don't miss the boat: towards a developmental nosology for disruptive mood dysregulation disorder in early childhood. J Am Acad Child Adolesc Psychiatry 2020;60(3):388–97.

21. Keenan K, Wakschlag LS. Are oppositional defiant and conduct disorder symptoms normative behaviors in preschoolers? A comparison of referred and nonreferred children. Am J Psychiatry 2004;161(2):356–8.

22. Cohen P, Cohen J, Brook J. An epidemiological study of disorders in late childhood and adolescence—II. Persistence of disorders. J Child Psychol Psychiatry 1993;34(6):869–77.

23. Lavigne JV, Arend R, Rosenbaum D, et al. Psychiatric disorders with onset in the preschool years: I. Stability of diagnoses. J Am Acad Child Adolesc Psychiatry 1998;37(12):1246–54.

24. Lavigne JV, Cicchetti C, Gibbons RD, et al. Oppositional defiant disorder with onset in preschool years: longitudinal stability and pathways to other disorders. J Am Acad Child Adolesc Psychiatry 2001;40(12):1393–400.

25. Harvey EA, Youngwirth SD, Thakar DA, et al. Predicting attention-deficit/hyperactivity disorder and oppositional defiant disorder from preschool diagnostic assessments. J Consult Clin Psychol 2009;77(2):349.

26. Hakulinen C, Jokela M, Hintsanen M, et al. Childhood family factors predict developmental trajectories of hostility and anger: a prospective study from childhood into middle adulthood. Psychol Med 2013;43(11):2417–26.
27. Lavigne JV, Bryant FB, Hopkins J, et al. Age 4 predictors of oppositional defiant disorder in early grammar school. J Clin Child Adolesc Psychol 2019;48(1): 93–107.
28. Burke JD, Loeber R, Lahey BB, et al. Developmental transitions among affective and behavioural disorders in adolescent boys. J Child Psychol Psychiatry 2005; 46:1200–10.
29. Hipwell AE, Stepp S, Feng X, et al. Impact of oppositional defiant disorder dimensions on the temporal ordering of conduct problems and depression across childhood and adolescence in girls. J Child Psychol Psychiatry 2011;52(10): 1099–108.
30. Burke JD, Hipwell AE, Loeber R. Dimensions of oppositional defiant disorder as predictors of depression and conduct disorder in preadolescent girls. J Am Acad Child Adolesc Psychiatry 2010;49(5):484–92.
31. Stringaris A, Goodman R. Three dimensions of oppositionality in youth. J Child Psychol Psychiatry 2009;50(3):216–23.
32. Stringaris A, Zavos H, Leibenluft E, et al. Adolescent irritability: phenotypic associations and genetic links with depressed mood. Am J Psychiatry 2012;169(1): 47–54.
33. Gomez R, Stavropoulos V. Oppositional defiant disorder dimensions: associations with traits of the multidimensional personality among adults. Psychiatr Q 2019;90:777–92.
34. Johnston OG, Cruess DG, Burke JD. Irritability and behavioral symptom dimensions of oppositional defiant disorder in young adults: associations with DSM-5 pathological personality traits. J Psychopathol Behav Assess 2020;42:424–35.
35. Herzhoff K, Tackett JL. Subfactors of oppositional defiant disorder: converging evidence from structural and latent class analyses. J Child Psychol Psychiatry 2016;57(1):18–29.
36. Ezpeleta L, Granero R, De La Osa N, et al. Dimensions of oppositional defiant disorder in 3-year-old preschoolers. J Child Psychol Psychiatry 2012;53(11): 1128–38.
37. Ezpeleta L, Granero R, de la Osa N, et al. Trajectories of oppositional defiant disorder irritability symptoms in preschool children. J Abnormal Child Psychol 2016; 44(1):115–28.
38. Faraone SV, Rostain AL, Blader J, et al. Practitioner review: emotional dysregulation in attention-deficit/hyperactivity disorder–implications for clinical recognition and intervention. J Child Psychol Psychiatry 2019;60(2):133–50.
39. Boylan K, Rowe R, Duku E, et al. Longitudinal profiles of girls' irritable, defiant and antagonistic oppositional symptoms: evidence for group based differences in symptom severity. J Abnormal Child Psychol 2017;45(6):1133–45.
40. Riglin L, Eyre O, Thapar AK, et al. Identifying novel types of irritability using a developmental genetic approach. Am J Psychiatry 2019;176(8):635–42.
41. Roberson-Nay R, Leibenluft E, Brotman MA, et al. Longitudinal stability of genetic and environmental influences on irritability: from childhood to young adulthood. Am J Psychiatry 2015;172(7):657–64.
42. Rowe R, Costello EJ, Angold A, et al. Developmental pathways in oppositional defiant disorder and conduct disorder. J Abnormal Psychol 2010;119(4):726–38.
43. Stringaris A, Cohen P, Pine DS, et al. Adult outcomes of youth irritability: a 20-year prospective community-based study. Am J Psychiatry 2009;166(9):1048–54.

44. Stringaris A, Goodman R. Longitudinal outcome of youth oppositionality: irritable, headstrong, and hurtful behaviors have distinctive predictions. J Am Acad Child Adolesc Psychiatry 2009;48(4):404–12.

45. Caprara GV, Paciello M, Gerbino M, et al. Individual differences conducive to aggression and violence: trajectories and correlates of irritability and hostile rumination through adolescence. Aggressive Behav 2007;33(4):359–74.

46. Krieger FV, Polanczyk GV, Goodman R, et al. Dimensions of oppositionality in a Brazilian community sample: testing the DSM-5 proposal and etiological links. J Am Acad Child Adolesc Psychiatry 2013;52(4):389–400.

47. Wesselhoeft R, Stringaris A, Sibbersen C, et al. Dimensions and subtypes of oppositionality and their relation to comorbidity and psychosocial characteristics. Eur Child Adolesc Psychiatry 2019;28(3):351–65.

48. Burke JD, Waldman I, Lahey BB. Predictive validity of childhood oppositional defiant disorder and conduct disorder: implications for DSM-V. J Abnormal Psychol 2010;119(4):739–51.

49. Wakschlag LS, Perlman SB, Blair RJ, et al. The neurodevelopmental basis of early childhood disruptive behavior: irritable and callous phenotypes as exemplars. Am J Psychiatry 2018;175(2):114–30.

50. Waldman ID, Rowe R, Boylan K, et al. External validation of a bifactor model of oppositional defiant disorder. Mol Psychiatry 2018;26(2):682–93.

51. Frick PJ, Ray JV, Thornton LC, et al. Can callous-unemotional traits enhance the understanding, diagnosis, and treatment of serious conduct problems in children and adolescents? A comprehensive review. Psychol Bull 2014;140(1):1.

52. Frick PJ, Ray JV, Thornton LC, et al. Annual research review: a developmental psychopathology approach to understanding callous-unemotional traits in children and adolescents with serious conduct problems. J Child Psychol Psychiatry 2014;55(6):532–48.

53. Gadow KD, Sprafkin J, Schneider J, et al. ODD, ADHD, versus ODD+ADHD in clinic and community adults. J Attention Disord 2007;11(3):374–83.

54. World Health Organization. International classification of diseases for mortality and morbidity statistics (11th Revision). 2018. Available at: https://icd.who.int/browse11/l-m/en. Accessed June 10, 2020.

55. Kumsta R, Sonuga-Barke E, Rutter M. Adolescent callous–unemotional traits and conduct disorder in adoptees exposed to severe early deprivation. Br J Psychiatry 2012;200(3):197–201.

56. Liu L, Chen W, Vitoratou S, et al. Is emotional lability distinct from "angry/irritable mood,""negative affect," or other subdimensions of oppositional defiant disorder in children with ADHD? J attention Disord 2019;23(8):859–68.

57. Burke JD. An affective dimension within oppositional defiant disorder symptoms among boys: personality and psychopathology outcomes into early adulthood. J Child Psychol Psychiatry 2012;53(11):1176–83.

58. Copeland WE, Shanahan L, Costello EJ, et al. Childhood and adolescent psychiatric disorders as predictors of young adult disorders. Arch Gen Psychiatry 2009; 66(7):764–72.

59. Dougherty LR, Smith VC, Bufferd SJ, et al. Preschool irritability: longitudinal associations with psychiatric disorders at age 6 and parental psychopathology. J Am Acad Child Adolesc Psychiatry 2013;52(12):1304–13.

60. Barry TD, Marcus DK, Barry CT, et al. The latent structure of oppositional defiant disorder in children and adults. J Psychiatr Res 2013;47(12):1932–9.

61. Boylan K, Vaillancourt T, Boyle M, *et al.* Comorbidity of internalizing disorders in children with oppositional defiant disorder. *Eur Child Adolesc Psychiatry* 2007:16;484–94.
62. Nock MK, Kazdin AE, Hiripi E, et al. Lifetime prevalence, correlates, and persistence of oppositional defiant disorder: results from the National Comorbidity Survey Replication. J Child Psychol Psychiatry 2007;48(7):703–13.
63. Orri M, Galera C, Turecki G, et al. Pathways of association between childhood irritability and adolescent suicidality. J Am Acad Child Adolesc Psychiatry 2019; 58(1):99–107.
64. Orri M, Galèra C, Turecki G, et al. Childhood irritability and depressive/anxious mood profiles, and adolescent suicidal ideation/attempt: a population-based cohort study 2018.
65. Orri M, Perret LC, Turecki G, et al. Association between irritability and suicide-related outcomes across the life-course. Systematic review of both community and clinical studies. J Affective Disord 2018;239:220–33.
66. Leadbeater BJ, Thompson KD, Gruppuso V. Co-occurring trajectories of symptoms of anxiety, depression, and oppositional defiance from adolescence to young adulthood. J Clin Child Adolesc Psychol 2012;41(6):719–30.
67. Johnston OG, Derella OJ, Burke JD. Identification of oppositional defiant disorder in young adult college students. J Psychopathol Behav Assess 2018;40(4): 563–72.
68. Canino G, Polanczyk G, Bauermeister JJ, et al. Does the prevalence of CD and ODD vary across cultures? Soc Psychiatry Psychiatr Epidemiol 2010;45(7): 695–704.
69. Leadbeater BJ, Homel J. Irritable and defiant sub-dimensions of ODD: their stability and prediction of internalizing symptoms and conduct problems from adolescence to young adulthood. J Abnormal Child Psychol 2015;43(3):407–21.
70. Thériault M-CG, Bécue J-C, Lespérance P, et al. Oppositional behavior and longitudinal predictions of early adulthood mental health problems in chronic tic disorders. Psychiatry Res 2018;266:301–8.

This Is Your Brain on Irritability

A Clinician's Guide to Understanding How We Know What We Know Now, and What We Need to Know in the Future, About Irritability in Children and Adolescents

Daniel P. Dickstein, MD[a,b],*, Christine M. Barthelemy[a,b],
Gracie A. Jenkins[a,b], Lena L.A. DeYoung[a,b], Anna C. Gilbert[c],
Petya Radoeva, MD, PhD[c], Kerri L. Kim, PhD[c],
Heather A. MacPherson, PhD[c]

KEYWORDS

- Irritability • Child • Adolescent • Neuroimaging • Behavior

KEY POINTS

- As with childhood leukemia, better understanding of brain/behavior mechanisms underlying psychiatric disorders involving irritability is important to improve how such problems are diagnosed and treated.
- This article strives to break down barriers that hinder clinicians' accessing and using this research, including explaining jargon and techniques.

INTRODUCTION

Irritability is the most common reason children are brought for psychiatric evaluation, including being a focus of more than 40% of pediatric emergency department visits for mental health and more than 20% of outpatient mental health visits.[1–4] Irritability is an explicit diagnostic criterion or associated symptom for multiple *Diagnostic and Statistical Manual of Mental Disorders* (*DSM*) diagnoses, including a manic episode in bipolar disorder (BD), major depressive episode in children, generalized anxiety disorder,

[a] PediMIND Program, Mclean Hospital, 115 Mill Street, Belmont, MA, USA; [b] Simches Center of Excellence in Child and Adolescent Psychiatry, McLean Hospital, Harvard Medical School; [c] Division of Child Psychiatry, Brown University (Prior PediMIND Program Members)
* Corresponding author. PediMIND Program, McLean Hospital, 115 Mill Street, Mail Stop 321, Belmont, MA 02478.
E-mail address: DDICKSTEIN@mclean.harvard.edu

Child Adolesc Psychiatric Clin N Am 30 (2021) 649–666
https://doi.org/10.1016/j.chc.2021.04.013
1056-4993/21/© 2021 Elsevier Inc. All rights reserved.

attention-deficit/hyperactivity disorder (ADHD), oppositional defiant disorder, and the new *DSM* (Fifth Edition) (*DSM-5*) disruptive mood dysregulation disorder (DMDD).[5] There is no well-validated, replicated biomarker (eg, scan or test) with sufficient sensitivity and specificity to guide clinicians in determining what disorder(s) involving irritability a child has, which may hinder treatment decisions. Childhood irritability is linked to decreased educational attainment and income, and greater risk for psychopathology and suicide.[2,6,7]

Over the past 20 years, research has advanced what is known about the brain and behavior mechanisms of disorders involving irritability. Too often, clinician's brains are turned off—rather than turned on—when they look at such articles, due to barriers to learning, including excessive jargon or complicated methods. This article seeks to address that observation, known as Dickstein's paradox, first by explaining the basic techniques. This is built on by providing examples of how those tools advance understanding of some *DSM* disorders involving irritability.

Greater access to this information may help professionals explain diagnostic and treatment choices to children and parents. Hopefully, in the future, these brain/behavior mechanisms are translated into better clinical care, as has already occured for childhood leukemia, where scans and tests routinely augment clinical care, resulting in decreased morbidity and mortality. Furthermore, by breaking down these barriers, the authors seek to inspire some clinicians to join research efforts—by joining extant research teams, launching their own studies, or recruiting participants for current studies.

TOOLS OF THE TRADE

First, the basics tools used for brain/behavior mechanism research are explained, including magnetic resonance imaging (MRI) and computerized behavioral tasks probing emotion or cognition.

Imaging

MRI has revolutionized health care; high-resolution pictures now can be obtained rapidly to aid diagnosis of clinical problems ranging from headache to appendicitis to cancer. MRI also has revolutionized research, especially in childhood psychopathology, because the same MRI machine can take 4 different types of pictures: (1) structural MRI, (2) functional MRI (fMRI), (3) diffusion tensor imaging (DTI) or diffusion spectral imaging, and (4) magnetic resonance spectroscopy (MRS) (**Table 1**).

Structural magnetic resonance imaging (brain = compass)

Structural MRI enables examination of brain structures, including the volume and shape of different structures, such as the amygdala, ventricles, and cortical thickness. The same noncontrast MRI often done clinically to evaluate causes of headaches is used for these research purposes.

How does structural MRI work? Think of the brain as a compass. Specifically, water is the most common substance in the brain, representing 80% by weight. Water (H_2O) is a polar molecule, with a north pole (with a pair of electrons on the oxygen atom) and a south pole (with 2 hydrogen atoms). Normally, water molecules in the brain rotate freely. In an MRI, the brain's water molecules line up along the length of the MRI tube (known as the bore) because the MRI scanner is a superconducting magnet 30,000-times stronger than the earth's magnetic field (if it is a 3T MRI). Noises during a structural MRI are radiofrequency pulses that push water molecules over, and the MRI measures how fast the water molecules rebound.

Table 1			
Magnetic resonance imaging basics			
Magnetic Resonance Imaging Type	**Analogy (Brain is like...)**	**Measures what**	**Main Outcomes**
Structural MRI	Compass	Structure	Volume, cortical thickness, shape
fMRI	Muscle	Activity with tasks and task-independent resting state	Activity and connectivity (synchronization of activation/deactivation)
DTI	Ziti	White matter integrity	FA RD MD AD
MRS	Chemicals	Neurometabolites	NAA Myo-inositol Choline Creatine GLX

To visualize this, stand up with one's hands stretched to the sky. The MRI radiofrequency noises push the person (the polar water molecule) over until the toes are touched. A T1 scan measures the longitudinal z-axis recovery (ie, how fast a person stands up). A T2 scan measures this recovery in the x-y plane (ie, how fast a person spins in a circle while standing upright). In a T1 scan, the brightest/white is white matter (because of fat content]) and then gray matter; cerebrospinal fluid (CSF) is darkest. In a T2 scan, CSF is brightest (mnemonic, T2 ~ H20 ~ "water white") and then gray matter; white matter is the darkest.

Other magnetic resonance imaging jargon
A 2-dimensional TV screen is made of pixels—squares with length and width. For a TV, the smaller and greater number of pixels, the better image quality of the TV. Similarly, MRIs take pictures of 3-dimensional objects, like a person's brain. The MRI equivalent of a pixel is called a "voxel"—or—volumetric pixel that has length, width, and height. When MRI articles refer to voxel size, they are conveying how big he 3-dimensional cubs are making up the brain picture. The smaller the voxel, the better the resolution of the MRI.

To look at a 3-dimensional brain on a 2-dimensional screen requires looking at the brain from 3 different angles, or planes. In **Fig. 1**, the coronal plane is looking through the back of someone's head, the axial plane is looking up through someone's feet toward the top of their head along the body's axis, and the sagittal plane is looking from the side (also known as the profile view).

Functional Magnetic Resonance Imaging: brain activity (brain = muscle)
fMRI allows examining brain activity. fMRI is not used clinically at present, although cardiology applications are growing. fMRI can be done with an accompanying cognitive or emotional task (also known as task-dependent fMRI) or when participants are at rest, not doing anything, known as resting state fMRI, or task-independent fMRI. Resting state fMRI is how the brain spends 95% of its energy.[8,9] Key outcomes from fMRI studies include areas of increased or decreased brain activity or changes in brain connectivity.

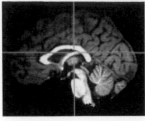 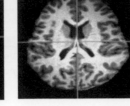 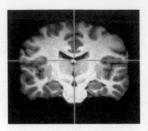

Sagittal Plane	Axial Plane	Coronal Plane
"Profile View"	"Look from feet to top of your head"	"Halo view"

Fig. 1. Basic MRI picture.

How does fMRI work? Think of the brain as a muscle. When running, more oxygen is extracted from the blood in the very active legs than the less active arms. The same is true for the brain—more active regions extract more oxygen than less active regions. Blood carries oxygen via the hemoglobin molecule that has an iron atom at its core. In the MRI magnetic field, deoxygenated hemoglobin from active brain areas (paramagnetic, attracted to magnetic fields) looks different from oxygenated hemoglobin from less active brain areas (diamagnetic, repelled from magnetic fields). Thus, fMRI measures brain activity as an index of the oxygenated to deoxygenated hemoglobin, also called the blood oxygen level–dependent response.

Diffusion tensor imaging: white matter integrity (brain = ziti)
DTI allows evaluating white matter integrity. DTI is used clinically for multiple sclerosis (MS) and brain cancer evaluations.

How does DTI work? Think of the brain as a collection of tubes, like ziti pasta—which represent neurons. DTI measures the movement of water (comprising 80% of the brain by weight). Water is more likely to move along the length of a neuron (or the ziti) than across the neuron. By tracking the diffusion (movement) of water along the lengths of neurons, DTI allows measuring the integrity of neurons.

Key DTI outcomes include (1) fractional anisotropy (FA) = extent to which diffusion is not random (an = not and isotropy = uniform movement in all direction); diffusion is increased in mature white matter or densely packed axons anf decreased in gray matter, CSF, or where there is demyelination like MS; (2) mean diffusivity (MD) = average amount of diffusion in a voxel; increased in axonal degeneration or demyelination and decreased in mature white matter; (3) radial diffusivity (RD) = diffusion/movement of water perpendicular to the major axis; increased in demyelination or axonal degeneration and decreased in mature white matter; and (4) axial diffusivity (AD) = diffusion/movement of water along the major axis of neurons; increased in mature white matter and decreased in gray matter.

Magnetic resonance imaging: neurometabolites (brain = collection of chemicals)
MRS measures brain chemicals (neurometabolites), related to brain function. MRS currently is used clinically in cancer diagnostics and treatment.

Key MRS outcomes include the following. N-acetylaspartate (NAA) is the most abundant chemical in mature neurons, representing 1/1000 of total brain weight. NAA is decreased in tumors and in MS. Glutamate/glutamine (GLX) often appears as a mixed result at MRI field strength of 3T or less, but GLX can be separated at 4T or higher into excitatory neurotransmitters glutamate (GLU) and glutamine (GLN). Creatine comes from energy metabolism, such as adenine triphosphate, and often MRS results are presented as a ratio of a single metabolite to creatine, that is, NAA/creatine. Choline represents neural membrane turnover and has been related to the increased adrenergic/decreased cholinergic imbalance theory of depression. Myo-inositol is related to the inositol phosphate intracellular second messenger cascade. Lithium's antimanic mechanism of action has been postulated to involve decreased mI.[10]

Computerized cognitive/emotional tasks

Computerized tasks or games test cognitive or emotional function. They can be administered on their own, to test behavioral performance (ie, reaction time or errors), or they can be coupled with either fMRI or electroencephalography (EEG), a technique also known as event-related potential, to test brain activity during those outcomes. Unfortunately, the human brain is wired neither for simplicity nor for *DSM*. Thus, most psychiatric disorders involve the interplay of several cognitive and emotional processes mediated by several brain areas.

Acknowledging this complexity is an important first step for clinicians in harnessing the brain science of mental illness—rather than allowing it to be an insurmountable barrier. **Table 2** explains some of the processes related to irritability and how researchers test them.

Reward processing is the response to pleasurable stimuli, possibly including winning/losing points or money or sensory reward (ie, the stimulus may taste, smell, sound, feel, or look good). The reward processing response may be cognitive, behavioral, or emotional and may be related to the seeking, receiving, or even anticipating getting the stimulus.

One aspect of reward processing is cognitive flexibility, defined as the ability to adapt to changing rewards and punishments. Reduced cognitive flexibility can trigger irritability. Cognitive flexibility can be measured with a reversal learning task, whereby participants must use trial-and-error learning to figure out which of 2 simultaneously presented stimuli are mostly correct (ie, mostly wins points) versus which is mostly wrong (ie, mostly loses points). Then, without warning, participants must adapt when the stimulus/reward relationship is reversed—that is, the previously correct/rewarded stimulus now is mostly punished (loses points), and the previously wrong/punished stimulus now is mostly rewarded (wins points). The Wisconsin Card Sorting Test (WCST) is a cognitive flexibility task familiar to many clinicians as part of psychoeducational testing for children. It requires children to adapt when the construct by which they are sorting a deck of cards changes, from color, to shape, to number, and so forth. Thus, cognitive flexibility involves attention and uses the dorsolateral prefrontal cortex (DLPFC)—an area near the temple—and reward, using the caudate and amygdala.

Another part of reward processing is frustrative nonreward (FNR), referring to the response stemming from blocked goal attainment. FNR is assessed with tasks using rigged feedback—that is, being told a response is wrong even though it was correct—to increase a participant's frustration, potentially triggering emotional responses, such as irritability or anger, and behavioral responses, such as verbal or physical aggression. Thus, rigged feedback ensures nonreward, because participants cannot earn reward no matter how hard they try. An example of an FNR task is the affective Posner task. The standard Posner task assesses attention, with participants indicating which side of the screen a target stimulus (blue square) appeared on when it was briefly

Table 2
Cognitive and emotional tasks used to study irritability

Construct	Definition	Tasks	Key Brain Areas
Reward processing–cognitive flexibility	Ability to adapt to changing rewards and punishments	Reversal learning: figure out which of 2 stimuli is rewarded and adapt when previously rewarded stimulus is now punished. The WCST: requires children to adapt when the construct by which they are sorting a deck of cards changes, from color to shape, to number, etc.	• DLPFC (attention processes) • Caudate and amygdala (reward processes)
Reward processing–FNR	Response stemming from blocked goal attainment; participants are told their responses are wrong, even though they are correct, and thus cannot maximize their receipt of reward no matter how hard they try.	Affective Posner: unlike the standard Posner task, where feedback is accurately tied to performance (WIN or LOSE based on participant's response), the affective Posner task uses rigged feedback, with participants told they LOSE or are TOO SLOW if even they were correct, to frustrate the person and cause irritability or anger.	
Response inhibition	Ability to stop a dominant, natural action	Go/no-go: do not press a button on no-go trials (1/3 of game) spread among the yes, press button, go trials (2/3 of game) Stroop interference task: identify color a word is printed in, not the word itself (if "red" is seen in blue ink, say "blue" [not "red"]).	• DLPFC • ACC (attention/planning) • Motor areas (striate, etc.)
Emotional face processing	Ability to identify what emotion someone's face is showing (eg, happy, angry, fear, neutral).	Diagnostic assessment of nonverbal accuracy: child and adult faces showing happy, sad, fear, and neutral	• Visual cortex • DLPFC • Hippocampus (memory area) • Amygdala (reward)

preceded by a cue stimulus (white square) that might hint at which side the target will appear on. Unlike the standard Posner task, where feedback is accurately tied to performance ("WIN" or "LOSE" based on participant's response), the affective Posner task uses rigged feedback, with participants told they "LOSE" or are "TOO SLOW" if even they were correct, to frustrate the person, inducing irritability or anger.

Response inhibition, referring to the ability to stop a dominant, natural action, is relevant to irritability as people become irritable if they make errors. Response inhibition can be tested by the go/no-go task, in which someone presses a button every time they see a star (which appears on 70% of trials) but to not press (inhibit the common response) if they see a moon (which appears on 30% of trials). Response inhibition also can be tested via the Stroop cognitive interference task, whereby someone is asked to identify the color a word is printed on. People are faster, and less likely to make errors, if the word and the color are the same ("green" printed in green) than if they are mis-matched ("green" printed in red). The latter requires the person to slow down and inhibit their tendency to say "green" and instead say "red." Response inhibition involves interplay from attention/planning areas, including the DLPFC and anterior cingulate cortex (ACC) (midline frontal part of the brain) and motor areas.

Emotional face processing, referring to the ability to recognize emotion displayed by someone's face, is relevant to irritability because it informs understanding of emotional responses, including irritability.[11] From birth, typically developing children are hard-wired to recognize their caregiver's emotions. Conversely, alterations in emotional face processing underlie some of the most serious forms of developmental disorders, including autism. Emotional face processing often is assessed using standardized picture sets of people, often actors, displaying particular types of emotions, for example, sad, angry, fear, and neutral. Participants may be asked to identify which emotion they think is being shown. Sometimes, morphed images are created, using computers to blend 2 different images in fixed ratios to see at what point can someone recognize the emotion has shifted, for example, going from 100% happy and 0% angry to 0% happy and 100% angry. Emotional face processing often involves contributions from visual cortex in the occipital lobe, attention/planning processes in the DLPFC (part of the brain near the outer edge of the eyebrow), reward areas of the amygdala, and memory areas of the hippocampus.

WHAT IS KNOWN ABOUT IRRITABILITY: NOW

Building on the guide to research tools used to advance understanding of the brain and behavior mechanisms underlying childhood irritability, what is known about these mechanisms in specific disorders is summarized. Potential clinical implications are noted and some study examples offered in **Table 3**.

Bipolar Disorder

BD youth have changes in a prefrontal cortex (PFC) striatal-amygdala circuit, mediating reward processing, response inhibition, and emotional face processing. These deficits have been found in multiple studies of BD youth and in some studies of youth at risk of BD by virtue of first-degree relatives with BD, suggesting that these may be trait deficits and distinct from what is seen in children with chronic irritability meeting research criteria for severe mood dysregulation (SMD).

Youth with BD demonstrate altered cognitive processing across many paradigms. For example, narrow phenotype BD youth, with distinct episodes of mania involving euphoria and often irritability, have impaired cognitive flexibility, making more errors on out-of-scanner reversal learning behavioral tasks compared with healthy controls. BD youth make more reversal errors than youth with other forms of psychopathology, including children with mood dysregulation disorder or children with severe mood dysregulation (SMD) (ie, chronic, nonepisodic irritability) and have been replicated in independent samples.[12-16] These deficits are not byproducts of mania itself, because they were observed during euthymia. Furthermore, they are not just a developmental phase, because they persist when participants with prospectively documented childhood-onset BD become adults.[17] fMRI shows BD youth have aberrant patterns

Table 3
Examples of brain/behavior research with children whose disorders involved irritability

Disorder	Construct	Study/Finding Example(s)	Clinical Implication
BD	Cognitive flexibility	Dickstein et al,[61] 2010: BD youth have the exact opposite fMRI activation during reversal learning than controls, with greater DLPFC and striatum fMRI activation than controls when reversing a stimulus/reward relationship.	BD involves PFC striatal-amygdala alterations in cognitive flexibility, reward processing, FNR, and response inhibition. Potentially explains why BD youth get irritable when they cannot adapt to situations or when things do not work out the way they expect
	FNR	Rich et al,[20] 2007: BD youth had altered P3 amplitude, reflecting impaired executive attention, compared with SMD and control youth, during the affective Posner task with rigged feedback paired with EEG.	Ongoing research to retrain the brain—to use computer games to build up these skills, and improve functioning, including cognitive flexibility.
	Reward	Singh et al,[19] 2012: BD youth have increased activation in the middle frontal gyrus and parietal cortex when anticipating losing money on a monetary incentive delay fMRI study.	
	Response inhibition	Leibenluft et al,[62] 2007: BD youth had less striatal and ventral PFC fMRI activation than controls during failed response inhibition.	
		Singh et al,[63] 2010: BD youth required greater fMRI activation in the DLPFC than controls to maintain similar accuracy during response inhibition no-go trials.	
		Weathers et al,[64] 2012: BD youths had decreased ACC fMRI activation during failed response inhibition compared with child controls and BD adults.	
	Emotional face processing	Deveney et al,[65] 2014: BD children and adults failed to activate the amygdala when making explicit and implicit ratings of how angry faces were during fMRI.	
		Bertocci et al,[66] 2019: greater fusiform gyrus activity during emotional face processing in combination with several other factors predicted irritability in Pittsburgh Bipolar Offspring Study and Longitudinal Assessment of Manic Symptoms Study in youth.	

		Findings	Interpretation
DMDD	Cognitive flexibility	Adleman et al,[18] 2011: SMD youth have significantly decreased inferior frontal gyrus fMRI activity during reversal learning vs BD and control youth.	DMDD involves PFC striatal dysfunction during reward, cognitive flexibility, and emotional face processing—different from BD youth with distinct episodes of euphoric mania. Ongoing work to reduce aberrant face processing to reduce irritability
	FNR	Tseng et al,[28] 2019: irritability in transdiagnostic sample of 52 DMDD, 42 ADHD, 42 anxious, and 61 control youth was positively correlated with increased DLPFC and caudate fMRI activity during rigged feedback on the affective Posner task.	
	Reward	Kessel et al,[27] 2016: preschool children with greater DMDD symptoms had greater positive response EEG response to reward on a monetary incentive delay task.	
	Emotional face processing	Stoddard et al,[29] 2016: DMDD youth misclassify ambiguous faces as angry rather than happy, and this may be trained, resulting in less irritability.	
ADHD	Reward	von Rhein et al,[33] 2015: unaffected siblings had similar increased fMRI activity at adolescents and young adults with ADHD in the ACC during the monetary incentive delay task. van Hulst et al,[32] 2017: increased ADHD symptoms correlates with decreased ventral striatal fMRI activity during reward anticipation on the monetary incentive delay task.	ADHD involves ~5 y delay in maturation of PFC striatal circuits mediating executive function (attention, planning, response inhibition), and reward. ADHD stimulant medications increase synaptic dopamine to improve reward-related behavior. Psychosocial treatments, including reward-based behavior modification, are important for ADHD but may be challenging as underlying circuits function differently in ADHD vs control youth.
	Response inhibition	Albajara Saenz et al,[36] 2020: ADHD youth had behavioral alterations in response inhibition on a stop-signal task, and increased right inferior parietal activation, whereas ASD youth had increased right frontal activation. Posner et al,[38] 2011: adolescents with ADHD scanned off their medications had impaired medial PFC activation during the emotional Stroop task. Administration of stimulant ADHD medication attenuated medial PFC activity to comparable levels as controls.	

(continued on next page)

Table 3
(continued)

Disorder	Construct	Study/Finding Example(s)	Clinical Implication
ASD	Reward	Scott-Van Zeeland et al,[47] 2010: ASD boys had greater activation than age/IQ-matched controls to monetary reward in the OFC and paracingulate gyrus but decreased activation than controls to social rewards in the ventral striatum.	ASD involves brain changes in all 4 lobes and the cerebellum—more globally than other disorders—potentially explaining more profound impairments. Studies trying to improve ASD symptoms, particularly in ASD adults, both building these cognitive skills and also studying potential for medications or preparations to augment improvements

of frontostriatal activity compared with controls during reversal learning tasks[14] and during reversal learning compared with youth with SMD.[18]

During reward processing, BD youth demonstrate increased middle frontal gyrus and parietal cortex activation when anticipating losing money but decreased inferior temporal gyrus and thalamus when anticipating winning money compared with controls.[19] In FNR studies using rigged, inaccurate feedback, BD youth are different from youth with SMD and controls. Pairing the affective Posner task with EEG showed that BD youth had altered P3 amplitude, reflecting impaired executive attention compared with SMD and control youths.[20] Another study using magnetoencephalography (EEG plus a task and a separate structural MRI) showed that BD youth had greater superior frontal activation and decreased insula activation after negative feedback compared with SMD and control youths.[21]

What are the clinical implications of these studies? They provide a potential mechanism for why BD youth get irritable when they cannot adapt to life situations or when things do not work out as they expect. Furthermore, they may explain why some forms of psychotherapy do not work well for BD youth. Specifically, behavior modification requires an intact reward processing system to adapt behavior to obtain rewards and to desire/anticipate reward. Cognitive-behavior therapy requires recognizing negative consequences of automatic thoughts/behaviors, such as losing out on rewarding relationships due to mindreading. Ongoing studies are determining if reversal learning cognitive remediation—that is, computer games to build up deficient reversal learning skills—can reduce BD symptoms in children as a potential brain mechanism–targeted treatment.[22]

Other MRI modalities further implicate the PFC amygdala-striatal circuit in pediatric BD. For example, increased resting state connectivity between the left basolateral amygdala and the left frontal pole/posterior cingulate distinguished BD versus SMD and control youth.[23] DTI studies show BD youth have alterations in white matter integrity, including reductions in FA and increases in RD versus controls, and DMDD youth had reduced FA and AD to the anterior corpus callosum, but the only difference between BD and DMDD youth was reduced FA in the corticospinal tract.[24] Together, these studies provide a cohesive understanding of the underlying deficits in emotional, reward, and cognitive processing observed in youth with BD.

Disruptive Mood Dysregulation Disorder

As discussed previously, and elsewhere in this 2-volume work, DMDD is a new diagnosis in *DSM-5* arising from research to answer whether BD in children uniquely presented as impairing irritability occurring so frequently it was chronic, as some investigators believed,[25] or if BD in children involved euphoria, as in adults.

A decade's worth of research has shown that SMD youth have a distinct longitudinal course and frontostriatal dysfunction during reward, cognitive flexibility, and emotional face processing compared with narrow phenotype BD youth.[26] Other research groups have shown that DMDD youth have frontostriatal alterations compared with typically developing controls. For example, children with more clinically significant DMDD symptoms at age 3 years old had greater EEG neural reactivity during a monetary reward task at age 9.[27] Some studies are beginning to look at the specificity of these alterations, whereas other studies are aggregating samples of youth with irritability transdiagnostically. For example, a transdiagnostic sample of children with DMDD, anxiety disorders, ADHD, or controls showed greater irritability was associated with increased DLPFC, inferior frontal gyrus, and caudate activation after frustration on the affective Posner task, a finding moderated by age, with stronger associations in younger children.[28]

What are the clinical implications of these brain/behavior mechanisms? For some youth with chronic irritability fitting SMD/DMDD criteria, these data show that this is not just a phase and may progress to depression in adulthood. Furthermore, studies for clinical translation are under way. For example, Stoddard and colleagues[29] identified that DMDD youth misclassified ambiguous faces as angry, rather than happy, and developed a computer game to retrain this balance point, which resulted in less irritability than pretraining.

Attention-deficit/Hyperactivity Disorder

Although irritability is not an explicit *DSM-5* symptom of ADHD, it is an associated feature possibly mediated by alterations in frontostriatal circuits mediating reward and also executive control and planning, including response inhibition.[30,31]

ADHD youth have deficits in reward processing, including often preferring small immediate rewards rather than larger delayed rewards. For example, children with ADHD have decreased ventral striatal fMRI activity during reward anticipation in children with ADHD symptoms, regardless of formal ADHD diagnosis.[32] Another fMRI study showed that both adolescents and young adults with ADHD and also their unaffected siblings had similar increased activity during the anticipation of monetary reward in frontal areas, including the ACC and anterior frontal cortex compared with controls, suggesting this may be a trait marker.[33] Other studies show that although ADHD youths have increased brain activity after they receive a reward or win money, including the ACC, an area mediating response to conflicting choices, whereas for control youths, brain activity decreased in both conditions.[34,35] These deficits merit comparison in youth with BD and DMDD.

Although an exhaustive review of executive function alterations in ADHD is beyond the scope of this article, a few recent articles highlight the consistency of these findings. For example, ADHD youth had behavioral alterations in response inhibition on a stop-signal task and increased right inferior parietal activation, whereas autism spectrum disorder (ASD) youth had increased right frontal activation.[36] Among 16,099 children with ADHD and their siblings, greater ADHD traits (regardless of diagnosis) are associated with decreased response inhibition, slower latency, and greater variability in performance, and response inhibition and ADHD traits are coheritable.[37] Finally, an fMRI study showed adolescents with ADHD scanned off their medications had impaired medial PFC activation during the emotional Stroop task, and that administration of stimulant ADHD medication attenuated medial PFC activity to comparable levels as controls.[38]

What are the clinical implications of these findings? Clinicians may find this research useful in explaining to patients, parents, and teachers why children with ADHD struggle with completing daily homework or chores, paying attention to schoolwork for prolonged time periods, or inhibiting their responses to look before they leap. They also explain some challenges of psychosocial treatments for ADHD, such as behavior modification and parent training, which require individuals to adapt their behavior to earn rewards—the exact systems that are impaired in ADHD. Yet other studies suggest how ADHD psychostimulants increase synaptic dopamine levels and improve reward-related behavior, including response inhibition and learning.[39] Finally, longitudinal structural MRI studies showing that children with ADHD have approximately a 5-year lag, but not permanent deficit, in the maturation of frontostriatal circuits compared with typically developing controls suggests a biological reason why for many, these treatments no longer may be needed as children become young adults, in contrast to more persistent or progressive mood syndromes.

Autism

Although irritability is not an explicit *DSM-5* diagnostic criterion for ASD, it is an associated feature, and there is a Food and Drug Administration indication for the use of atypical neuroleptics to treat irritability associated with ASD. Irritability in ASD often results when ASD diagnostic core features (eg, deficits in social relationships, communication, or restricted repetitive behaviors and interests) cannot be accommodated, such as when preferred food, clothing, people, or schedules are unavailable or must change. This is in distinction to DMDD, where irritability is chronic (ie, nearly every day) without specific trigger, and in distinction to manic or major depressive episodes when irritability occurs during a shift from baseline euthymic mood and accompanied by other symptoms.

Unlike BD, DMDD, and ADHD, ASD involves brain changes affecting all 4 lobes and the cerebellum, and by structural, functional, and diffusion imaging techniques.[40–42] Substantial work has evaluated emotional face processing in ASD, given that ASD involved impaired social-emotional reciprocity.[43–46]

With respect to reward processing in ASD, the social motivation hypothesis posits that individuals with ASD find social stimuli less rewarding than typically developing children. This hypothesis emanates from work separately examining fMRI responses to both social and monetary rewards. ASD boys had greater activation than age/IQ-matched controls to monetary reward in the orbitofrontal cortex (OFC) but decreased activation than controls to social rewards in the ventral striatum.[47] A meta-analysis of reward processing fMRI studies in ASD (n = 259) and control (n = 246) participants, showed aberrant processing of both social and nonsocial rewards in the striatum, including the caudate, partially linked to restricted interests.[48]

Cognitive flexibility is important to ASD core symptoms of restricted range of interests and repetitive behaviors.[49] Although to the best of the authors' knowledge, there are no published fMRI studies of cognitive flexibility children with ASD, 2 studies have demonstrated adults with ASD have increased parietal activity during fMRI tasks requiring cognitive flexibility and switching.[50,51] A meta-analysis of cognitive performance in ASD (n = 2137) to control (n = 2185) participants found the greatest mean effect size was for set shifting and moderate effect sizes for perseverative errors.[52] Others have shown that ASD children had higher switch cost, meaning they responded much slower on switch trials than on maintain trials[53] or made more perseverative errors on the WCST and more errors on switch versus maintain trials on the switch task than controls.[54] A third study showed that unaffected first-degree relatives of ASD probands made more perseverative errors on the WCST than controls, suggesting impaired cognitive flexibility may be an inherited ASD trait.[55]

Response inhibition in ASD potentially is linked to repetitive behaviors and restricted range of interests. For example, adults with ASD have impaired inhibition of prepotent responses and/or altered fMRI activity in regions mediating response inhibition, such as the ACC, on tasks including the go/no-go task or visual saccade tasks, the latter requiring participants to inhibit the natural response of looking at novel stimuli appearing in one's visual fields.[56,57]

What are the clinical implications of these findings? Clinicians may find such information useful when explaining the profound nature of ASD impairments, given neuroimaging findings in all 4 lobes and the cerebellum. Clinical translations into potential treatments are under way. For example, a recent double-blind placebo-controlled fMRI study showed citalopram administration normalized aberrant inferior frontal activation in adults with ASD during a response inhibition task.[58] Similarly, ongoing research is evaluating oxytocin—a naturally occurring neuropeptide produced by the hypothalamus, released by the posterior pituitary, and which plays a role in social bonding and reproduction—as a potential targeted treatment to assist reward processing and social skills impairments in people with ASD.[59,60]

WHAT IS NEEDED TO KNOW ABOUT IRRITABILITY: THE FUTURE

Hopefully the future can bring greater understanding of the brain/behavior mechanisms underlying irritability that can be translated into meaningful advances in clinical care. Following the example of childhood leukemia, in the future, the authors hope that when a parent, clinician, or teacher is concerned about a child's irritability causing problems at home, school, or with peers, their clinical history augmented by a scan or test might confirm with 95% certainty which diagnosis the child has and can guide the most efficacious treatment.

Progress comes from research that examines brain/behavior mechanisms underlying *DSM*-defined psychopathology involving irritability, whereas other studies start with the brain first—testing how patterns of brain/behavior dysfunction cluster children and what symptoms and strengths they have.

This work will be transformative only if everyone—clinicians, parents, educators, and policymakers—joins forces by breaking down barriers to harness current knowledge, fueling future discovery.

SUMMARY

Breaking down barriers limiting clinicians' use of current knowledge about the brain/behavior mechanisms underlying psychiatric disorders involving irritability allows them to use this information when explaining diagnoses and treatments to families. Transformative improvement in child mental health care will require collaboration between clinicians, parents, and researchers who can harness mechanism-oriented research—for example, by using scans and tests that assess these brain/behavior mechanisms to augment clinical diagnostic processes, making them more specific, or by developing treatments that target underlying brain/behavior mechanisms. This will lead to a brighter tomorrow for today's children, as already has occurred in mechanism-augmented clinical care for children with leukemia, transforming it from the past, with almost certain mortality, to now 95% 5-year survival.

ACKNOWLEDGMENT

Received National Institute of Mental Health (NIMH)/National Institutes of Health (NIH) funding from (R01MH111542) Brain/Behavior Mechanisms of Irritability and Cognitive Flexibility in Children, (K24MH110402) Mid-career Mentorship and Research in Imaging-related Patient Oriented Research, (R01MH110379) Non-suicidal Self-Injury in Children: Brain/behavior Alterations and Risk for Suicidal Behavior, and Charles Hood Foundation Major Grant Brain/behavior Mechanisms of Irritability and Suicide in Children and Adolescents. I have no other support for my work or non-grant research funding besides NIH/NIMH and Foundations.

REFERENCES

1. Peterson BS, Zhang H, Santa Lucia R, et al. Risk factors for presenting problems in child psychiatric emergencies. J Am Acad Child Adolesc Psychiatry 1996; 35(9):1162–73.

2. Stringaris A, Cohen P, Pine DS, et al. Adult outcomes of youth irritability: a 20-year prospective community-based study. Am J Psychiatry 2009;166(9):1048–54.

3. Kelly C, Molcho M, Doyle P, et al. Psychosomatic symptoms among schoolchildren. IntJ AdolescMedHealth 2010;22(2):229–35.

4. Collishaw S, Maughan B, Natarajan L, et al. Trends in adolescent emotional problems in England: a comparison of two national cohorts twenty years apart. J Child Psychol Psychiatry 2010;51(8):885–94.

5. American Psychiatric Association. Diagnostic and Statistical manual of mental disorders, Vol 5. Arlington, VA: American Psychiatric Association; 2013.

6. Leibenluft E, Cohen P, Gorrindo T, et al. Chronic versus episodic irritability in youth: a community-based, longitudinal study of clinical and diagnostic associations. J Child Adolesc Psychopharmacol 2006;16(4):456–66.

7. Pickles A, Aglan A, Collishaw S, et al. Predictors of suicidality across the life span: the Isle of Wight study. Psychol Med 2010;40(9):1453–66.

8. Raichle ME, Gusnard DA. Intrinsic brain activity sets the stage for expression of motivated behavior. J Comp Neurol 2005;493(1):167–76.

9. Fox MD, Snyder AZ, Vincent JL, et al. The human brain is intrinsically organized into dynamic, anticorrelated functional networks. Proc Natl Acad Sci U S A 2005; 102(27):9673–8.

10. Moore GJ, Bebchuk JM, Hasanat K, et al. Lithium increases N-acetyl-aspartate in the human brain: in vivo evidence in support of bcl-2's neurotrophic effects? Biol Psychiatry 2000;48(1):1–8.

11. Vuilleumier P, Pourtois G. Distributed and interactive brain mechanisms during emotion face perception: evidence from functional neuroimaging. Neuropsychologia 2007;45(1):174–94.

12. Dickstein DP, Treland JE, Snow J, et al. Neuropsychological performance in pediatric bipolar disorder. Biol Psychiatry 2004;55(1):32–9.

13. Gorrindo T, Blair RJ, Budhani S, et al. Deficits on a probabilistic response-reversal task in patients with pediatric bipolar disorder. Am J Psychiatry 2005;162(10): 1975–7.

14. Dickstein DP, Finger EC, Brotman MA, et al. Impaired probabilistic reversal learning in youths with mood and anxiety disorders. Psychol Med 2010;40(7): 1089–100.

15. Dickstein DP, Axelson D, Weissman AB, et al. Cognitive flexibility and performance in children and adolescents with threshold and sub-threshold bipolar disorder. Eur Child Adolesc Psychiatry 2016;25(6):625–38.

16. Frías Á, Dickstein DP, Merranko J, et al. Longitudinal cognitive trajectories and associated clinical variables in youth with bipolar disorder. Bipolar Disord 2017; 19(4):273–84.

17. Wegbreit E, Cushman GK, Weissman AB, et al. Reversal-learning deficits in childhood-onset bipolar disorder across the transition from childhood to young adulthood. J Affect Disord 2016;203:46–54.

18. Adleman NE, Kayser R, Dickstein D, et al. Neural correlates of reversal learning in severe mood dysregulation and pediatric bipolar disorder. J Am Acad Child Adolesc Psychiatry 2011;50(11):1173–85.e1172.

19. Singh MK, Chang KD, Kelley RG, et al. Reward processing in adolescents with bipolar I disorder. J Am Acad Child Adolesc Psychiatry 2013;52(1):68–83.

20. Rich BA, Schmajuk M, Perez-Edgar KE, et al. Different psychophysiological and behavioral responses elicited by frustration in pediatric bipolar disorder and severe mood dysregulation. Am J Psychiatry 2007;164(2):309–17.

21. Rich BA, Carver FW, Holroyd T, et al. Different neural pathways to negative affect in youth with pediatric bipolar disorder and severe mood dysregulation. J Psychiatr Res 2011;45(10):1283–94.
22. Dickstein DP, Cushman GK, Kim KL, et al. Cognitive remediation: potential novel brain-based treatment for bipolar disorder in children and adolescents. CNS Spectr 2015;20(4):382–90.
23. Stoddard J, Hsu D, Reynolds RC, et al. Aberrant amygdala intrinsic functional connectivity distinguishes youths with bipolar disorder from those with severe mood dysregulation. Psychiatry Res 2015;231(2):120–5.
24. Linke JO, Adleman NE, Sarlls J, et al. White matter microstructure in pediatric bipolar disorder and disruptive mood dysregulation disorder. J Am Acad Child Adolesc Psychiatry 2019.
25. Wozniak J, Biederman J, Richards JA. Diagnostic and therapeutic dilemmas in the management of pediatric-onset bipolar disorder. J Clin Psychiatry 2001; 62(Suppl 14):10–5.
26. Biederman J, Klein RG, Pine DS, et al. Resolved: mania is mistaken for ADHD in prepubertal children. J Amacadchild Adolescpsychiatry 1998;37(10):1091–6.
27. Kessel EM, Dougherty LR, Kujawa A, et al. Longitudinal associations between preschool disruptive mood dysregulation disorder symptoms and neural reactivity to monetary reward during preadolescence. J Child Adolesc Psychopharmacol 2016;26(2):131–7.
28. Tseng WL, Deveney CM, Stoddard J, et al. Brain mechanisms of attention orienting following frustration: associations with irritability and age in youths. Am J Psychiatry 2019;176(1):67–76.
29. Stoddard J, Sharif-Askary B, Harkins EA, et al. An open pilot study of training hostile interpretation bias to treat disruptive mood dysregulation disorder. J Child Adolesc Psychopharmacol 2016;26(1):49–57.
30. Castellanos FX, Lee PP, Sharp W, et al. Developmental trajectories of brain volume abnormalities in children and adolescents with attention-deficit/hyperactivity disorder. JAMA 2002;288(14):1740–8.
31. Shaw P, Eckstrand K, Sharp W, et al. Attention-deficit/hyperactivity disorder is characterized by a delay in cortical maturation. Proc Natl Acad Sci U S A 2007;104(49):19649–54.
32. van Hulst BM, de Zeeuw P, Bos DJ, et al. Children with ADHD symptoms show decreased activity in ventral striatum during the anticipation of reward, irrespective of ADHD diagnosis. J Child Psychol Psychiatry 2017;58(2):206–14.
33. von Rhein D, Cools R, Zwiers MP, et al. Increased neural responses to reward in adolescents and young adults with attention-deficit/hyperactivity disorder and their unaffected siblings. J Am Acad Child Adolesc Psychiatry 2015;54(5): 394–402.
34. Holroyd CB, Baker TE, Kerns KA, et al. Electrophysiological evidence of atypical motivation and reward processing in children with attention-deficit hyperactivity disorder. Neuropsychologia 2008;46(8):2234–42.
35. Umemoto A, Lukie CN, Kerns KA, et al. Impaired reward processing by anterior cingulate cortex in children with attention deficit hyperactivity disorder. Cogn Affect Behav Neurosci 2014;14(2):698–714.
36. Albajara Saenz A, Septier M, Van Schuerbeek P, et al. ADHD and ASD: distinct brain patterns of inhibition-related activation? Transl Psychiatry 2020;10(1):24.
37. Crosbie J, Arnold P, Paterson A, et al. Response inhibition and ADHD traits: correlates and heritability in a community sample. J Abnorm Child Psychol 2013; 41(3):497–507.

38. Posner J, Maia TV, Fair D, et al. The attenuation of dysfunctional emotional processing with stimulant medication: an fMRI study of adolescents with ADHD. Psychiatry Res 2011;193(3):151–60.

39. Luman M, Papanikolau A, Oosterlaan J. The Unique and combined effects of reinforcement and methylphenidate on temporal information processing in attention-deficit/hyperactivity disorder. J Clin Psychopharmacol 2015;35(4): 414–21.

40. Nickl-Jockschat T, Habel U, Michel TM, et al. Brain structure anomalies in autism spectrum disorder–a meta-analysis of VBM studies using anatomic likelihood estimation. Hum Brain Mapp 2012;33(6):1470–89.

41. Philip RC, Dauvermann MR, Whalley HC, et al. A systematic review and meta-analysis of the fMRI investigation of autism spectrum disorders. Neurosci Biobehav Rev 2012;36(2):901–42.

42. Dickstein DP, Pescosolido MF, Reidy BL, et al. Developmental meta-analysis of the functional neural correlates of autism spectrum disorders. J Am Acad Child Adolesc Psychiatry 2013;52(3):279–289 e216.

43. Schultz RT, Gauthier I, Klin A, et al. Abnormal ventral temporal cortical activity during face discrimination among individuals with autism and Asperger syndrome. Arch Gen Psychiatry 2000;57(4):331–40.

44. Klin A, Jones W, Schultz R, et al. Visual fixation patterns during viewing of naturalistic social situations as predictors of social competence in individuals with autism. Arch Gen Psychiatry 2002;59(9):809–16.

45. Klin A, Jones W. Attributing social and physical meaning to ambiguous visual displays in individuals with higher-functioning autism spectrum disorders. Brain Cogn 2006;61(1):40–53.

46. Weng SJ, Carrasco M, Swartz JR, et al. Neural activation to emotional faces in adolescents with autism spectrum disorders. J Child Psychol Psychiatry 2011; 52(3):296–305.

47. Scott-Van Zeeland AA, Dapretto M, Ghahremani DG, et al. Reward processing in autism. Autism Res 2010;3(2):53–67.

48. Clements CC, Zoltowski AR, Yankowitz LD, et al. Evaluation of the social motivation hypothesis of autism: a systematic review and meta-analysis. JAMA Psychiatry 2018;75(8):797–808.

49. Lopez BR, Lincoln AJ, Ozonoff S, et al. Examining the relationship between executive functions and restricted, repetitive symptoms of Autistic Disorder. J Autism Dev Disord 2005;35(4):445–60.

50. Schmitz N, Rubia K, Daly E, et al. Neural correlates of executive function in autistic spectrum disorders. Biol Psychiatry 2006;59(1):7–16.

51. Latinus M, Clery H, Andersson F, et al. Inflexibility in Autism Spectrum Disorder: need for certainty and atypical emotion processing share the blame. Brain Cogn 2019;136:103599.

52. Leung RC, Zakzanis KK. Brief report: cognitive flexibility in autism spectrum disorders: a quantitative review. J Autism Dev Disord 2014;44(10):2628–45.

53. Van Eylen LB B, Steyaert J, Evers K, et al. Cognitive flexibility in autism spectrum disorder: explaining the inconsistencies? Res Autism Spectr Disord 2011;5(4): 1390–401.

54. Van Eylen L, Boets B, Steyaert J, et al. Executive functioning in autism spectrum disorders: influence of task and sample characteristics and relation to symptom severity. Eur Child Adolesc Psychiatry 2015;24(11):1399–417.

55. Van Eylen L, Boets B, Cosemans N, et al. Executive functioning and local-global visual processing: candidate endophenotypes for autism spectrum disorder? J Child Psychol Psychiatry 2017;58(3):258–69.
56. Kana RK, Keller TA, Minshew NJ, et al. Inhibitory control in high-functioning autism: decreased activation and underconnectivity in inhibition networks. Biol Psychiatry 2007;62(3):198–206.
57. Agam Y, Joseph RM, Barton JJ, et al. Reduced cognitive control of response inhibition by the anterior cingulate cortex in autism spectrum disorders. Neuroimage 2010;52(1):336–47.
58. Wichers RH, Findon JL, Jelsma A, et al. Modulation of brain activation during executive functioning in autism with citalopram. Transl Psychiatry 2019;9(1):286.
59. Stavropoulos KK, Carver LJ. Research review: social motivation and oxytocin in autism–implications for joint attention development and intervention. J Child Psychol Psychiatry 2013;54(6):603–18.
60. Preckel K, Kanske P, Singer T, et al. Clinical trial of modulatory effects of oxytocin treatment on higher-order social cognition in autism spectrum disorder: a randomized, placebo-controlled, double-blind and crossover trial. BMC Psychiatry 2016;16(1):329.
61. Dickstein DP, Finger EC, Skup M, et al. Altered neural function in pediatric bipolar disorder during reversal learning. Bipolar Disord 2010;12(7):707–19.
62. Leibenluft E, Rich BA, Vinton DT, et al. Neural circuitry engaged during unsuccessful motor inhibition in pediatric bipolar disorder. Am J Psychiatry 2007; 164(1):52–60.
63. Singh MK, Chang KD, Mazaika P, et al. Neural correlates of response inhibition in pediatric bipolar disorder. J Child Adolesc Psychopharmacol 2010;20(1):15–24.
64. Weathers JD, Stringaris A, Deveney CM, et al. A developmental study of the neural circuitry mediating motor inhibition in bipolar disorder. Am J Psychiatry 2012; 169(6):633–41.
65. Deveney CM, Brotman MA, Thomas LA, et al. Neural response during explicit and implicit face processing varies developmentally in bipolar disorder. Soc Cogn Affect Neurosci 2014;9(12):1984–92.
66. Bertocci MA, Hanford L, Manelis A, et al. Clinical, cortical thickness and neural activity predictors of future affective lability in youth at risk for bipolar disorder: initial discovery and independent sample replication. Mol Psychiatry 2019; 24(12):1856–67.

Chronic Irritability in Youth
A Reprise on Challenges and Opportunities Toward Meeting Unmet Clinical Needs

Ellen Leibenluft, MD*, Katharina Kircanski, PhD

KEYWORDS

- Irritability • Children and adolescents • Frustrative nonreward
- Emotion dysregulation • Disruptive mood dysregulation disorder
- Attention-deficit hyperactivity disorder • Anxiety
- Functional magnetic resonance imaging

KEY POINTS

- Irritability is a subtype of emotion dysregulation that is characterized by increased proneness to anger, relative to peers, and is a suitable focus for translational research.
- Chronic, severe irritability is not a pediatric presentation of bipolar disorder. Instead, it is longitudinally associated with unipolar depression and anxiety and genetically associated with unipolar depression, anxiety, and attention-deficit hyperactivity disorder.
- Frustrative nonreward is a construct that can be evaluated across species to understand mechanisms underlying irritability.
- Research on brain mechanisms mediating aberrant responses to frustration in youth can guide the development of novel interventions.

INTRODUCTION

Emotion dysregulation is one of, if not the, most common reason that youth are brought to psychiatric care. The impact of emotion dysregulation is experienced, not only by youth, but also as by their families, as described in the parent perspective by Pavlov-Blum that opens volume I.[1] This commentary adopts a translational perspective on one subtype of emotion dysregulation, irritability. A translational perspective is key to elucidating pathophysiological mechanisms of irritability; elucidating such mechanisms is, in turn, central to the development of novel, personalized interventions.

We first focus on challenges and an opportunity that arise when studying irritability from a translational perspective. One *translational challenge* concerns defining the construct of interest.

Section on Mood Dysregulation and Neuroscience, Intramural Research Program, National Institute of Mental Health, Building 15K, MSC 2670, Bethesda, MD 20892-2670, USA
* Corresponding author.
E-mail address: leibs@mail.nih.gov

Child Adolesc Psychiatric Clin N Am 30 (2021) 667–683
https://doi.org/10.1016/j.chc.2021.04.014
1056-4993/21/Published by Elsevier Inc.

For example, in a volume on emotion dysregulation, why focus specifically on irritability? Our discussion here complements the work presented by Connor and Doerfler and Althoff and Ametti.[1] We "drill down" into the construct of irritability; our working definition of irritability is "elevated proneness to anger, relative to peers."[2] We discuss external validity of irritability and differing, but closely associated, variations in its presentation (ie, phasic vs tonic irritability). We then discuss the related challenge that, at least in clinical populations, irritability rarely occurs alone. In youth selected specifically for severe irritability (ie, those with disruptive mood dysregulation disorder [DMDD]), the most common comorbid diagnoses are anxiety disorders and attention-deficit hyperactivity disorder (ADHD). It is important to identify shared versus unique mechanisms among irritability, anxiety, and ADHD in order to predict the course of children presenting with complex combinations of these phenotypes and guide the development of personalized treatments. Here, our discussion complements the Blader, Walkup and colleagues, and Weisbrot and Carlson articles.[1]

We then turn to basic mechanisms afforded by a focus on irritability, namely the utility of the construct of frustrative nonreward (FNR) in studying the neural mechanisms of severe irritability in youth. FNR is a construct and behavioral paradigm developed first in rodents and studied in nonhuman primates and humans.[3] In a heuristic model of irritability published in 2017,[2] we posited that irritability can be understood as aberrant responses to frustration and to threat. We focus specifically on studies of frustration and include a discussion of the implications of this work for the development of novel interventions.

TRANSLATIONAL CHALLENGES IN STUDYING IRRITABILITY
Defining Irritability and Overlapping Constructs

Multiple constructs and definitions have been used to capture the clinically important severe dysregulation that is the focus of this special edition (eg, Spring and Carlson, Keluskar and colleagues, Ashurova and colleagues, Keeshin and colleagues, Benton and colleagues, and Sharma and McClellan).[1] See **Fig. 1** for one conceptualization of

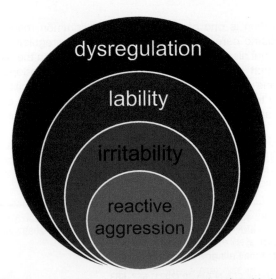

Fig. 1. Select overlapping constructs used to describe emotional and behavioral dysregulation. The figure highlights the increasing specificity and narrow scope of the constructs. See text for definition and discussion of each construct.

some of these constructs. Dysregulation itself, sometimes operationalized using the Children's Behavior Checklist (CBCL) Dysregulation Profile, is one construct, encompassing dysfunction across emotional, behavioral, and attentional domains (see Connor and Doerfler and Althoff and Ametti, volume I).[1] Lability and irritability are narrower, as their definition is based on emotion and mood, with associated behavior seen as secondary. Lability can be defined as abnormally frequent shifts into both negative and positive emotions and moods. It features prominently in the literature on bipolar disorder (BD), where euphoric mood is associated with hedonic behaviors. Also, the clinical observation that youth with ADHD may have uncontrollable bouts of "silliness" sparked interest in emotional lability in ADHD and was sometimes viewed as supporting a diagnosis of mania in these youth.[4–6]

Irritability has had multiple definitions and conceptualizations; for a thorough review, see Toohey and DiGiuseppe.[7] One parsimonious conceptualization specifies that, like lability, irritability is characterized by frequent and marked shifts of mood and emotion, but in irritability the shifts are only into a negative mood state, specifically anger. Behavioral outputs of irritability can then include explosive temper outbursts and reactive aggression (see Spring and Carlson and Connor and Doerfler, volume I).[1]

Our group's working definition of irritability is "elevated propensity to anger, relative to peers."[2] This definition is admittedly imperfect and likely to require modification as we learn more. The definition was influenced by the conceptualization in **Fig. 1**; our aim was to be narrow and specific enough to enable us to frame tractable research questions while being broad enough to encompass important clinical phenomena. Importantly, because our research aims at identifying brain mechanisms of irritability, we wanted a construct that allows for translational bridges, as this does in linking to anger, aggression, frustration, and threat.[2] We wanted a dimensional construct that encompasses psychopathology. Our definition does not allow for "normative irritability," which can be seen as a limitation, nor does it specify a threshold for "elevated." Also, arguably the definition conflates mood and emotion, and its conceptualization of behavior as secondary to mood and emotion needs to be confirmed by further research.

External Validity of the Irritability Construct

How useful is the irritability construct in furthering clinically meaningful research? To assess this, we use the framework for "external validity" developed Dr Kenneth Kendler[8] for the Diagnostic and Statistical Manual of Mental Disorders, Fifth Revision (DSM-5) process. External validity was defined as reliably providing relevant clinical information. Six high-priority validators were defined: (1) familial aggregation and/or co-aggregation (eg, family, twin, or adoption studies); (2) biological markers (eg, molecular genetics, neural substrates); (3) degree or nature of functional impairment; (4) diagnostic stability; (5) course of illness; and (6) response to treatment. Although these criteria were designed to assess categorical diagnostic constructs, here we apply them to the dimensional construct of irritability. The question is whether knowing if an individual is relatively high or low on trait irritability provides useful cross-sectional and predictive information. Because, in clinical samples, irritability rarely occurs alone (see later in this article), the goal of these studies is to identify associations with irritability specifically, rather than with comorbid traits or diagnoses.

First, in terms of *familial aggregation*, family studies show a link between parental (especially maternal) depression and child irritability, with the causal arrows usually being bidirectional.[9–11] Perhaps more compellingly, twin studies show the heritability of irritability to be in the moderate range (ie, approximately 0.3–0.6), similar to anxiety and unipolar depressive disorders.[12–17] Thus, there appears to be good evidence for familial aggregation.

Second, regarding *biological markers*, for irritability as for all other psychological traits and psychiatric diagnoses, the search for biomarkers remains ongoing and aspirational; hopefully the research described later in this article and other ongoing work further this effort.

Third, there is good evidence that irritability can be *impairing* in multiple domains (home, school, peers).[18,19] Further, comorbid irritability is associated with increased impairment in youth with illnesses such as anxiety or ADHD.[20,21] Youth irritability appears to be associated with impairment into early adulthood, again after controlling for other symptoms.[22]

The fourth criterion for external validity, *stability*, was articulated for DSM-5 in terms of stability of categorical diagnoses; here we focus primarily on evidence for stability of the dimensional trait. In a large, community-based twin sample (N = 1431 pairs) with 1-year follow-up, there was moderate stability for both the categorical and dimensional formulations of DMDD/irritability.[15] However, other evidence suggests that dimensionally operationalized trait irritability may be more stable than categorical DMDD. For example, in a 2-year to 4-year follow-up of 200 youth with severe mood dysregulation (SMD, the precursor phenotype to DMDD[23]) in community treatment, the % meeting SMD criteria declined from 100% at baseline (mean age 11.6 ± 2.6 years) to 49% at 2 years and 40% at 4 years, indicating poor stability.[24] However, throughout the follow-up period, youth remained moderately impaired, with markedly stable Clinical Global Impression (CGI) SMD and CGI overall impairment ratings. Notably, more than 80% continued to receive psychotropic medications and more than 20% had been hospitalized. Major limitations of this study include poor retention, possibly introducing bias. Similar results were found in a smaller (N = 36) and younger (ages 6–9 years) sample.[25] Of note, however, some studies do not find good stability, even for dimensionally assessed irritability.[26,27]

The decreased stability of categorical versus dimensional approaches to irritability may reflect arbitrary and nondevelopmentally sensitive thresholds for the category. Indeed, in a community-based sample of preschoolers (N = 425, mean age = 4.7 years), dimensional measures were used to derive a severity cutoff to identify potentially concerning irritability. A 2-item measure identified diagnostic status at baseline and persistent irritability, diagnoses, and impairment at follow-up (mean = 2.9 years), showing good stability.[19]

Studies that use latent class longitudinal approaches to differentiate trajectories of irritability can provide more detailed information about stability. These studies identify classes of youth that differ in the developmental course of their irritability. The most common class (ie, the normative trajectory) shows decreasing irritability from preschool through adolescence.[28–30] Classes can be compared on clinical as well as neural features,[29] and can be useful in future studies of staging and prognostication. Classes of particular interest to clinicians include youth with persistently moderate to high irritability.

The fifth external validity criterion is *course of illness*. Applying this criterion to a dimensional trait, one can ask whether irritability is associated with an increased risk for the emergence of specific symptoms or diagnoses over time. As noted previously, longitudinal research conducted in the context of questions about irritability and pediatric BD demonstrated an association between childhood irritability and increased risk for unipolar depression and anxiety disorders (for a meta-analysis, see Vidal-Ribas and colleagues[31]). Twin studies suggest that this longitudinal association is, in part, genetically mediated.[12–17] In addition, multiple studies show longitudinal associations between the irritable dimension of oppositional defiant disorder and risk for unipolar depression and anxiety (see Burke, volume II).[1] However, the literature is not entirely consistent, as studies that differ in methodology and sampling find more protean longitudinal associations between childhood irritability and future psychopathology.[32,33] Future research parsing the heterogeneity of irritability (eg, threat-based vs reward-based irritability and tonic vs phasic irritability, see later in this article) may allow for more personalized and accurate predictions. It is also important to note longitudinal associations between earlier irritability and later suicidality (see Benton and colleagues, volume I),[1,22,30,34] and new data showing associations between irritability and suicidality in depressed adults.[35]

Finally, does the presence of irritability predict *treatment response*? Few studies specify irritability as an outcome, and adequate measurement of irritability is perhaps the most important area for future research to facilitate the development of novel treatments (see Carlson and Singh, volume I/II introductions, and Wozniak and colleagues, Patino and DelBello, Volume II).[1] A post hoc analysis of the MTA study on the treatment of ADHD found that methylphenidate (MPH) decreased irritability in youth with ADHD.[36] Although this effect was not attributable to the effect of MPH on ADHD symptoms, it is unknown whether stimulant medication would reduce irritability in youth without ADHD. As mentioned previously, a trial of MPH plus citalopram versus MPH versus placebo showed promising results,[37] and again the effect of treatment on irritability was not secondary to effects on anxiety or depression. Further, in adults with major depressive disorder (MDD), decreased irritability early in SSRI treatment was a favorable predictor of remission[35] and data suggest that, in depressed adults, sertraline decreases irritability independent of its effect on depression.[38] Thus, there is emerging evidence that irritability itself may respond to specific treatment interventions.

There is also evidence for specific psychotherapeutic interventions in school (Mattison and colleagues, volume II), inpatient (Chua and colleagues, volume II), residential (Huefner and colleagues, volume II), and outpatient (Waxmonsky and colleagues, Singh and colleagues, Fristad and colleagues, volume II) settings.[1] A recent analysis of youth (N = 81) with severe irritability found that those treated with Modular Approach to Therapy for Children with Anxiety, Depression, Traumatic Stress, or Conduct Problems (MATCH), a modular, transdiagnostic, behavioral/cognitive-behavioral intervention, had faster improvement than those who received standard manualized treatments (SMT) or usual care (UC). SMT and MATCH both surpassed UC in irritability reduction (effect size = 0.49) (see Evans and colleagues, volume II).[1] A trial of dialectical behavior therapy in pre-adolescents (N = 43) also showed feasibility and preliminary efficacy in youth with DMDD.[39]

In summary, how would we assess the external validity of irritability? The data provide at least moderate support for familial aggregation and impairment. There is modest to moderate evidence for stability of the dimensional trait and the ability of irritability to predict future clinical course. Given the paucity of research, there are only suggestive data for specific treatment responses, and currently there is no clear evidence for specific biological markers. We conclude that this qualitative analysis suggests sufficient external validity for the construct to justify future research, although quantitative, systematic assessment is warranted. From the research and clinical perspective, we suggest that priority be placed on longitudinal designs to ascertain stability and prediction of clinical course, systematic treatment trials, and discovering biological markers that might facilitate both diagnosis and the development of novel interventions.

Tonic versus Phasic Irritability

Although irritability is a narrower construct than some others in **Fig. 1**, it is nonetheless complex. As discussed in Spring and Carlson (volume I),[1] the importance of distinguishing chronic irritability from irritability occurring in the context of a depressive or manic mood episode contributed to confusion regarding the diagnosis of pediatric BD. However, even within the context of chronic irritability, there is phenomenological variation, including in the form of tonic and phasic irritability.

Our first attempt to operationalize irritability occurred when we specified criteria for the SMD phenotype.[23] These served as inclusion criteria for studies differentiating youth with "classic," episodic BD from those with the controversial phenotype of chronic severe irritability, operationalized as SMD. In defining SMD, we specified 2 types of irritability: phasic (ie, developmentally inappropriate temper outbursts) and tonic (ie, chronically grumpy, angry mood between outbursts). This differentiation was done on clinical grounds, with the observation that some children (anecdotally, often children with ADHD with comorbid oppositional defiant disorder) have normal mood between outbursts. In studies contrasting chronically irritable youth to those with clear, episodic BD, we wanted to limit the chronically irritable group to youth who had, not only extreme and frequent temper outbursts, but also a persistent mood disorder between outbursts. This chronically irritable mood contributed to their receiving the diagnosis of BD and to severe impairment, making them a more suitable match for the youth with "classic" BD.

A major question is whether tonic and phasic irritability are distinct constructs with differential mechanisms and predictions (see Vidal-Ribas and Stringaris and Spring and Carlson, volume I, and Burke and colleagues, volume II).[1] Indeed, in assessing the 2 constructs, tonic irritability is frequently assessed by asking about the ease of precipitating an outburst, so in practice it can be difficult to rate the 2 constructs independently. Parenthetically, the DMDD criteria for tonic irritability is modeled on the "A" criterion for MDD; both require that the abnormal mood be present most of the day, nearly every day, and these 2 diagnoses both received "questionable" kappas in the DSM-5 field trials.[40] Whether this low reliability is due to specific challenges associated with assessing chronic mood abnormalities is a question deserving of further research.

In both clinical and community samples, tonic and phasic irritability are highly correlated. In a sample of 489 youth including healthy subjects, DMDD youth, ADHD youth, and youth with irritability symptoms not meeting the DMDD threshold, the correlation between phasic and tonic irritability was 0.79 (Cardinale and colleagues, in press).[41] In the Great Smoky Mountain community sample (N = 1420, ages 9–16 years), 51.4% of subjects reported phasic irritability (ie, a tantrum at least once in the previous 3 months), 28.3% tonic irritability, and 22.8% both.[42] Overlap was high, and tonic irritability rarely occurred without phasic irritability. Thus, research attempting to dissociate the two requires large samples with adequate representation in the discordant cells.

Nonetheless, there is preliminary genetic, comorbidity, and treatment evidence supporting differentiation of the 2 constructs. In each instance, phasic irritability appears to carry stronger predictions than does tonic irritability, perhaps reflecting greater reliability in assessment. Regarding genetic evidence, a study of 1431 twin pairs, aged 8 to 17, found that, compared with tonic irritability, phasic irritability was somewhat more stable and heritable and contributed more to a latent variable designed to capture the DMDD phenotype.[15] Further, only half the genetic variance of tonic irritability was shared with phasic irritability. Regarding comorbidity, in the sample of 489 youth oversampled for irritability and ADHD described previously, high comorbid ADHD symptoms were associated with greater phasic irritability than were moderate levels of ADHD symptoms, whereas there was no differences between groups in tonic symptoms (Cardinale and colleagues, in press).[41] These results complement recent work on an "irritable subtype" of ADHD by focusing attention on youth with ADHD and phasic irritability.[43] Finally, regarding treatment, in the open stimulant-only phase of the citalopram + MPH trial described previously, MPH reduced temper outbursts and ADHD symptoms, but not irritable mood between outbursts.[37] Thus, there is some preliminary evidence that phasic and tonic irritability may differ in treatment response.

Preliminary ecological momentary assessment (EMA) data suggest that the use of mobile technology may advance research on the differentiation of phasic versus tonic irritability while also clarifying informant effects that impact on the assessment of irritability and other childhood psychopathology.[44] In EMA, parents and children are prompted simultaneously several times a day on their smart-phones to answer questions about the child's mood, behavior, sleep, and other relevant variables. This acquisition of real time, contemporaneous ratings from parent and child holds the promise of circumventing the well-known biases inherent in retrospective report and of clarifying informant effects. Preliminary data in 62 youth who sought treatment for irritability (eg, DMDD or sub-DMDD) and/or ADHD indicate (1) an informant effect whereby parents report more symptoms than do youth; (2) evidence that child and parent data are independently informative in predicting temper outbursts; (3) good agreement between clinician characterization of child's irritability (based on retrospective parent and child report) and EMA measures; and (4) evidence that tonic and phasic irritability are dissociable dimensions (Chue and colleagues and Naim and colleagues, unpublished, 2020). Ultimately, self- and parent-reported EMA data can be paired with measures of the child's physiology (eg, heart rate variability, skin conductance response, actigraphy), also acquired through mobile technology, with the goal of predicting temper outbursts and, when an impending outburst is detected, delivering to the child's smartphone prompts to engage in a therapeutic intervention. Smart phone and sensor measurements may be particularly useful in the development of novel primary and secondary preventive interventions as reviewed by Singh and colleagues in volume II.[1]

Further research on possible distinctions between tonic and phasic irritability could facilitate more personalized medication approaches and prognoses. In addition, such research could have important pathophysiological and theoretic implications. That is, the phasic irritability construct can be conceptualized as an evoked response to a motivationally important stimulus (eg, a frustrating or threatening event), and is thus consistent with definitions of *emotion* in the affective neuroscience literature. In contrast, tonic irritability is a longer-duration *mood*, less tightly tied to a specific precipitant. Also, the most salient features of phasic irritability are the *behaviors* associated with a temper outburst, although it is also associated with angry emotion. Tonic irritability, in contrast, is defined in terms of *mood*, although one would also expect to see associated behaviors. Identifying biological hallmarks of these different constructs is important for future work on irritability.

Common Comorbidities: Anxiety and Attention-Deficit Hyperactivity Disorder

Clinicians know that irritability rarely presents alone; the articles in Volume I discuss in detail the many childhood psychopathologies that co-occur with irritability. We focus on 2 of the most common co-occurring diagnoses: anxiety disorders and ADHD (see Blader and also Walkup and colleagues, volume I).[1] In a recent sample of 191 youth with DMDD that we recruited, 72% met criteria for ADHD and 46% met criteria for an anxiety disorder (Cardinale and colleagues, unpublished data). As noted previously, in research designed to elucidate the pathophysiology of irritability, it is important to use recruitment and analytical strategies designed to identify common versus unique pathophysiological mechanisms for example, dimensional approaches in transdiagnostic samples enriched for the phenotypes of interest. Also, because comorbidity is the rule rather than the exception in psychiatry, there is now consider-able interest in statistical approaches that can dissociate such mechanisms, for example, bifactor modeling, network analyses, and latent profile analyses.[45]

Anxiety and irritability share psychological commonalities, that is, both can be viewed as high-arousal, negative valence responses to threat.[2] They differ, however, in the nature of the response, that is, avoidance for anxiety and approach (eg, increased motoric activity, yelling) for irritability. Both anxious and irritable youth show an attention bias toward threat.[46,47] In a functional MRI (fMRI) study of attention bias to threat in youth with anxiety, DMDD, ADHD, or no diagnosis (N = 197), we used bifactor modeling to differentiate neural activity associated specifically with parent-rated irritability, child-rated irritability, or parent-rated and child-rated anxiety, or with a shared common factor of negative affectivity.[48] (Notably, although parent-rated and child-rated anxiety loaded on one factor, parent-rated and child-rated irritability did not, indicating a marked informant effect.) The major associations were between neural activity and parent-related irritability and between neural connectivity and anxiety. Specifically, parent-reported irritability was associated with abnormally increased amygdala, insula, and dorsolateral prefrontal cortex activity when subjects were asked to focus their attention away from threat. In studies that do not consider irritability, abnormal activity in these regions has been reported in association with anxiety,[49–51] demonstrating the importance of considering both traits simultaneously.

Considerable research has focused on emotion dysregulation in ADHD. Mirroring the previous discussion of overlapping constructs, emotionality has been operational-ized in multiple ways in the ADHD literature, including deficient emotional self-regulation, emotional impulsiveness, and irritability.[5] The question of whether such emotion dysregulation should be conceptualized as a core construct of ADHD, a co-morbidity, or characteristic of an ADHD subtype has been the subject of considerable theoretic and empirical work (see Blader, volume I).[1,5,43,52]

In this context, it is important to note literature emerging on associations between genetic risk for ADHD and emotional dysregulation. As noted previously, several twin studies have found genetic associations among unipolar depression, anxiety, and irritability. In a complementary literature, recent studies in samples enriched for ADHD use polygenic risk scores (PRS) to investigate genetic associations among irritability, ADHD, and MDD. PRS quantify genetic risk based on the presence of single nucleotide polymorphisms associated with an illness or trait.[53]

Two recent studies have provocative findings. Riglin and colleagues[54] used PRS and longitudinal trajectories of irritability to identify 2 irritability subtypes in a commu-nity sample (N = 7924). The first subtype, early-onset irritability, was predominately male and associated with childhood ADHD and ADHD PRS. The second subtype, adolescent-onset irritability, was predominately female and associated with adoles-cent depression and PRS for MDD. This highlights the importance of considering possible sex, as well as age, effects in studies of irritability. Second, Nigg and col-leagues[5] studied ADHD and MDD PRS in a sample of 514 patients with ADHD and without ADHD. This study conceptualized emotion dysregulation in the context of temperament, specifically irritability and surgency, with the latter being a temperament defined as positive valence emotion dysregulation (eg, impulsivity, sensation-seeking). They found that ADHD PRS score was associated with both irritability and surgency. This finding would suggest that ADHD PRS is associated with lability, shifts into both positive and negative valence states, rather than simply the negative valence states characterized by irritability (see **Fig. 1**). More detailed phenotyping of these mood states would be required to identify their precise time course that is, whether positive and negative mood states occur concurrently or simultaneously (as in mixed states), and the role of tonic versus phasic irritability. In any case, these early studies, and the ones above of anxiety and irritability, demonstrate the importance of identifying unique versus shared mechanisms between irritability and other co-occurring illnesses and traits. We can expect to see considerably more research in this important and emerging area.[46–48]

Irritability and the Diagnostic and Statistical Manual of Mental Disorders, Fifth Revision

As described in Volume I, major changes were introduced in DSM-5 in response to increased rates of youth receiving the diagnosis of BD, coupled with data suggesting that this increase might be attributable to the unavailability of a more appropriate DSM diagnosis for youth with very severe, chronic irritability (see Spring and Carlson, volume I).[1] The most controversial change was the introduction of DMDD into the diagnostic manual. There are many valid criticisms of this action, with Evans and colleagues[55] providing a cogent and informative critique.

An important critique of DMDD is its overlap with ODD. Indeed, there are 3 diagnoses for which youth can qualify based primarily on their irritability or associated behavior: ODD, DMDD, and intermittent explosive disorder. Notably, the ODD diagnosis contains 2 dimensions, irritability and headstrong/defiant, that are dissociable in their longitudinal predictions and possibly in their genetic associations and treatment response (see Vidal-Ribas and Stringaris, volume I; Burke and colleagues, volume II).[1] The implications of these 2 commonly co-occurring dimensions for the ODD, DMDD, and IED diagnoses should be considered. A major consideration for the field concerns how these 3 diagnoses can be rationalized and integrated in the DSM.

A second major critique of DMDD is that thresholds for the frequency and severity of both outbursts and between-outburst mood were not derived empirically. Indeed, a necessary step in integrating ODD, IED, and DMDD is the acquisition of population-based data to guide the development of empirical thresholds for pathologic irritability. With an appreciation of the developmental context in which these outbursts occur (see Crowell and also Dougherty and colleagues, Volume II),[1] important examples of such work are in a birth cohort of 9-year-old to 11-year-old youth,[18] and in preschoolers.[56] Importantly, the latter work, along with other work[25] challenges limiting the DMDD diagnosis to children older than 6 years. Specifically, this work demonstrates than non-normative temper outbursts can be identified in preschoolers while illustrating the importance of developmentally sensitive criteria for irritability-based diagnoses.[57]

Translational Opportunity: Frustrative Nonreward

The irritability construct provides important translational opportunities in its links to threat and frustration, 2 processes that can be modeled across species. Whereas our group's *clinical* definition of irritability formed the basis for the preceding discussion, here we focus on our *neuroscientific* conceptualization of irritability, that is, aberrant approach responses to frustration or threat.[2] Specifically, this section focuses on using frustration tasks and fMRI to study individual differences in neural responses to frustration and thereby elucidate pathophysiological mechanisms of irritability (for a broader review, see Dickstein and colleagues, volume II).[1]

Irritability and Frustrative Nonreward

The FNR paradigm was defined by Amsel in 1958.[3] In recent adaptations,[58] rats are conditioned via instrumental learning to expect that, if they push a lever when a cue light is illuminated, they will receive a food reward. Then, the rat presses the lever when the light is on and yet no food is delivered, that is, the expected reward is withheld, goal attainment is blocked, and frustration is induced (**Fig. 2A**). Amsel[3] noted that the normative response to frustration included increased motor activity and increased aggression. The FNR paradigm has been used in studies of rodents, nonhuman primates, and humans. Ongoing translational research bridges work on frustration in rodents and nonhuman primates to research on irritability in youth.

Our proposed model hypothesizes that irritable youth have exaggerated emotional and behavioral responses to FNR (**Fig. 2B**).[2] That is, when they experience blocked goal attainment, irritable youth experience a more marked high-arousal, negative affective state (ie, frustration, anger) than do their nonirritable peers. Related to this exaggerated emotional response, irritable youth show more extreme increases in motor activity and aggression, thus displaying developmentally inappropriate temper outbursts. These exaggerated responses could be due to deficits in instrumental learning, either because irritable youth have difficulty learning contingencies (deficits in the process of instrumental learning at baseline and/or when frustrated) or because their maladaptive behavior is rewarded (there are deficits in the content of instrumental learning, in that having an emotional outburst results in receiving the desired reward). In addition, aberrant behavioral responses could be initiated by

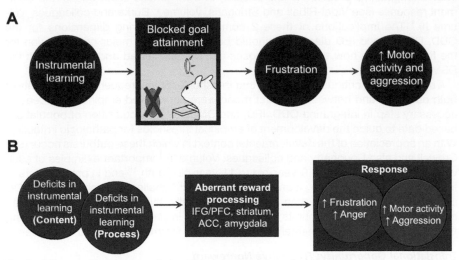

Fig. 2. (A) A representation of the FNR paradigm first described by Amsel in 1958[3] and adapted by Burokas and colleagues in 2012.[58] Rodents are conditioned to expect food reward if the lever is pressed when the cue light is on. Frustration is then induced by withholding reward even if the lever is pressed at the correct time (blocked goal attainment). The emotional state of frustration is associated with increased motor activity and aggression, relative to baseline. (B) Brotman and colleagues[2] proposed a translational model for clinically relevant irritability in youth that includes an adaptation of Amsel's[3] FNR paradigm.[3] Whereas Amsel's model[3] describes a normative response to frustration, Brotman and colleagues[2] suggest deficits that may contribute to an irritable child's exaggerated and maladaptive response to frustration. These deficits may include aberrant instrumental learning or reward processing (see text). These aberrancies, in turn, result in an exaggerated emotional response (ie, increased anger and frustration in response to blocked goal attainment) and maladaptive behavior in the form of pathologically increased motor activity and aggression (ie, a temper outburst).

exaggerated neural responses in the form of the prediction error that encodes the failure to receive an expected reward, or the receipt of an unanticipated punishment (**Fig. 3**).[59]

Importantly, the translational perspective of FNR identifies potential targets for novel interventions (see **Fig. 3**, an adaptation of our original model focused specifically on treatment targets). These targets include the deficits in instrumental learning noted previously, some of which are addressed by parent training.[60] In addition, we now also highlight potential deficits in cognitive control (eg, motor inhibition, attention shifting) that might contribute to the inability to modulate responses to FNR.[61] These targets have been incorporated into a novel treatment, currently being tested, that combines exposure-based techniques to frustrating stimuli with parent training techniques.[59]

Frustrative Nonreward and Functional MRI

Although the literature is relatively limited, FNR paradigms have been used in normative and non-normative adult and pediatric samples, in behavioral, electroencephalogram, and fMRI studies (for a review, see Leibenluft[61]). The specific results of these studies must be viewed as preliminary, given small samples, methodological differences, and the lack of replication attempts. The discussion that follows will focus on the largest clinical fMRI study of frustration, with a focus not only on the results, but also on methods and complexities in this line of research.

The largest study of FNR in youth included 195 subjects (ages 12.9 ± 2.4 years) with DMDD, anxiety disorders, ADHD, or no diagnosis; thus, there was a range of irritability in the sample.[62] The study used an adaptation of the Posner attention paradigm

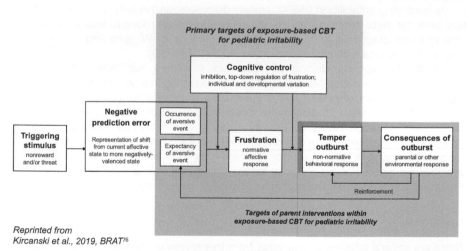

Reprinted from
Kircanski et al., 2019, BRAT[76]

Fig. 3. Exposure-targeted model of pediatric irritability. Visual representation of proposed proximal processes that surround a clinically significant temper outburst in pediatric irritability, typically occurring within a timescale of minutes. White boxes denote key constructs in bold text. Within each box, additional text briefly describes the construct. Arrows denote direct or moderating influences of these components on one another. Boxes encompassed by red background indicate the primary targets of exposure-based cognitive behavioral therapy for irritability. Boxes encompassed by blue background indicate targets of parent interventions within this CBT. (For interpretation of the references to color in this figure legend, the reader is referred to the Web version of this article.) (Reprinted with permission from Ref.[59])

modified to induce frustration.[62–64] During the Posner attentional task, children are told that they will receive money for each correct response and lose money for each response that is incorrect or too slow (instrumental learning).

In the first block, children are given accurate feedback. Because the task is easy, they typically achieve 90% accuracy and receive frequent reward. The next block is rigged: on 60% of correctly completed trials, the child receives feedback that their response is too slow, and they lose most of the money won in the first block. fMRI analysis compares neural activity when the child completes the attentional task on the "N+1" trial following frustrating versus nonfrustrating feedback. This contrast examines the clinically important question of whether attentional control differs in the frustrated versus nonfrustrated state, and whether such changes are associated with irritability. The statistical analysis focused on associations between irritability and neural activity on these 2 contrasts, controlling for the effects of anxiety or ADHD.

We found relatively strong associations between irritability and neural activity during the N+1 trial, that is, when performing the attentional task after frustrating versus nonfrustrating feedback. We highlight 3 clinically relevant aspects of the findings. First, increased irritability was associated with increased frontal-striatal activation in the anterior cingulate cortex, dorsolateral prefrontal cortex, inferior frontal gyrus, and caudate. These regions are implicated in cognitive control functions including motor inhibition and attentional control, suggesting the potential importance of such processes in potential treatment interventions. Second, some findings were most marked in younger subjects, indicating developmental effects on the neural mechanisms of irritability. And third, the findings associated with irritability were present across diagnostic categories (DMDD, anxiety disorders, ADHD); importantly, analyses based on diagnostic categories did not yield significant findings. This suggests that the mechanisms mediating irritability in DMDD, anxiety disorders, and ADHD are similar, consistent with the data noted previously showing genetic and longitudinal associations among these diagnoses (in contrast, see the findings of Wiggins and colleagues[65] where associations with irritability differed in DMDD vs BD).

Each fMRI paradigm, including each frustration paradigm, has limitations, so we use complementary frustration tasks that differ. For example, in a second frustration task, the order of frustration versus nonfrustration blocks is randomized, and a third task is designed to test whether irritable youth have deficits in instrumental learning at baseline and/or after frustration. Finally, our model suggests that irritability can be associated with aberrant responses to threat or frustration. This begs the question of whether there is heterogeneity among irritable youth (or adults) in the form of threat versus frustration-sensitive subtypes. We are currently testing this question in a study integrating data from a sample of youth who have completed both threat and frustration fMRI paradigms.

SUMMARY

There are several take-away messages from this review of irritability, viewed particularly from a translational perspective. First, irritability is one of many constructs that can be used to study emotion dysregulation. It has reasonable external validity, with more data accumulating regarding its biology, genetics, and response to specific treatments. Further, it has good longitudinal stability and ability to predict clinical course, and these validators are being examined with increasingly sophisticated statistical techniques. Importantly, to the extent that irritability is conceptualized as aberrant responses to frustration and/or threat, it is amenable to cross-species research, that is, responses to both frustration and threat can be assessed in humans and animals using parallel tasks.

Research suggests that phasic irritability (temper outbursts) may be a distinct construct from tonic irritability (grouchy mood between outbursts). Important questions include whether these constructs have differential longitudinal outcomes or response to treatment, and the degree to which the severity of the tantrums in terms of behavior, duration, or pervasiveness impacts on outcome or treatment response. EMA may help answer these questions, given the difficulty of differentiating tonic versus phasic irritability by retrospective report. Such research could complement data from large epidemiologic studies, and from samples enriched for irritability. Epidemiologic studies are needed to determine thresholds for clinically significant irritability and enable the rationalization and integration of irritability-related diagnoses in the DSM.

The hypothesis that irritability reflects exaggerated negative responses to frustration suggests that standardized tasks that induce frustration can be used to study the neural mechanisms mediating irritability in youth. Such studies suggest associations between increased irritability and increased fronto-striatal activity when children attempt to complete an attentional task immediately after frustration. This work informs the development of a novel psychotherapeutic approach to irritability, currently being tested. The therapeutic approach includes the child experiencing graded exposure to frustration and learning to increase his or her cognitive control capabilities in order to be able to inhibit temper outbursts. Concurrently, parents receive training teaching them to reward the child's positive, but not negative, behavior.

Chronic irritability in youth is associated with severe impairment and adverse outcomes, and there is also considerable burden on their families. Hopefully, careful and systematic conceptualization and research focused on their emotional and behavioral difficulties will ultimately help to alleviate the considerable suffering of these children and their families.

DISCLOSURE

The work is funded by the Intramural Research Program of the National Institute of Mental Health.

REFERENCES

1. Carlson GA, Singh MK, editors. Emotion dysregulation in children: Part I and Part II (child and adolescent psychiatric clinics). Elsevier; 2021.
2. Brotman MA, Kircanski K, Stringaris A, et al. Irritability in youths: a translational model. Am J Psychiatry 2017;174(6):520–32.
3. Amsel A. The role of frustrative nonreward in noncontinuous reward situations. Psychol Bull 1958;55(2):102–19.
4. Hulvershorn LA, Mennes M, Castellanos FX, et al. Abnormal amygdala functional connectivity associated with emotional lability in children with attention-deficit/ hyperactivity disorder. J Am Acad Child Adolesc Psychiatry 2014;53(3): 351–61.e1.
5. Nigg JT, Karalunas SL, Gustafsson HC, et al. Evaluating chronic emotional dysregulation and irritability in relation to ADHD and depression genetic risk in children with ADHD. J Child Psychol Psychiatry 2020;61(2):205–14.
6. Vogel AC, Jackson JJ, Barch DM, et al. Excitability and irritability in preschoolers predicts later psychopathology: the importance of positive and negative emotion dysregulation. Dev Psychopathol 2019;31(3):1067–83.
7. Toohey MJ, DiGiuseppe R. Defining and measuring irritability: construct clarification and differentiation. Clin Psychol Rev 2017;53:93–108.

8. Kendler KS. A history of the DSM-5 scientific review committee. Psychol Med 2013;43(9):1793–800.

9. Whelan YM, Leibenluft E, Stringaris A, et al. Pathways from maternal depressive symptoms to adolescent depressive symptoms: the unique contribution of irritability symptoms. J Child Psychol Psychiatry 2015;56(10):1092–100.

10. Eyre O, Langley K, Stringaris A, et al. Irritability in ADHD: associations with depression liability. J Affect Disord 2017;215:281–7.

11. Rice F, Sellers R, Hammerton G, et al. Antecedents of new-onset major depressive disorder in children and adolescents at high familial risk. JAMA Psychiatry 2017;74(2):153.

12. Stringaris A, Zavos H, Leibenluft E, et al. Adolescent irritability: phenotypic associations and genetic links with depressed mood. Am J Psychiatry 2012;169(1): 47–54.

13. Roberson-Nay R, Leibenluft E, Brotman MA, et al. Longitudinal stability of genetic and environmental influences on irritability: from childhood to young adulthood. Am J Psychiatry 2015;172(7):657–64.

14. Savage J, Verhulst B, Copeland W, et al. A genetically informed study of the longitudinal relation between irritability and anxious/depressed symptoms. J Am Acad Child Adolesc Psychiatry 2015;54(5):377–84.

15. Moore AA, Lapato DM, Brotman MA, et al. Heritability, stability, and prevalence of tonic and phasic irritability as indicators of disruptive mood dysregulation disorder. J Child Psychol Psychiatry 2019;60(9):1032–41.

16. Mikolajewski AJ, Taylor J, Iacono WG. Oppositional defiant disorder dimensions: genetic influences and risk for later psychopathology. J Child Psychol Psychiatry 2017;58(6):702–10.

17. Waldman ID, Rowe R, Boylan K, et al. External validation of a bifactor model of oppositional defiant disorder. Mol Psychiatry 2018;26(2):682–93.

18. Laporte PP, Matijasevich A, Munhoz TN, et al. Disruptive mood dysregulation disorder: symptomatic and syndromic thresholds and diagnostic operationalization. J Am Acad Child Adolesc Psychiatry 2020;60(2):286–95.

19. Wiggins JL, Briggs-Gowan MJ, Estabrook R, et al. Identifying clinically significant irritability in early childhood. J Am Acad Child Adolesc Psychiatry 2018;57(3): 191–9.e2.

20. Cornacchio D, Crum KI, Coxe S, et al. Irritability and severity of anxious symptomatology among youth with anxiety disorders. J Am Acad Child Adolesc Psychiatry 2016;55(1):54–61.

21. Galera C, Orri M, Vergunst F, et al. Developmental profiles of childhood attention-deficit/hyperactivity disorder and irritability: association with adolescent mental health, functional impairment, and suicidal outcomes. J Child Psychol Psychiatry 2021;62(2):232–43.

22. Stringaris A, Cohen P, Pine DS, et al. Adult outcomes of youth irritability: a 20-year prospective community-based study. Am J Psychiatry 2009;166(9):1048–54.

23. Leibenluft E, Charney DS, Towbin KE, et al. Defining clinical phenotypes of Juvenile mania. Am J Psychiatry 2003;160(3):430–7.

24. Deveney CM, Hommer RE, Reeves E, et al. A prospective study of severe irritability in youths: 2- and 4-year follow-up. Depress Anxiety 2015;32(5):364–72.

25. Dougherty LR, Barrios CS, Carlson GA, et al. Predictors of later psychopathology in young children with disruptive mood dysregulation disorder. J Child Adolesc Psychopharmacol 2017;27(5):396–402.

26. Mayes SD, Mathiowetz C, Kokotovich C, et al. Stability of disruptive mood dysregulation disorder symptoms (Irritable-Angry mood and temper outbursts)

throughout childhood and adolescence in a general population sample. J Abnorm Child Psychol 2015;43(8):1543–9.

27. Axelson D, Findling RL, Fristad MA, et al. Examining the proposed disruptive mood dysregulation disorder diagnosis in children in the longitudinal assessment of manic symptoms study. J Clin Psychiatry 2012;73(10):1342–50.

28. Wiggins JL, Mitchell C, Stringaris A, et al. Developmental trajectories of irritability and bidirectional associations with maternal depression. J Am Acad Child Adolesc Psychiatry 2014;53(11):1191–205.e4.

29. Pagliaccio D, Pine DS, Barch DM, et al. Irritability trajectories, cortical thickness, and clinical outcomes in a sample enriched for preschool depression. J Am Acad Child Adolesc Psychiatry 2018;57(5):336–42.e6.

30. Orri M, Galera C, Turecki G, et al. Pathways of association between childhood irritability and adolescent suicidality. J Am Acad Child Adolesc Psychiatry 2019; 58(1):99–107.e3.

31. Vidal-Ribas P, Brotman MA, Valdivieso I, et al. The status of irritability in psychiatry: a conceptual and quantitative review. J Am Acad Child Adolesc Psychiatry 2016;55(7):556–70.

32. Althoff RR, Verhulst FC, Rettew DC, et al. Adult outcomes of childhood dysregulation: a 14-year follow-up study. J Am Acad Child Adolesc Psychiatry 2010; 49(11):1105–16.e1.

33. Hawes MT, Carlson GA, Finsaas MC, et al. Dimensions of irritability in adolescents: longitudinal associations with psychopathology in adulthood. Psychol Med 2020;50(16):2759–67.

34. Pickles A, Aglan A, Collishaw S, et al. Predictors of suicidality across the life span: the Isle of Wight study. Psychol Med 2010;40(9):1453–66.

35. Jha MK, Minhajuddin A, Chin Fatt C, et al. Association between irritability and suicidal ideation in three clinical trials of adults with major depressive disorder. Neuropsychopharmacology 2020;45(13):2147–54.

36. Fernández de la Cruz L, Simonoff E, McGough JJ, et al. Treatment of children with attention-deficit/hyperactivity disorder (ADHD) and irritability: results from the multimodal treatment study of children with ADHD (MTA). J Am Acad Child Adolesc Psychiatry 2015;54(1):62–70.e3.

37. Towbin K, Vidal-Ribas P, Brotman MA, et al. A double-blind randomized placebo-controlled trial of citalopram adjunctive to stimulant medication in youth with chronic severe irritability. J Am Acad Child Adolesc Psychiatry 2020;59(3): 350–61.

38. Jha MK, Minhajuddin A, Chin Fatt C, et al. Improvements in irritability with sertraline versus placebo: findings from the EMBARC study. J Affect Disord 2020; 275:44–7.

39. Perepletchikova F, Nathanson D, Axelrod SR, et al. Randomized clinical trial of dialectical behavior therapy for preadolescent children with disruptive mood dysregulation disorder: feasibility and outcomes. J Am Acad Child Adolesc Psychiatry 2017;56(10):832–40.

40. Regier DA, Narrow WE, Clarke DE, et al. DSM-5 field trials in the United States and Canada, Part II: test-retest reliability of selected categorical diagnoses. Am J Psychiatry 2013;170(1):59–70.

41. Cardinale EM, Freitag GF, Brotman MA, et al. Phasic versus tonic irritability: differential associations with ADHD symptoms. J Am Acad Child Adolesc Psychiatry. In press.

42. Copeland WE, Brotman MA, Costello EJ. Normative irritability in youth: developmental findings from the Great Smoky mountains study. J Am Acad Child Adolesc Psychiatry 2015;54(8):635–42.

43. Karalunas SL, Gustafsson HC, Fair D, et al. Do we need an irritable subtype of ADHD? Replication and extension of a promising temperament profile approach to ADHD subtyping. Psychol Assess 2019;31(2):236–47.

44. De Los Reyes A, Augenstein TM, Wang M, et al. The validity of the multi-informant approach to assessing child and adolescent mental health. Psychol Bull 2015; 141(4):858–900.

45. Satterthwaite TD, Feczko E, Kaczkurkin AN, et al. Parsing psychiatric heterogeneity through common and unique circuit-level deficits. Biol Psychiatry 2020; 88(1):4–5.

46. Hommer RE, Meyer A, Stoddard J, et al. Attention bias to threat faces in severe mood dysregulation. Depress Anxiety 2014;31(7):559–65. https://doi.org/10. 1002/da.22145.

47. Salum GA, Mogg K, Bradley BP, et al. Association between irritability and bias in attention orienting to threat in children and adolescents. J Child Psychol Psychiatry 2017;58(5):595–602.

48. Kircanski K, White LK, Tseng W-L, et al. A latent variable approach to differentiating neural mechanisms of irritability and anxiety in youth. JAMA Psychiatry 2018;75(6):631.

49. Fu X, Taber-Thomas BC, Pérez-Edgar K. Frontolimbic functioning during threat-related attention: relations to early behavioral inhibition and anxiety in children. Biol Psychol 2017;122:98–109.

50. Monk CS, Nelson EE, McClure EB, et al. Ventrolateral prefrontal cortex activation and attentional bias in response to angry faces in adolescents with generalized anxiety disorder. Am J Psychiatry 2006;163(6):1091–7.

51. Monk CS, Telzer EH, Mogg K, et al. Amygdala and ventrolateral prefrontal cortex activation to masked angry faces in children and adolescents with generalized anxiety disorder. Arch Gen Psychiatry 2008;65(5):568.

52. Barkley R. Deficient emotional self-regulation: a core component of attention-deficit/hyperactivity disorder. J ADHD Relat Disord 2010;1:5–37.

53. Lewis CM, Vassos E. Polygenic risk scores: from research tools to clinical instruments. Genome Med 2020;12:44.

54. Riglin L, Eyre O, Thapar AK, et al. Identifying novel types of irritability using a developmental genetic approach. Am J Psychiatry 2019;176(8):635–42.

55. Evans SC, Burke JD, Roberts MC, et al. Irritability in child and adolescent psychopathology: an integrative review for ICD-11. Clin Psychol Rev 2017;53:29–45.

56. Lee Wiggins J, Briggs-Gowan MJ, Brotman MA, et al. Don't miss the boat: towards a developmental Nosology for disruptive mood dysregulation disorder in early childhood. J Am Acad Child Adolesc Psychiatry 2020;60(3):388–97.

57. Wakschlag LS, Estabrook R, Petitclerc A, et al. Clinical implications of a dimensional approach: the normal: abnormal spectrum of early irritability. J Am Acad Child Adolesc Psychiatry 2015;54(8):626–34.

58. Burokas A, Gutiérrez-Cuesta J, Martín-García E, et al. Operant model of frustrated expected reward in mice. Addict Biol 2012;17(4):770–82.

59. Kircanski K, Craske MG, Averbeck BB, et al. Exposure therapy for pediatric irritability: theory and potential mechanisms. Behav Res Ther 2019;118:141–9.

60. Kazdin A. Parent management training: treatment for oppositional, aggressive, and antisocial behavior in children and adolescents. England: Oxford University Press; 2005.

61. Leibenluft E. Pediatric irritability: a systems neuroscience approach. Trends Cogn Sci 2017;21(4):277–89.
62. Tseng W-L, Deveney CM, Stoddard J, et al. Brain mechanisms of attention orienting following frustration: associations with irritability and age in youths. Am J Psychiatry 2018;176(1):67–76.
63. Tseng W-L, Moroney E, Machlin L, et al. Test-retest reliability and validity of a frustration paradigm and irritability measures. J Affect Disord 2017;212:38–45.
64. Deveney CM. Reward processing and irritability in young adults. Biol Psychol 2019;143:1–9.
65. Wiggins JL, Brotman MA, Adleman NE, et al. Neural correlates of irritability in disruptive mood dysregulation and bipolar disorders. Am J Psychiatry 2016;173(7):722–30.

Moving?

Make sure your subscription moves with you!

To notify us of your new address, find your **Clinics Account Number** (located on your mailing label above your name), and contact customer service at:

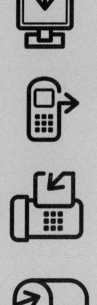

Email: journalscustomerservice-usa@elsevier.com

800-654-2452 (subscribers in the U.S. & Canada)
314-447-8871 (subscribers outside of the U.S. & Canada)

Fax number: 314-447-8029

Elsevier Health Sciences Division
Subscription Customer Service
3251 Riverport Lane
Maryland Heights, MO 63043

*To ensure uninterrupted delivery of your subscription, please notify us at least 4 weeks in advance of move.

ELSEVIER

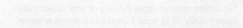

Printed and bound by CPI Group (UK) Ltd, Croydon, CR0 4YY

03/10/2024

01040404-0006